Apraxia of Speech:

Physiology, Acoustics, Linguistics, Management

Apraxia of Speech:

Physiology, Acoustics, Linguistics, Management

Edited by

John C. Rosenbek, PhD
VA Medical Center
Madison, Wisconsin

Malcolm R. McNeil, PhD
University of Wisconsin
Madison, Wisconsin

Arnold E. Aronson, PhD
The Mayo Clinic
Rochester, Minnesota

COLLEGE-HILL PRESS, San Diego, California

College-Hill Press
4284 41st Street
San Diego, California 92105

Library of Congress Cataloging in Publication Data

Main entry under title:

Apraxia of speech.

Includes bibliographies and index.
1. Apraxia—Addresses, essays, lectures.
2. Darley, Frederic L. I. Rosenbek, John C. II. McNeil, Malcolm Ray, III. Aronson, Arnold Elvin [DNLM: 1. Apraxia, WL 340 A654]
RC394.A75A67 1984 616.85'52 83-14392

ISBN 0-933014-08-2

Contents

Contributors

Arnold E. Aronson, PhD
Mayo Clinic
Rochester, MN 55901

John C. Booth, PhD
Program in Communicative Disorders
Elborn College
University of Western Ontario
London, Ontario, Canada N6G lHl

Joe R. Brown, MD
1784 Alta Vista
Vista, CA 92083

Steven E. Deutsch, PhD
Speech Pathology Section (126)
VA Medical Center
5901 E. 7th Street
Long Beach, CA 90822

Joseph R. Duffy, PhD
Department of Communication
Disorders
University of Massachusetts
Amherst, MA 01003

Carol A. Gawle, MA
Department of Communication
Disorders
University of Massachusetts
Amherst, MA 01003

Montonobu Itoh, PhD
Tokoyo Metropolitan Institute
of Gerontology
Tokyo, Japan

Eric Keller, PhD
Département de linguistique
Université du Québec àMontréal
C.P. 8888
Montréal, Qué. Canada H3C 3P8

Raymond Kent, PhD
Department of Communication Disorders
University of Wisconsin — Madison
1975 Willow Drive
Madison, WI 53706

Andrew Kertesz, MD, FRCP
Department of Clinical Neurological Sciences
Saint Joseph's Hospital
London, Ontario, Canada NGA 4V2

Leonard L. LaPointe, PhD
Audiology & Speech Pathology
VA Medical Center
Gainesville, FL 32602

Herbert A. Leeper, Jr., PhD
Program in Communicative Disorders
Elborn College
University of Western Ontario
London, Ontario, Canada N6G lHl

Thomas P. Marquardt, PhD
Department of Speech Communication
University of Texas
Austin, TX 78712

Malcolm R. McNeil, PhD
Department of Communicative Disorders
Speech Motor Control Laboratories
University of Wisconsin
Madison, WI 53706

John C. Rosenbek, PhD
Audiology & Speech Pathology
VA Medical Center
2500 Overlook Terrace
Madison, WI 53705

Sumiko Sasanuma, PhD
Yokohama National University
Tokyo Metropolitan Institute of Gerontology
Tokyo, Japan

Cynthia M. Shewan, PhD
Program in Communicative Disorders
Elborn College
University of Western Ontario
London, Ontario, Canada N6G lHl

Harvey Sussman, PhD
Department of Speech Communication
University of Texas
Austin, TX 78712

Robert T. Wertz, PhD
Audiology & Speech Pathology
VA Medical Center
150 Muir Road
Martinez, CA 94553

Dedication

This book and companion text on the dysarthrias have grown from two perceived needs. The first is a need to provide a state of science review of the nature, assessment, and treatment of apraxia of speech, along with the most prominent current research by the leading researchers in the field. This need has been addressed by providing a major review and projective essay preceding the original data-based contributions on apraxia of speech.

The second, and equally important need grew from a desire to honor the time-unlimited contributions to motor speech disorders made by Dr. Frederic L. Darley on his formal retirement. His colleagues and his pre- and postdoctoral fellows at the Mayo Clinic initiated this tribute. In order to provide recognition of his profound impact on the field of motor speech disorders, on dysarthric and apraxic persons, and on all of us, this book is dedicated to him. Its scope reflects neither the trails traveled nor the passages opened by Dr. Darley. However, this book does reflect the fervor, diversity of approaches and the intellectual honesty needed to address motor speech disorders. This fervor, diversity and honesty he champions.

John C. Rosenbek
Malcolm R. McNeil
Arnold E. Aronson

Acknowledgments

We wish to acknowledge Debra Shimon, Brenda Kleinheinz, Kathy Lindgren, and Marilyn Parnell for their editorial and secretarial support. This work was in part supported by Grants NS 18797-01 and NS 13274-071 from the National Institute of Neurological and Communicative Disorders and Stroke.

Preface

Abnormalities of motor speech have long been used as clues to the type of neurologic dysfunction and as an aid to neurologic diagnosis. However, prior to 1969 there were few organized studies of the specific deviations of speech in various motor system disorders. At that time, Darley and colleagues identified, defined, and rated the deviant sounds encountered in dysarthrias of varied types. Subsequently, the perceptual characteristics of apraxia of speech were defined. It was concluded that the observed abnormalities of motor speech were determined by the part of the motor system that was impaired and the resultant specific neuromuscular defect (weakness, slowness, hypertonus, etc.). These abnormalities of motor speech should be verifiable by measurements of physiologic and neural functioning.

This book and the companion volume on the dysarthrias are an outgrowth and extension of those stated principles. This text opens with an overview of apraxia of speech, providing background information and furnishing a perspective. Subsequent contributions are devoted to specifics, with an emphasis on information derived from measurements of physiologic, acoustic, linguistic, or anatomic alterations in apraxia of speech. The final contributions are devoted to treatment.

Joe R. Brown, MD
Vista, CA

1

Apraxia of Speech: An Overview and Some Perspectives

John C. Rosenbek
Ray D. Kent
Leonard L. LaPointe

The subject of apraxia of speech has been bathed in controversy for over 120 years. Salient characteristics of the syndrome, explanation of the underlying nature of the disorder, and the very label itself have spawned debate and sometimes desk-pounding argument. Clearly we have made progress. The media bombard us with the revelation that we are a "high-tech" society, and that ever more sophisticated breakthroughs allow us to understand the world and the creatures that walk and crawl it. We are impressed by advances that promise to bring us just a bit closer to resolution of some of the puzzles that have eluded us. This is particularly true of the problems revolving around the brain and behavior. Although the brain, the only organ capable of studying itself, has been regarded as one of the classic scientific frontiers, few contemporary neuroscientists view it as the forbidding "black hole" of bygone days. In fact, as Lewis Thomas suggests, "neurobiologists can do all sorts of things in their investigations, and the brain is an organ different from what it seemed twenty-five years ago... Nobody has the feeling any longer, as we used to believe, that we can never find out how the brain works" (Thomas, 1979, p. 139).

This note of optimism about neuroscience in general probably can be filtered down to neuropathology and communication disorders as well.

Recent advances in fiberscopics, wide-band spectrogram analysis, and advanced electromyographic techniques may signal a path to clearer understanding, and ultimately better management of the disorder of apraxia of speech.

Although the path may be demarcated, the trip remains. This essay documents some of the previous travelers and attempts some reasonable speculation as to where the trail may wind. We have a little clearer feel for the disorder than did our forebearers, but some of the old arguments about nomenclature, symptomatology, and nature revisit us with the frequency of shuffling in-laws.

EARLY MODELS AND THE LESSONS OF HISTORY

The debate is not new. We can reason fairly assuredly that clans in caves were not bothered over whether the grunts that fell from the mouths of their head-injured hairy friends were phonetic or phonemic. After a few years differing views on the nature of brain damage and speech disruption emerged. "Neurologists, philosophers, linguists, and educators have blunted their lances on this problem for centuries" (Joynt, 1975, pp. 51-52). And in the 18th and 19th centuries, when more and more attention was focused on cerebral localization, particularly as it regarded speech production, debate flourished. As Marx points out, "discussions on language theory in the 18th century were polemics on a purely philosophical basis, men of letters, poets, philosophers, and the theologians argued their individual points of view, and this was continued throughout the next century" (Marx, 1966, p. 329). The halls of the Anthropological Society in Paris were a great rallying place for some of the most heated philosophical arguments of the 19th century. The heavy intellects from across the continent and beyond would gather there to wrestle the burning issues. Some of these discussions turned into systolic-raising shouting matches that resulted in invitations to settle the debated point by dueling pistols or, at the very least, leg wrestling. One of the hottest issues discussed at that time was the idea of speech as a localized function. One of the strongest advocates of this view, which seemed to arise from Franz Joseph Gall's overextended views of phrenology, was the influential Dean of Medicine, Professor Jean-Baptiste Bouillaud. As early as 1825 Bouillaud adopted Gall's views of the plurality of cerebral organs and called the anterior lobes the "legislative organs of speech" (Riese, 1947). Bouillaud distinguished, for the first time, the faculty to create words as signs of ideas and retain them in memory from the faculty to articulate them. According to

Bouillaud, loss of speech might be due to impairment of either of these faculties. Therein lie some of the early seeds of controversy about apraxia of speech which persist to this day.

Riese highlighted an early landmark on the nature of certain related speech disorders. He remarked, "In 1820 Lordat described "alalia," a disorder of the synergy of the muscles used for speech" (Riese, 1947, p. 322). Of course, this "disorder of synergy" could be either apraxic speech or dysarthria, and this notion of disynergy or discoordination is receiving increased attention in contemporary revisions of the definition of speech apraxia.

Despite the advocacy of Bouillaud, the relationship of speech and cerebral localization was not widely accepted until the issue was reintroduced to repeated sessions of the Anthropological Society of Paris by the 36-year-old son of a mirror maker, Ernest Auburtin. Some writers have called April 4, 1861 the most important single date (so far) in the study of brain and language (Critchley, 1970). On this date and at subsequent meetings Auburtin argued, rebutted, and interpreted published pathological reports on speech and cerebral localization. He also presented dramatic evidence himself, with the unprecedented experiment of observing the effects on speech of pressing a spatula on the undamaged anterior lobes of a patient who had completely shot away the frontal bone in a suicide attempt.

Auburtin's contributions are somewhat overshadowed by those of Paul Broca who was a newly elected secretary of the Anthropological Society during the time of Auburtin's presentations to the group. Broca proceeded to present information on his two classic cases, LeBorgne and LeLong. Broca felt he was not only implicating a specific cerebral area as responsible for the speech behavior he had observed, but also presented some very specific views on the nature of the impaired speech. Assuming a correct translation, Broca's words are:

> There are cases in which all the muscles — including those which subserve phonation and articulation — are under voluntary control, the auditory apparatus is intact, and the general faculty of language remains unaffected, but in which nevertheless, a cerebral lesion abolishes articulate speech. It seems to me that this loss of speech in patients who are neither paralyzed or demented is singular enough to warrant a special designation; therefore, I shall name this symptom *aphemia* because these patients lack only the ability to articulate words. (Rottenberg & Hochberg, 1977, p. 137)

Of course, Broca's interpretations subsequently have both come under fire and have been exalted. Whether or not those early patients and Broca's descriptions of aphemia are accurate descriptions of apraxia of speech remains moot. Time and lost data do not allow conclusive statements to be made. Questions of whether or not the disorder described by Broca was morphosyntactic impairment rather than disruption of execution of movement sequences were raised from the onset. According to Riese,

> He (Broca) left it open whether aphemia might be intellectual in origin and due to a loss of memory of the articulatory movements or whether it is but a type of locomotor ataxia, limited to the mechanism presiding over articulatory movements; but he was more in favor of the first interpretation. (Riese, 1947, p. 324)

Further interpretations of Broca's work are offered by Hughlings Jackson, who warned against the use of terms as "memoire de moyens de coordination," because they recall distinct faculties. Jackson presents his interpretation of what Broca *really* meant by supposing: "M. Broca means by memory of words the connection [that] the seats of motor impulses (coordinating centres or whatever they may be called) for words have with that other part or the nervous system (whatever and wherever it may be) which set them a-going" (Jackson, 1915, p. 55).

These cases are of historical import in tracing the evolution of thought about cerebral damage and subsequent disruptions of speech, and Bouillaud and Auburtin deserve as much recognition for their courageous early views as does Paul Broca. These historic vignettes that outline the evolution of the concept of apraxia of speech are presented more thoroughly in Wertz, LaPointe, and Rosenbek (1984).

Tracing the concept of apraxia of speech through the conceptual and creative filters of several generations is more than an academic exercise. Not only can we more fully appreciate the nature of contemporary controversy, but we discover that precedent exists for our views and for the views of those who disagree with us. Clarity and inspiration for future tasks are not impotent reasons for appreciating the stream of scientific history. Another compelling reason for touching this history is extremely relevant to this volume. Darley, in his early formulations of the advocacy of distinction between aphasia and apraxia of speech, cites the early case presentations of Broca as examples of a disorder not exactly the same as aphasia.

DARLEY'S INFLUENCE

In one of his earlier public advocacies for distinguishing apraxia of speech from other disorders, Darley discussed at some length what he considered to be some important gaps in our knowledge and understanding of neurogenic speech and language impairments. He stated in the proceedings of a conference held at Princeton, New Jersey in November of 1965:

> Another [distinction] relates to behaviors which have traditionally gone by the name of aphasia but which are distinguishable from it. When we review the behavior that Broca described, which has since gone by the name of motor aphasia, many of us believe it should be called by a name other than aphasia because it is in a different, nonlinguistic dimension. One of the latest to point this out is Wepman in 1955 and again in a revised statement in 1960. The gropings of the motor aphasic patient for correct positioning of his articulators, his clumsiness in finding the correct pattern of movement to produce a polysyllabic word, his near misses phonemically, and his retrials are predominant. And in the kind of patient I am talking about, they are coupled, as Broca pointed out, with no reduction in auditory comprehension and no disability in expressing himself fluently in writing. In other words, his performance represents no cross-modality impairment in the use of language symbols but a specific modality-bound deficit, better labeled an apraxia, to be exact, an oral verbal apraxia." (Darley, 1967, p. 236)

This quote is from the subsequently published proceedings of that conference, titled *Brain Mechanisms Underlying Speech and Language* (Millikan & Darley, 1967). Darley has modified his label selection since that conference, but it serves as a contemporary milestone in the study of the disorder from several reasons. First, Darley convinced a number of his colleagues that the distinctions he advocated were important and, second, his attention to this distinctive disorder spawned a groundswell of renewed research interest.

Johns and LaPointe (1976) also trace the history of the evolution of the term apraxia of speech, including some of Darley's early rationale for distinguishing the disorder from aphasia. Johns and LaPointe quote Darley as stating he and his colleagues at the Mayo Clinic feel that,

> The identification of this disorder (apraxia of speech) as distinct from dysarthria and aphasia is extremely important both for the neurologist and the speech pathologist, but especially for the speech pathologist since management of the disorder is quite different from the management of aphasia. (Johns & LaPointe, 1976, p. 173)

The 1960s brought a wave of descriptive research in apraxia of speech. Darley inspired students and colleagues and, in addition to earlier descriptive research by Critchley (1952), Fry (1959), and Shankweiler and Harris (1966), a host of doctoral dissertations on neurogenic phonological impairment emerged at about the same time. Studies by Johns (1968), LaPointe (1969), Larimore (1970), and Trost (1970) attempted to blaze the descriptive trail of the disorder.. Though broad phonetic transcription was used in these early perceptual studies, they provided a base for understanding the nature of the disorder and the impetus for more refined study. Much of this early effort at defining the symptomatology of the condition is traced by Johns & LaPointe (1976).

THE ICONOCLASTS

While the early response to Darley's pleas may have resembled the religious fervor and singularity of purpose reserved for earlier American migrations to the promised valleys of the West, not everyone joined the trek. Some writers were adamant in their rejection of the term apraxia of speech (Martin, 1974), and others failed to embrace it with any sincerity of affection.

Others recognized the disorder, appear to reject the term, but equivocate a bit as their argument progresses. For example, Kertesz states,

> Recently, interest in aphemia or cortical dysarthria has been renewed by Darley (1964) and other speech pathologists, who have popularized the term 'apraxia of speech' or 'verbal apraxia' to identify a purely motor speech disorder, distinct from dysarthria and often seen in association with aphasia Darley (1964) and Johns and Lapointe [sic] (1976) emphasize the necessity to separate this entity from the rest of the aphasias, from the point of view of therapy. The relationship of Broca's aphasia to apraxia of speech remains controversial. Geschwind (1965), DeRenzi *et al.* (1966) and Heilman (1973) suggest that Broca's aphasia and facial apraxia may vary independently. Many cases of marked 'verbal apraxia' have comprehension deficit, and the articulatory disorder is similar to the phonemic paraphasias seen in other aphasics. Yet there are some patients in whom the articulatory disorder is distinctive enough to justify nosologic separation. (Kertesz, 1979, p. 3)

Kertesz has tempered some of his early rejection in this area and in this volume he documents "verbal apraxia" in several cases with subcortical pathology. He still appears resistant to viewing cortically based apraxia as simply a "motor" phenomenon, however. He argues that the integrated functions of language transcend mere descriptive levels, such as articulation or phonemic selection, and suggests it is unlikely central lesions that result in verbal apraxia affect only motor function. It is difficult to reconcile that stand with the existence of a well-documented cortically based dysarthria, as in pseudobulbar palsy.

Heilman (1979) also disavows the concept of apraxia of speech and argues, as does Kertesz, that nonfluent speech, and, in fact, the fluent speech of the conduction aphasic, can exist with or without the presence of a buccofacial or nonverbal apraxia of the oral mechanism. These authors seem to argue that since patients who have difficulty programming movements necessary for speech can be found with *no* coexisting or underlying buccofacial apraxia, the designation "apraxia of speech" is untenable. This is essentially a straw man argument. None of the advocates of apraxia of speech build their case on the necessity of an underlying and therefore hierarchially causal buccofacial apraxia. Darley and other advocates of apraxia of speech readily admit that the mechanisms controlling volitional speech movements and nonspeech oral movements may well be quite separate. To dismiss the term and condition of apraxia of speech on such grounds is to ignore the literature which outlines the rationale for its selection (Darley, Aronson, & Brown, 1975; Johns & LaPointe, 1976).

QUESTIONS IN SEARCH OF ANSWERS

As outlined here and treated in considerably more detail in Wertz, LaPointe, and Rosenbek (in press), a variety of questions, confusions, and curiosities have shadowed the study of the disorder. Some of them recur. Many have never disappeared or been satisfactorily answered. Some of the questions that have spawned the controversy surrounding the disorder include:

Does apraxia of speech exist as a separate entity? Is it merely a type of aphasia? How adequate is our definition? Is it a speech or language disorder? Where do speech and language overlap? Is is a disturbance at the phonologic level or simply disrupted articulation? What is the difference between articulation and phonologic disruption? Are phonologic rules violated?

Is it phonetic or phonemic? Can all phonologic disruptions be clearly classified as either phonetic or phonemic? Is it a performance or a competence deficit? Does it affect surface structure or deep structure? Is it purely a motor speech disorder? How interdependent are certain motor and linguistic phenomena? Is it all motor or partly sensory-perceptual? What role does ongoing sensory-perceptual feedback have in it? What role does unconscious afference have in it? What role does seriation play in the disorder? What role does the parietal lobe play? Is the disorder different in the parietal lobe? What is the role of subcortical structure on the disorder? Does one treatment type help more than others? What difference does it make that meaning and length have an influence? How is it related to slips of the tongue? Is the disorder merely intensification of normal tendencies? How does thought affect it? Is it a variety of dysarthria? What part does mistiming and incoordination play in the disorder? Is it a form of ataxic dysarthria? Do *types* of apraxia of speech exist? Does the condition change its nature over time? How is it behaviorally distinctive from aphasia and the dysarthrias? Is it treatable? Should it be treated differently at different times? Will it go away if left alone? Why is it so often seen with aphasia? Does it truly exist in pure culture? If it is a motor programming disorder, how do you measure programming? What is programming? Does the neuromuscular movement disorder just exist in parallel to the phonological encoding problem? Is it primarily a selection and sequencing problem? Is it primarily an initiation problem? Is it speech specific? Are there analogues in other movement disruptions? Is it related to errors on the typewriter or piano? Is the essential nature of it masked in very severe cases? Is it a disconnection phenomenon? What part does disrupted input play? Is it syntagmatic or paradigmatic? What is volitional movement? What is error "variability"? Is there a difference between sequencing and transitionalizing? What are the nonlinguistic behavioral characteristics of the disorder? Why is all of this important?

These are only a few of the issues with which professionals have grappled at conferences and workshops, with students, and in this volume.

LESSER'S CONTRIBUTION

Ruth Lesser (1978) has written a remarkably clear synthesis of the controversy surrounding apraxia of speech. She presents a linguist's perspective but impregnates the controversy with the fairness of other views and shores her arguments with some of the experimental evidence that is available.

The levels of organization and explanation of the disorder are categorized by Lesser (1978) into three divisions:

(1.) The Neuromuscular Approach — This is the approach which emphasizes articulation and prosodic problems in terms of a breakdown in the complicated neuromuscular organization needed for controlled initiation and sequencing of speech sounds.

(2.) The Phonological Encoding Approach — This approach considers phonological disorders to be encoding disturbances which follow lawful linguistic patterns, rather than neuromuscular disruption.

(3.) The Central Phonological Approach — This approach considers the breakdown as being one of central phonological organization traceable in both speech and comprehension.

As suggested earlier, the term apraxia of speech is not universally acceptable and Lesser presents some of the arguments on both sides of the issue. First, she discusses the necessary distinction of phonetic versus phonemic differences. This distinction has been discussed as well by Goodglass (1975), and in a later portion of this essay. He proposed that phonemic errors are errors of programming entire, well-articulated phonemes while phonetic failures are best conceived of as involving the organization of motor commands.

Lesser (1978) draws from the work of Lecours and his colleagues (Lecours, Dordain & Lhermitte, 1970; Lecours & Lhermitte, 1976) to explain and amplify the phonetic level of organization. These French researchers have conceived of a variety of processes that result in phonetic realization, including what they call the "third articulation"; a level that involves the choice of a number of discrete actions of muscles of the oral apparatus plus their cotemporal integration into speech sounds. They also describe the "second articulation" (Lesser calls it the phonemic level) which involves the selection of phonemes and their serial integration into more complex segments. Lesser suggests that this view permits us to make distinctions among phonological impairments and to isolate a phonetic disorder, with its characteristic distorted sounds, allophonic variants, or sounds which are not part of the inventory of the native language. For other speakers, who supposedly deviate only at the phonemic level, phonemic transcription without diacritical markings is sufficient to capture their errors, since the sounds they produce are "well articulated" and acceptable to the phonemic inventory, but may be inappropriate to context and presumably differ from their intended realization. Intent is sometimes very difficult to discern, however, although context and careful preparation of speech-eliciting stimuli can aid us in this determination. Lesser suggests that this distinction, phonetic from phonemic, is one that may escape by using such a broad classification as "apraxia of speech", and may be a disadvantage of the label. Use of the label, however, has never negated the necessity for careful and complete behavioral and linguistic description of phonological behavior, for therein lies the core of relevant treatment, as well as an understanding of the nature of the condition. Most of the people who subscribe to the use of "apraxia of speech" realize fully that the disorder can be characterized by a mosaic of phonetic, phonemic, and nonlinguistic behaviors. The precise ratio and nature of the ingredients in this phonological and behavioral mixture is no doubt influenced by lesion and time, but exactly how and in what ways are still unclear.

Lesser also points out that those who use the term "apraxia of speech" sometimes do so with different emphases. Some, such as Darley et al. (1975), emphasize faulty programming of movements of the articulators. Control and coordination of the muscles required for speech are compromised when the left or dominant hemisphere, which assumes the lead in selecting and sending the messages for speech movements, is damaged.

Lesser summarizes some of the beliefs of those who view *Apraxia of Speech as a Neuromuscular Phenomenon*. The proponents of this perspective conclude that:

(1.) A neuromuscular coordination system specific to language and probably under unilateral dominance regulates speech.

(2.) A person with the disorder is assumed to have intact "intention to speak," with phonological shapes of the words mapped out but not yet realized, and the prime difficulty is in translation of these shapes into coordinated patterns of articulatory movements for phonetic realization.

(3.) Linguistic factors can influence phonological integrity with regularity, but only in the sense of the degree to which successful coordination is achieved.

(4.) The disorder is specific to the production of speech and implications in other modalities are as yet undocumented.

(5.) Syntactic and semantic disorders coexist only as the result of neighborhood lesions compromising separate systems, and the disorder is specific to phonological speech production.

In her summary of the *Phonological Encoding Approach*, Lesser advances the arguments of Blumstein (1973) and of Martin and Rigrodsky (1974) as well as others. Blumstein's primary conclusions from her study of phonological disturbances in aphasic speech are:

(1.) Errors are not inconsistent and can be described according to a system.

(2.) The linguistic constructs of distinctive features and markedness can be used in describing this systematic phonological disruption.

(3.) All types of aphasia showed similar patterns of phonological errors.

Blumstein's finding of the essential homogeneity of phonological errors in the main types of aphasia, coupled with the findings of Poncet, Degos, Deloche, and Lecours (1972) and other researchers, leads Lesser to suggest that phonological disorders in aphasia can be best described in terms of the utilization of a linguistic encoding system rather than principally in terms of neuromuscular difficulties.

In support of a *Central Phonological Deficit Approach*, Lesser cites a series of studies on comprehension and phonemic discrimination. In addition, the arguments of Schnitzer (1971) are presented as evidence of a central linguistic deficit. Schnitzer concluded from a comprehensive analysis of the responses of one aphasic patient that the characteristics of the errors demonstrate not only the violation of the rules of generative phonology but also "account for widespread and seemingly random phonetic-level errors."

Blumstein (1974), however, has suggested that the errors of Schnitzer's patient were limited to reading aloud and may be explainable in terms of reading strategies rather than by violations of phonetic output rules.

Lesser concludes her discussion of approaches to the controversies involved in phonological disorders by suggesting that the systematic linguistic nature of phonological errors in speech weakens the case for phonemic disorders being principally disruptions of neuromotor programming for speech. She also states that the case for their being disorders specifically of linguistic encoding that exist without disruption of perception or comprehension has not yet been refuted. She concludes, "taken together these observations suggest that not only the phonetic but the phonemic level of language operates at a relatively peripheral part of the language system" (Lesser, 1978, p. 182).

Several areas of controversy have been explored by Buckingham in a chapter he titles "Explanation for the concept of apraxia of speech" (Buckingham, 1981). He outlines his views on the reasons for some of the confusion surrounding the disorder and proposes that "certain phonological functions as understood by linguistics operate *in parallel with* and at a distinct level from the hierarchically organized sensory-motor practic functions of the brain" (Buckingham, 1981, p. 271). He feels much of the confusion surrounding the disorder is at the level of explanation and not at the level of data. Buckingham postulates and reviews the historical precedent and contemporary evidence for two different neuroanatomical explanations for apraxia; center lesion and disconnection. Buckingham develops an insightful critique of both positions, reviews the contributions of contemporary studies on voice onset time, pleads for more careful description of both the linguistic parameters and the behavioral context in which they occur, and aptly concludes, "whether or not one of these explanations will generally come to be accepted over the other, only time will tell" (Buckingham, 1981, p. 297). Both notions are discussed later in this essay.

This has been a presentation of some of the historic and contemporary controversy surrounding the disorder of apraxia of speech. Future research and interpretation will no doubt clarify issues and answer some questions. Equally certain is that the process of scientific inquiry will open new avenues of controversy and generate further hypothesis testing. We hope to do the same with this essay.

To that end, subsequent portions of this essay outline our attitudes about the disorder's definition, nature, clinical diagnosis, and treatment. A substantive portion of all these sections is given over to contemporary acoustic data. Mostly they were written as answers to selected questions raised in the first section of this essay and to guide future research.

ON DEFINITIONS

The definition of apraxia of speech as an impairment of motor programming can create certain difficulties from both clinical and theoretical perspectives. Motor programs are a hypothetical, and currently controversial, idea in motor control (Reed, 1982). Particularly with respect to limb movements, several objections have been thrown against the strict version of the motor programming hypothesis, viz., that a preplanned pattern of movement commands is executed without reliance on afferent information generated during performance of the movements. Another difficulty with the motor programming definition of apraxia of speech is that we do not have a universally recognized clinical tool to measure impaired capacity for motor programming. Such an impairment is strictly inferential and the basis for its determination must be explicitly stated so that the impairment in motor programming can be distinguished from other neuropathologies. If the idea of motor program is stated too abstractly, then it might be difficult to distinguish apraxia of speech from an aphasic impairment (which is exactly the position that Martin, 1974, took). In order that the term "motor programming impairment" can be made experimentally and clinically verifiable, the content of the motor program must be specified (cf. Kent, 1981). Otherwise, it is not clear what aspects of motor control are part of a program and what aspects are not specified in the program.

Darley's (1969) definition, published somewhat later than his original definition summarized in the previous historical review, indicated the content of a speech motor program to include positioning and sequencing of the articulators. He defined apraxia of speech as "an articulatory disorder resulting from impairment, as a result of brain damage, of the capacity to program the positioning of speech musculature and the sequencing of muscle movements for the volitional production of phonemes" (cited by Deal & Darley, 1972, p. 639). So far the definition would not exclude the dysarthrias, particularly if one believes along with Grimm and Nashner (1978) that conditions like certain of of the dysarthrias may be grouped together as program disorders. Darley continued his definition by noting that, "The speech musculature does not show significant weakness, slowness, or incoordination when used for reflex and automatic acts." Finally, he added, "prosodic alterations may be associated with the articulatory problem, perhaps in compensation for it." The semantic kernel of this three-sentence definition seems to be that apraxia of speech is an impaired capacity to form vocal tract configurations and to make transitions between vocal configurations for volitional speech production, in the absence of motor impairments for other actions using the same musculature. This last phrase is critical for it distinguishes apraxia of speech from the dysarthrias. Even for those dysarthrias that might be called motor program disorders (by analogy to the motor program disorders described by Grimm & Nashner, 1978) impaired movement generally is observed for all contexts and purposes of that movement.

Anyone undertaking the task of defining a speech or language impairment is well-advised to read Crystal's (1982) paper in which he suggests a lexicographer's analysis of terms used in the literature of speech and language disorders. He considers by way of example definitions of apraxia of speech by Martin (1974) and of developmental articulatory apraxia by Morley (1972). Lexicographic analysis can help us to formulate more rigorous and less ambiguous definitions, or at the least to be more aware of the assumptions underlying our definitions. The definition offered above indicates that the observable symptoms of apraxia of speech are failures to make appropriate vocal tract configurations for sounds and to effect transitions between these configurations. The impairment was observed during attempts at volitional, purposive speech production, and to a lesser degree, if at all, during automatic or reflexive speech. In addition, the definition states that the motor impairment applies to speech only, and not to nonspeech tasks using the musculature of the speech apparatus. Practically (that is, clinically) speaking, this definition is adequate for diagnostic purposes if it can be agreed as to what constitutes evidence of impaired capacity to form vocal tract configurations and to make transitions between configurations. There might be some disagreement about the relative prominence of substitution errors versus distortion errors; about the centrality of prosodic abnormalities in characterizing the disorder; about site of lesion; about the importance of establishing hierarchies of difficulty for different types of phonetic or linguistic material, and so on. These questions are not solved by fiat and will be considered in some detail in the balance of this chapter. Many of these questions have to do with the nature of apraxia of speech, a topic to which we turn next.

THE NATURE OF APRAXIA OF SPEECH

Perceptual Descriptions of Articulatory Errors

Darley (1982) describes apraxia of speech as a disorder in which the "patient has trouble speaking because of a cerebral lesion that prevents his executing voluntarily and on command the complex motor activities involved in speaking, despite the fact that muscle strength is undiminished" (p. 10). Darley lists 13 descriptive properties of apraxia of speech which nicely summarize the perceptual characterizations of this disorder.

These properties are briefly summarized below (see Darley's book for supporting citations).

(1.) Articulatory errors increase as the presumed complexity or difficulty of the speech motor task increases. Thus, errors increase in the order: vowels, singleton consonants, consonant clusters.

(2.) Initial consonants are more often in error than consonants in other positions.

(3.) Both a consistency effect and an adaptation effect are observed as an apraxic patient repeatedly reads the same material. That is, although errors tend to occur in the same places in the text, the overall number of errors declines on successive readings.

(4.) The frequency of errors for phonemes is related to the frequency of occurrence of phonemes in the language, with fewer errors for frequently occurring phonemes.

(5.) Distinctive feature analyses of substitution errors in apraxia of speech reveal variable relationships between errors and targets. Most substitutions involve one or two feature errors, which indicates that substitutions preserve some properties of the target sound.

(6.) Sequential errors of prepositioning, postpositioning, and metathesis account for a small part (less than 10% of the total errors). Prepositioning errors are the dominant type of sequencing error.

(7.) Automatic and reactive speech production tends to be much better than volitional-purposive speech production.

(8.) Articulatory errors occur more frequently during imitative performance than during spontaneous speech. Repetitive responses of some subjects have remarkably long latencies.

(9.) Articulation errors increase with word length.

(10.) Articulatory errors during oral reading are more likely to occur on words carrying greater propositionality or greater linguistic or psychologic weight. Relevant factors include: grammatical class, difficulty of initial phoneme, position in the sentence, and word length.

(11.) Mode of stimulus presentation can affect stimulus performance, with better results for live presentation by a visible examiner than for tape recorded or printed stimuli.

(12.) Probability of an eventual correct performance is higher for repeated trials of a word than for a single trial after multiple presentations of the word.

(13.) Articulatory performance is *unaffected* by the following visual, auditory and psychological variables: availability of visual monitoring by mirror; masking noise to reduce or prevent perception of errors; provision of a delay before attempting an imitative response; instructional set (especially expectation of difficulty); availability of rhythmic auditory stimulation (metronome).

Acoustic and Physiological Descriptions

Kent and Rosenbek (1983) conclude from an acoustic study of seven apraxic subjects that the disorder is characterized by a variety of segmental and prosodic abnormalities including: slow speaking rate with prolongations of transitions, steady states, and intersyllable pauses; reduced intensity variation across syllables in an utterance, slow and inaccurate movements of the articulators; discoordination of voicing with other articulations; initiation difficulties; and errors of selection or sequencing of segments. Prolongations of segments were especially marked for longer utterances, and the slowed speaking rate typically took one of two major forms. The first of these, *articulatory prolongation,* is defined as a lengthening of steady-state segments and the intervening transitions. The second, *syllable segregation*, is defined as a pattern of temporally separated or isolated syllables. The reduced range of intensity variation from syllable to syllable was part of an overall weakening of prosodic contrast which included occasional failure of vowel reduction (i.e., inappropriately long durations of unstressed vowel targets) and fractured f_0 contours over sentence-length utterances. Acoustic transitions between steady-state targets frequently were lengthened in comparison to normal speech and sometimes evidenced plateaus as though the gestures were interrupted and then resumed after a brief delay. Discoordination of voicing with supralaryngeal articulation was observed especially for stop and fricative segments. For example, in a word like *shush*, voicing for the vowel segment sometimes began before the end of the frication for the initial fricative and ceased too early with respect to the final fricative. Initiation difficulties were expressed as prolongations of initial segments and as interrupted vocal patterns occuring on the first sound of an utterance.

The significance of the prosodic abnormalities is open to question. Darley (1969; 1982) seems to favor the idea that prosodic alterations are compensations for the more primary articulatory impairment or, at most, that such alterations are accompaniments of the articulatory impairment. One reason for the uncertainty about prosodic dimensions is that they have not been described as carefully as the articulatory component of the apraxic syndrome. Another reason, we believe, is that prosodic (or suprasegmental) and segmental aspects are not as easily separated in the neuropathologies as they are in general linguistics (Kent & Rosenbek, 1983). For example, if slowness of movement is a hallmark feature of apraxia of speech, then a prosodic deviance in the form of reduced speaking rate logically follows. A related interpretive problem is that the direct effects of a lesion are not easily distinguished from compensations for the impairment (Kent, Netsell, & Abbs, 1979).

The overall prosodic picture from the results of Kent and Rosenbek (1983) is that apraxia of speech tends to be associated with a slow speaking rate (with lengthening of both transitions and steady states of the acoustic signal) and a flattening of prosodic contrast among syllables. This prosodic flattening was especially evident in the intensity envelope of speech, for which the apraxic subjects showed smaller syllable-to-syllable variations than did normal speakers. This intensity effect could have been related to the slower speaking rate of the apraxic subjects. Kent and Rosenbek did not observe consistent differences in the fundamental frequency contour (f_0) of apraxic and normal speakers, although individual apraxic subjects produced abnormal patterns. Terminal fall (decreasing f_0 on the final word or syllable of an utterance) was reliably produced by the apraxic subjects, an observation which led Kent and Rosenbek to conclude that this prosodic feature may be highly robust and therefore resistant to all but devastating brain damage. Because of the large interspeaker variability, it was difficult to assess the presence or absence of declination (or f_0"downdrift"), which has been invested with psycholinguistic significance by several writers (Cooper & Sorensen, 1977, 1981; Pierrehumbert, 1979; Sorensen & Cooper, 1980; Thorsen, 1980). Presumably, declination, which is perceived as a long-term fall of the medium pitch line during a sentence, varies with utterance duration, syntactic bracketing, and sentence type. Accordingly, this prosodic feature is of interest in neuropathologies of speech and language as a possible indicator of linguistic integrity and/or preprogramming capacity. Given the difficulty of assessing declination in some patients with apraxia of speech and given various doubts about its relevance to psycholinguistic factors and mechanisms of preprogramming (Cohen, Collier, & Hart, 1982), it seems prudent to leave the matter to further investigation.

Itoh and Sasanuma (this volume, Chap. 5) conclude that at the base of the symptom complex called "apraxia of speech" is a faulty programming of the speech musculature. They go on to suggest that the "most natural and reasonable end-products of this underlying deficit are (phonetic) distortions." They believe that distortions occur more frequently than the literature indicates, especially because perceptual factors bias toward the perception of substitutions (change of phonemic category) rather than distortions (within category variations). Two of us (Kent & Rosenbek, 1983) have argued in similar fashion and will not belabor this particular point here.

Unfortunately, the phonetic habits we use in describing our data often shape our results and conclusions more than we might like. For example, we read in Keller's paper (this volume, Chap. 8) that one form of simplification is "the insertion of uncalled-for phonemes (such as intrusive schwas)." The problem here is that the intrusive schwa generously supplied by our auditory system is not necessarily, indeed in all likelihood is not, a phoneme. We may often tend to perceive schwas when articulatory transitions are slow, irregular, or otherwise deviant from the normal dynamic pattern. But we should not imply that these schwas are intrusive phonemes operating in the phonology of the speaker; more correctly, they are intrusive schwas operating in the auditory perceptual systems of the listener. Frequently, what we hear as schwas are not well-defined, brief steady states, but rather intervals of continuous articulatory change (Shriberg & Kent, 1982). We must guard against the phonemic (segmental) overinterpretation of slow, labored, or irregular articulatory transitions. What we are inclined to hear as intrusive segments often might be more appropriately understood as misguided or poorly regulated transitions between targets.

Difficulty with articulatory transitions is evidenced not only by the slowness and discoordination of articulatory movements comprising transitions, but perhaps as well by increased durations and other abnormalities of the steady-state segments intervening between transitions. That is, the disturbed mechanism may adjust for the difficulty in making appropriate transitions by slowing the overall rate of motor performance. Increased durations of the steady-state segments may allow more time for the planning and initiation of upcoming transitions. Difficulties in retrieval and execution frequently affect behavioral components immediately preceding the event causing the difficulty. Thus, Butterworth (1979) reported that neologisms in jargon aphasia were found to follow pauses, so that pauses can be taken as evidence of a word-finding difficulty even before the neologism is uttered. In similar fashion, lengthening of steady-state segments (particularly vowels and consonantal constrictions) may indicate not so much a difficulty with the prolonged segment as a difficulty with the upcoming segment or the transition to it. This idea may reconcile Duffy and Gawle's finding (this volume, Chap. 6) of shorter than normal vowel durations in apraxic productions of imitated consonant-vowel-consonant (CVC) utterances with other results showing that apraxic vowels are longer than normal vowels for word or sentence length utterances (Ryalls, 1981; Kent & Rosenbek, 1983). CVC utterances, by virtue of their relative simplicity, may not present to the apraxic speaker the degree of difficulty that longer, more complex utterances present. The CVC syllable involves few transitions and very likely no major transitions involving the tongue body (the major articulator for vowel-to-vowel transitions).

It would be predicted from speech production models that posit a parallel but coordinated production of vowels and consonants (Fowler, 1980) that CVC utterances would be simpler motorically than utterances involving both consonantal and vowel changes. CVC utterances require only a single vowel (tongue body) adjustment, which is often anticipated during (coproduced with, in Fowler's terms) the syllable-initial consonant. Because the vowel gesture is basically accomplished at syllable onset, and because the vowel target is not followed by another vowel target (thus another tongue body transition), lengthening of the vowel segment of CVCs is not expected.

Phonetic transitions, that is, transitions between the presumed phonetic targets in an output string, are accomplished by movements of one or more articulators. These component movements can be timed to occur synchronously or sequentially (Kent, 1983), depending on the nature of the transition and its acoustic-perceptual impact. Data reported by Itoh, Sasanuma, and Ushijima (1979) and by Itoh and Sasanuma (this volume, Chap. 5) indicate that apraxia of speech is associated with a breakdown of the normally tight temporal patterning of two or more component movements in a transition. Speech is ultimately describable temporally (in the physical sense of time) not as a sequence of perceived phonetic segments, but as a sequence of component movements, the timing of which ensures the transmission of the desired linguistic message. A mistiming of the component movements can result in a marked perceptual change, indeed one large enough to qualify as a substitutional error. Itoh, Sasanuma, and Ushijima (1979) described how the mistiming of two articulatory movements (velar movement and tongue tip movement) can generate a deviation recognized perceptually as a substitution of /d/ for /n/.

Ryalls (1981) interpreted acoustic data on vowel production to mean that motor aphasic subjects had "a problem in motor implementation of an appropriate phonemic selection" and also "a deficit in the internal phonemic representation" (p. 365). Because Ryalls' conclusions speak directly to a major issue in understanding apraxia of speech (Keller, this volume, Chap. 8), his data and conclusions merit a closer look. Ryalls inferred the problem in motor implementation (which he also described as "a deficit in phonetic realization" (p. 365), from data showing a greater variability in formant patterns for the subjects with motor aphasia than for normal speakers. This greater variability was observed even when the two groups did not differ in their mean formant frequency values: "aphasic patients produced more variability in formant productions than did normals for the F1 of the vowel /ɔ/, and the F2 of the vowel /ɛ/, in spite of no difference in the means" (p. 368). Ryalls' conclusion that the subjects with motor aphasia could not maintain a stable phonetic output should be viewed in the light that he reported group statistics. A stronger case could have been made if it could be shown that the motor aphasic subjects had greater individual variability *across time* than did the normal speakers. Unfortunately, group data on formant frequencies are affected by several variables, such as differences in size of the vocal tract, dialect, and speaking rate. Assessments of stability of production are more appropriately made by observing intra-individual variability in repeated productions of a target (Eguchi & Hirsh, 1969; Kent & Forner, 1980).

Ryalls' second conclusion, that of "a deficit in internal phonemic representation" (which he alternatively phrased as a "phonetic disintegration of the phonemic targets," p. 365) also is based on arguable evidence, viz., that the mean formant frequency values differed significantly between the two groups for some of the vowels. As noted above, formant frequencies for any given vowel are determined by the dimensions of a speaker's vocal tract, by dialectal factors, by speaking rate, and several other variables. Any one of these could contribute to the differences in mean formant frequency reported by Ryalls. Furthermore, Ryall's discussion of these data is self-contradictory. He stated on page 368 that "The change in mean F1 and F2 values resulted in an /ɑ/ which was raised and fronted for the aphasic patients," but then later commented that the aphasic patients' "productions of the vowel /ɑ/ were significantly backed and lowered (higher F1 and lower F2, respectively" (p. 373). Generally speaking, the F1 frequency varies with tongue height and the F2 frequency varies with advancement, or just the opposite of Ryalls' statement. Given these several interpretative problems and inconsistencies, we cannot agree with Ryalls' conclusions at least not on the basis of the data he presented.

Dimensions of Phonetic Deterioration: Feature Unmarking and Simplification as Entropic Decay

Markedness (naturalness) analyses indicate that errors in apraxic speech are similar to patterns observed in children's speech development (Klich, Ireland, & Weidner, 1979; Marquardt, Reinhart, & Peterson, 1979). One interpretation of this result is that apraxia of speech is a kind of developmental regression, or a falling back to an earlier developmental phase. But this is not the only, nor most useful, interpretation. Another interpretation rests on Bailey's (1982) observation that, "Connatural feature-unmarkings are to language what entropy is to thermodynamics" (p. 154). A few words of explanation are in order. First, *connatural* refers to bioneurologically motivated developments occuring in a language that is isolated from other systems (as opposed to *abnatural* developments that result from interlanguage contact). Second, feature-unmarking denotes a phonetic change in the direction of naturalness. Third, entropy is the uniform, random, high-probability distribution of unconnected molecules that the second law of thermodynamics holds to be the ultimate state of any closed system. The linguistic analogue of entropy is a totally unmarked (maximally natural) language system.[1]

The deterioration of phonetic patterns in apraxia of speech (or in any other disorder tending toward feature-unmarking) is an entropic change, that is, a change toward the most predictable states or outcomes. Unmarked features are determined largely by studies of speech development in children and by studies of language change. It is not surprising that certain speech and language disorders should result in phonetic patterns like those seen in young children's speech. Indeed, the more remarkable outcome would be negentropic change (toward feature marking). Possibly, feature-unmarking in neuropathologies reflects a relaxation or weakening of the analytic, sociocommunicational functions of language. As these functions are impaired, entropic changes in the form of connatural feature-unmarkings will accelerate. The entropic hypothesis is one answer to Keller's question "what cognitive or motoric aspect of unmarked sounds causes them to be easier to produce than marked sounds under conditions of speech neuropathology?" (It should be kept in mind that naturalness does not necessarily imply ease or reduced difficulty of articulation. For example, /s/ is a relatively unmarked consonant, but it is a relatively late sound to be mastered by children and is often judged difficult to produce.)

Naturalness is one factor that influences articulatory patterns in apraxia of speech. Keller's data on the dual hypotheses of simplification and gesture reduction may represent similar dimensions (or complementary aspects) of phonologic or articulatory deterioration. Keller further proposes that the two hypotheses may be married into a single "ease of transition" hypothesis, which predicts that apraxic and aphasic speakers will use fewer "difficult" transitions and will reduce the "trajectories" of transitions they do produce. Given that the result provided fairly strong support for the simplification hypothesis but at best moderate support for the gesture reduction hypothesis, we should perhaps be reluctant to accept the combined "ease of transition" hypothesis. The fact that both reduction *and* extension were observed for Broca's and conduction aphasic subjects is reason to be cautious about a premature acceptance of the idea that these subjects reduce the "trajectory" of articulatory transitions.

Perhaps Keller's ideas are elaborations of the notion of naturalness in phonetic production. Furthermore, perhaps determinations of naturalness point to a major dimension of phonologic or phonetic change in neuropathologies, namely, an entropic deterioration in which natural (unmarked) states tend to replace unnatural (marked) states. Feature-unmarking is not necessarily evidence of developmental regression but rather a kind of phonetic decay (entropic change) which lies at the root of both developmental phonetic patterns and phonetic patterns in some neuropathologies.

How Many Apraxias Are There?

Many questions remain about how apraxia of speech relates to oral apraxia and how both of these relate to the traditional apraxias such as ideational, ideomotor, and limb-kinetic apraxias. Is apraxia of speech a form of limb-kinetic apraxia? Does apraxia of speech take only one form, or are there types of apraxia of speech? Buckingham (1979) concluded that, "all the center-lesion theories of apraxia usually admit of one or more distinct 'apraxias of speech'" (p. 215). For example, Buckingham notes that both Luria and Jason Brown refer (implicitly if not explicitly) to kinetic, ideomotor, and ideational apraxias of speech. If different forms of apraxia of speech are to be recognized, then the problem of syndrome delineation goes far beyond the matter of simply differentiating apraxia of speech from the aphasias and the dysarthrias. Johns and LaPointe (1976) regard apraxia of speech as a kind of limb-kinetic apraxia of the speech musculature, although as Buckingham points out, they may mention complications which might lead to the recognition of an apraxic syndrome based primarily on sensory-perceptual deficits rather than a motor impairment per se. (See Deutsch in this volume, Chap. 4, for further discussion.)

Uncertainties also surround the relationship of oral apraxia to ideomotor limb apraxia. Poeck, Lehmkuhl, and Willmes (1982) stated that the "great majority of patients with (ideomotor) limb apraxia have also oral apraxia in the form of bucco-facial movements'' (p. 1125). They regarded this correlation to be inconsistent with Geschwind's (1975) opinion that patients with ideomotor apraxia can perform axial (whole body or midline structure) movements. However, because Geschwind excepted oral movements from this general principle, Poeck et al. also examined axial movements more in keeping with Geschwind's notion (e.g., rolling both eyes upward, moving the head or shoulders, walking). They determined that even these axial movements frequently were impaired in the patients with ideomotor apraxia. Thus, axial or whole-body movements may not be spared in ideomotor apraxia, and oral movements may be affected similarly to movements of other midline structures.

Distinctions among the ideational, ideomotor, and limb-kinetic forms of apraxia could have profound implications for description, explanation, and treatment of an apraxic impairment. For example, Lehmkuhl and Poeck (1981) concluded that ideational apraxia, in contrast to ideomotor apraxia, ''is not characterized by defective motor programming but that it is a disturbance in the conceptual organization of actions'' (p. 157). The essential difference between the two forms of apraxia is shown by their dissimilar performances in a task of distinguishing correct and incorrect gestures in photographs. Patients with ideomotor apraxia perform quite well but patients with ideational apraxia fare poorly.

Many writers on motor performance distinguish the plan or goal of a behavior from its serial order. Locke (1978) offered this concise statement: ''This plan, or prediction, constitutes the intent of the organism. And the serial order of behavior is determined by the intent'' (p. 114). Thus, we might imagine errors in planning to be distinct from errors in serial ordering, which in turn could be distinct from errors in execution or implementation. Whether or not these three types of errors are useful in describing apraxia of speech is a matter of some disagreement.

Clinicoanatomic Studies of Apraxia of Speech

Clinicoanatomic studies do not always yield a clear picture of the correlation between functional impairment and structural damage. Marquardt and Sussman's paper in this volume (Chap. 3) is further testimony to the difficulties in this area of investigation. A major issue is the suitability of the various methods used to describe regions of brain damage. A number of techniques have been used: computed tomography, pertechnetate brain scanning, angiography, pathology, and regional cerebral blood flow (and nuclear magnetic resonance soon may be added to the list). The different techniques do not necessarily yield the same information about location or size of lesion. We will not take the time here for an extensive review of the pertinent literature, but point instead to an example. Metter, Wasterlain, Kuhl, Hanson, and Phelps (1981) investigated the correlations among clinical studies, anatomy (as described by computerized tomography, CT), and metabolism (monitored by positron emission computed tomography using F-2-fluoro-2-deoxy-D-glucose) in five aphasic patients. Results showed reduction of local cerebral metabolic activity in an area larger than the area of infarction demonstrated by CT. Moreover, a metabolic lesion discovered in one patient and judged to be the cause of the aphasic impairment, was not apparent by CT.

There has been a general, or statistical, success in localizing lesions for major types of aphasia, e.g., demonstration of anterior lesions for Broca's (nonfluent) aphasia and posterior lesions for Wernicke's (fluent) aphasia (Basso, Salvolini, & Vignolo, 1979; Blunk, DeBlesser, Willmes, & Zeumer, 1981; Mazzucchi & Vignolo, 1979; Noel, Bain, Collard, & Huvelle, 1980). However, exceptions even to this general pattern have been reported. In addition, some refinements to the traditional picture should be noted: studies indicate that damage to the insular cortex often may be associated with nonfluent aphasia or with apraxic syndromes (see review of studies in Kent, in press-a). Another complication is that broad categories such as fluent versus nonfluent aphasia may disguise significant clinical variations within a broad category of impairment. Cappa, Cavalotti, and Vignolo (1981) reported that two types of fluent aphasia were associated with different lesion sites. One type with predominantly lexical errors was associated with damage to regions nearer the lateral fissure (the perisylvian areas), whereas another type with predominantly phonemic errors was correlated with damage to regions more remote from the lateral fissure (the marginal areas). Similarly, with respect to anterior syndromes, Tonkonogy and Goodglass (1981) concluded from studies of two patients with expressive disorders that word-finding difficulties are associated with lesions of posterior F3 and that articulatory disorders are associated with lesions of the rolandic operculum.

How does apraxia of speech stand with respect to the three broad divisions of brain structure and function, namely, anterior versus posterior, left versus right hemisphere, and cortical versus subcortical? It must be acknowledged at the outset that these divisions and the implied dichotomies can be highly misleading. Nevertheless, these divisions bear on the disorder of apraxia of speech, if for no other reason than that the traditional centerist theory places the underlying damage primarily to the anterior regions of the left (dominant) hemisphere. Our consideration begins with relevant evidence of functional hemispheric asymmetry.

The literature on lateralization of the brain is formidable and it does not permit simple characterizations of left-hemisphere function versus right-hemisphere function (a brief review of the complications is offered in Kent, in press-a). However, it is useful to denote certain tendencies of lateral preference as "hemispheric advantages" which frequently show a complementary pattern (thus, hemispheric functional contrasts have been described as verbal/nonverbal, analytic/holistic, serial/parallel, focal/diffuse, algebraic/geometric, propositional/affective, and so on). While recognizing that any such complementary advantages are not without exception, we believe that these functional descriptions have a certain value in understanding the neural organization of behavior. The functional contrast we wish to use here is closely related to the analytic/holistic description, except that in our usage we do not mean to imply that the right hemisphere with its presumed advantage in holistic processing is incapable of operations in the temporal domain (particularly for the more slowly varying time patterns such as those required for processing of prosody, vocally conveyed emotion, or voice recognition). We do not endorse the idea that the right hemisphere is nonverbal or mute, although it might have somewhat different linguistic propensities than the left.

The preferred analytic mode of the left hemisphere seems to take two major forms: sequences and hierarchies. Both of these require the explicit nature of analysis: differentiation into constituents. Although there is a large risk in the overinterpretation of apparent hemispheric specializations (more properly called complementary advantages), there is substantial evidence that sequential and hierarchical arrangements are more the work of the dominant (left) hemisphere rather than the right. Part of the evidence is that the left hemisphere seems to be capable of a finer temporal resolution than the right (Mills & Rollman, 1979; Divenyi & Efron, 1979; Hammond, 1982). Why this should be so is not clear, but Seldon's (1981a, 1981b) work indicates that the left hemisphere might be cytoarchitectonically biased to favor precise temporal processing. When the arrangements of columnar clusters of neuron somata are compared for the left and right human auditory cortices, both the column diameters and their intercolumn spacing are larger for the left, which Seldon (1981b) sees as favoring the left-hemisphere processing of rapid auditory patterns. If this asymmetry is genetically determined, then the left hemisphere is more likely than the right to attract control of behavior requiring fine temporal resolution (therefore speech perception and production). (It is interesting that Walker, 1980, concluded from a review of studies on lateralization in the vertebrate brain that the strongest evidence of hemispheric lateralization exists for humans and birds, both of which have highly developed vocalization abilities. Thus, vocalization ability may be the primary factor in conditioning functional asymmetry of the cerebral hemispheres.)

A left-hemisphere capacity for processing of hierarchical structure is indicated by the work of Grossman (1980). In his experiments, subjects with Broca's aphasia were asked to construct nonlinguistic, hierarchical tree structures. Their poor performance on this task was interpreted to mean that they forgot the hierarchical organization of the visuospatial material and relied instead on a chainlike strategy. That is, damage to Broca's area results in impairment of the processing of hierarchical structure. Some investigators have proposed that the supplementary motor area is similarly involved in the planning of sequential or hierarchical behavior (Kornhuber, 1980; Kirzinger & Jurgens, 1982; Eccles, 1982). This hypothesis is supported by the observation of Roland, Larsen, Lassen and Skinhoj (1980) that local cerebral blood flow in the supplementary motor area increased not only during the execution of finger movements but also during the *imagined* performance of these movements. Furthermore, the increases in blood flow were reported for *complex* motor sequences, but not for a simple tapping task.

It appears, then, that various regions of the left hemisphere are vested with the capacity for the processing of temporal sequence or hierarchical structure (analytic processing). Damage to these areas results in deficits in managing sequential or hierarchical information, the primary characteristics of anterior (nonfluent) aphasia, oral apraxia, and apraxia of speech. Conceivably, the symptoms of apraxia of speech relate primarily to impairment of sequential (temporal) processing, whereas nonfluent aphasia involves primarily (or additionally) an impairment of hierarchical information processing (thus agrammatism).

It is significant that apraxia of speech is not accompanied by marked impairments of auditory perception. This discrepancy between productive and perceptual capabilities may indicate that the left-hemisphere advantage for temporal processing is not based on a single "center" of temporal resolution. Interestingly, a similar hemispheric size asymmetry seems to apply to both the posterior speech region (Geschwind & Levitsky, 1968; Galaburda, Sanides & Geschwind, 1978) and the anterior speech region (Falzi, Perrone, & Vignolo, 1982). Both of these size asymmetries are opposite to what may be an overall hemispheric size asymmetry for the mammalian brian: Data for humans (Crichton-Browne, 1880) and rat, mouse, rabbit, and cat (Kolb, Sutherland, Nonneman, & Wishaw, 1982) show a larger right hemisphere, by total surface or weight measurements.

The dissociation of productive and perceptual capability in apraxia of speech stands in conflict with prediction based on Ojemann and Mateer's (1979) discovery of a cortical region with allied functions of phoneme identification and orofacial motor sequencing. This area was determined in cortical stimulation studies (during craniotomy) in which stimulation of the area in question interfered with the subject's performance in tasks of phoneme identification and nonverbal orofacial movements. Ojemann & Mateer regarded this area as a possible cortical center for the motor theory of speech perception. However, the strong perceptual-motor linkage implied by the stimulation studies are not born out in lesion studies, for which independent deficits of speech perception and orofacial motor sequencing frequently have been noted. Other explanations of Ojemann's data have been suggested (Kent, in press-b), but even if the idea of a common region for speech perception and orofacial movement is not confirmed, Ojemann's results fall into the general pattern discussed above, viz., regions of the left hemisphere are implicated in temporal resolution and temporal sequence.

Although apraxia of speech typically is thought to result from cortical damage, it is becoming clear that many types of impairment traditionally associated with cortical dysfunction may result as well from subcortical lesions. We learn from Kertesz' paper in this volume (Chap. 2) that "the subcortical lesions of the striatum are specifically associated with prominent verbal apraxia without many other features of aphasia in the more acute stages of stroke." Furthermore, Kertesz reports that except for differences in severity, the cortical syndrome often is indistinguishable from the subcortical syndrome. These findings fit into a general pattern of the recent literature in which some aphasic impairments have been associated with predominantly subcortical lesions (Ojemann, 1976; Damasio, Damasio, Rizzo, Varney, & Gersh, 1981; Jonas, 1981; Naeser, Alexander, Helm-Estabrooks, Levins, Laughlin, & Geschwind, 1982; Naeser, 1982). For example, Naeser (1982) reported a similarity in language deficit (primarily reduced fluency with good comprehension) between patients with cortical Broca's aphasia and a patient with a subcortical anterior-superior capsular/putaminal lesion. In addition, she observed the same syndrome of fluent speech but impaired language comprehension in patients with cortical Wernicke's aphasia and a patient with posterior capsular/putaminal damage. These observations may confirm Brown's (1979) hypothesis that the fluent–nonfluent distinction that usefully differentiates posterior and anterior aphasias resulting from cortical lesions would similarly apply at the subcortical level (Kent, in press-a).

Reports such as that of Kertesz give us reason to be very careful in making site-of-lesion statements as part of the definition of apraxia of speech. These reports also must be considered in proposing or evaluating models of the apraxic impairment. Many of these models are strictly cortically based. Mlcoch and Noll (1980), elaborating a model presented by Darley, Aronson, and Brown (1975), proposed a model of speech production involving five primary components: an auditory speech processor located at the midtemporal lobe of the dominant cerebral hemisphere; a central language processor in the angular gyrus region; an articulatory coder in the oral-facial region of the postcentral gyrus; a motor speech programmer located at the inferior portion of the third frontal convolution; and the primary motor area of the oral-facial region of the precentral gyrus. Mlcoch and Noll suggested that damage to components in the posterior region, particularly the articulatory coder and speech processor, will result in selectional speech errors, whereas damage to anterior components, especially the motor speech programmer, will lead to sequencing impairments (errors of anticipation, sequencing, and incoordination).

Notwithstanding the long tradition of placing linguistic capacities within cortical structures, we should hold open the possibility that subcortical lesions will impair a variety of language and motor functions. If movements for speech are progressively elaborated in the nervous system, at both cortical and subcortical levels, then we may have to consider models along the lines of Thach's (1975, p. 240) description: "A command for movement . . . occurs in cerebral association cortex and then sequentially feeds through pons, dentate, VA-VL thalamus, and motor cortex, gaining specifications at each stage." A similar kind of functional neural organization may be a feature of coalition models of motor control (to be discussed).

The anterior-posterior dimension of brain damage figures strongly in many considerations of aphasic impairment. Although apraxia of speech has been regarded by some to reflect damage to anterior regions, others hold that the site of lesion at least flirts with the anterior-posterior boundary, if not lying within posterior areas proper (Buckingham, 1979). A disconnectionist view of the disorder is compatible with damage to any part of the brain that may be thought of as a connecting pathway between brain centers. Thus, apraxia of speech could be thought of as an impairment of information transmission between posterior and anterior centers, rather than as a direct result of damage to either an anterior or posterior center. Different hypotheses as to site of lesion can be identified with the centerist school of thought. Darley, Aronson, and Brown (1975) proposed that apraxia of speech results from impairment of a motor speech programmer based anatomically in Broca's area. However, Mlcoch and Noll (1980) hypothesized that apraxic errors reflect damage to both anterior and posterior areas (as reviewed above). Evidence from both stimulation mapping (Ojemann & Mateer, 1979) and lesion studies of oral apraxia (Tognola & Vignolo, 1980) indicate that sequencing impairments are associated with a rather large area of cortex including frontal, parietal, and temporal cortex. A rather similar region is implicated in fluent aphasia characterized by predominantly phonemic errors (Cappa, Cavalotti, & Vignolo, 1981). Another variation of the centerist theory might be that both selectional (phoneme retrieval) processes and motor sequential processes are vested in roughly the same area—the perisylvian cortex.

THEORY AND EXPLANATORY CONCEPTS

Our efforts here are not intended to describe what we believe to be the best theory or explanation of apraxia of speech, but rather to consider different theories or explanations that have been offered. The coverage will not be exhaustive, and no doubt someone's favorite theory will be excluded from discussion. Our choice of theories is constrained somewhat by our definition of apraxia of speech and by the nature of the contributed papers in the volume. The ones that are discussed represent different theoretical approaches to apraxic disorders.

Reed (1982) argued that traditional distinctions in motor control such as central versus peripheral, open loop versus closed loop, and even motor versus sensory are no longer tenable. Among the concepts and theories he rejects are several that have been favorites in discussions of apraxic disorders. One such concept is the *motor program*, or a central command pattern for generating a given pattern of movement. Reed summarizes the evidence against motor programs in two categories: studies of the sensorimotor integration of simple movements, and studies of the limitations of central programming to generate adaptive movements. Regarding the first class of studies, it is clear that reflexes and other simple or triggered responses are organized in such a way that they can be adapted to changing circumstances—a conclusion which runs counter to any idea of fixed movement patterns emanating from a central programmer. The second class of studies is less conclusive and more difficult to present in brief form. Suffice it to say that centrally preprogrammed movements do not appear to be capable of adjusting to perturbations of the movement itself as well as to postural perturbations. We will not try to summarize Reed's lengthy discussions of the failings of traditional concepts of motor control but simply point to his paper to indicate that many established ideas are coming under serious re-examination.

Centers, Coalitions, or Stages?

Centerists versus connectionists. The two traditional schools of thought in the explanation of apraxia of speech are identified by Buckingham (1979) as the "centerist" and "connectionist" positions as we noted earlier in this essay. The center lesion theory holds that the impairment results from damage to a cortical center responsible for the formulation or programming of speech. The disconnectionist theory posits that functional centers or zones are somehow disconnected (in the words of Geschwind, 1975, p. 190: "The explanation . . . tries to account for all the apraxias on the basis of disconnection of the areas in which the command is comprehended from those areas where the command is carried out." Both the centerist and disconnectionist positions hold that functional centers exist; the major difference between them is that the centerist school believes that the disorder of apraxia is the result of damage directly to a functional center, whereas the disconnectionist school maintains that apraxia may be the consequence of a disconnection between functional centers, interrupting the flow of information needed for the adequate control of behavior.[2]

Coalition model. An alternative model, which we term here the "coalition model," is based on the idea that behavior emerges from functional coalitions of neural sructures, which may cross traditional boundaries such as that between cortical and subcortical levels. One version of this model has been described by Kelso and Tuller (1981) who discuss it with particular reference to apraxic disturbances, including apraxia of speech. The coalition model has been favored in some systems theory approaches to social or political organizations. The basic idea is that groups of people who share some but not all goals form coalitions to accomplish objectives of mutual advantage. The coalitions thus formed are not permanent, indeed may not survive beyond an issue or two, but change as a function of the constituent groups. By analogy, sets of neural structures may function together to accomplish certain objectives, but any one constituent structure may also participate in still other coalitions.

Kelso and Tuller argue that the coalition model overcomes some of the serious limitations of the hierarchical model of motor control. Among these limitations are the unidirectionality of information flow in hierarchical systems, the principle of linear transitivity in hierarchical networks (which essentially states that functions at subordinate levels are dictated by higher levels), and the context independence of hierarchically organized systems. The coalition model offers multidirectional information flow, circular transitivity, and context dependency of action. The coalition model is based on the recognition that the relation between an individual and the environment is specific to the behavioral goal, and movement dynamics are constrained by this relation. An advantage of coalitional organization of motor processes is that some properties that cannot be ascribed to any part of a complex structure emerge from the cooperation and interaction of the various substructures. These *emergent properties* can accomplish important functions but need not be identified with any one neural structure operating independently. Thus, some desirable properties may become evident by operation of certain coalitions but disappear when these coalitions are fractionated. Kelso and Tuller link the coalition model to evidence that speech articulation may be organized in terms of functional units (Kent, Carney, & Severeid,

1974) and that apraxia of speech exhibits a disruption of normally invariant timing patterns among articulators (Itoh et al., 1978; Freeman et al., 1978).

Multistage or multilevel model. Some writers have described stages, levels or sequences of processing, as alternatives to the idea of centers of processing or command preparation. Requin (1980) discusses stages of motor organization in the nervous system:

> In this rapidly developing perspective of a behavioral neurophysiology, a structural and functional organization of motor systems, which presents some analogy to the serial processing stage models of psychologists, is progressively emerging. A privileged axis would be formed by a) a first stage, starting in the association cortical areas and ending in the neocerebellum, responsible for the action ''project'' definition, b) a second stage, starting in the neocerebellum and ending in the precentral motor cortex, where the motor program is selected and build [sic], c) a third stage, starting in the motor cortex and ended by motoneuron activation, accounting for movement execution. (p. 376)

Basically, these three stages can be called planning, programming, and execution. No one of these functions or operations is identified with a single brain center but rather each involves the participation of several neural structures.

Brown (1975, 1979) is among those who propose a neural organization of speech and language in terms of stages or levels rather than functional centers connected by pathways of information transfer. Brown rejects the centers of traditional neuropsychology and argues for levels of organization in which cognitive processing is carried through different stages. He disputes the traditional notion of neural pathways and proposes instead that the actual function of these connections is to accomplish a temporal linkage of transformations that occur at different points in a ''microgenetic sequence.''

Brain centers as continuously optimized neural connectivities. Although the traditional conception of brain centers is that they represent a fixed network of neurons dedicated to some function (for example, sequencing of phonetic segments), recent work in neurophysiology by Merzenich and associates (Merzenich, 1983) indicates that cortical somatosensory representation is dynamic and performance oriented. For example, somatosensory representation changes for the monkey's hand following temporary denervation, amputation of fingers, or bandaging of the hand. If the same property of functional dynamism applies to various parts of the cortex, then it might be better to think of functional centers not as invariant connections of neurons but as connectivity patterns that are continually subject to reassignment and revision. Thus, an important property of the brain would be its ability to reformulate neuronal connections to achieve optimal or efficient control of function. In other words, the brain would assume autoregulatory (self-organizing) properties in which the process of organization is not distinct from the product of organization.

The idea of floating or dynamic functional centers would have significant implications for recovery of function and for the understanding of functional impairment following brain damage. Because neuroanatomic constraints impose limitations on the degree to which functions can be reassigned to neuronal networks after a part of the brain is damaged, recovery of function may not be possible even with dynamic centers. Persistent impairment would be especially likely if a lesion affected a part of the brain with severely limited capacity for dynamic reassignment of connectivity patterns. To take a hypothetical situation, suppose that the final motor pathway were damaged beyond the brain's capability to establish new functional connections. In the face of this neural bottleneck, other centers would have to continue to work through the impaired system and may be even further hindered if dynamic reorganization itself has gone awry in the damaged brain tissue, causing variations in functional connections that are essentially unpredictable to the other brain centers that must operate through the damaged center. In such a situation, there would be little recourse but to send signals to the damaged center, and thus commit frequent errors, which might be corrected on successive attempts after the nature of the error is fully evident in the behavioral response.

The kind of brain center envisaged here represents a dynamically optimized functional representation in which neuronal connectivities are revised and adapted to performance variables. Self-organizational properties should apply to the damaged brain as well as to the normal brain, except that flexibility will be diminished in accord with the location and size of lesion. Performance of the brain-damaged patient would be expected to change over time as a consequence of the adaptive representation in the brain. If we assume that the brain has evolved toward maximal flexibility of representation, then a further possibility of neural organization is the coalition of dynamically optimized representations (centers). Each such center would be organized to optimize a certain function or set of functions (for example, the sequencing of articulatory movements for speech), but would cooperate with other centers possibly in a coalitional strategy that offers the advantage of emergent properties (a term discussed above which can be defined briefly as a property which comes about from the interaction of substructures in a larger organization).

Motor Program Models

A major difficulty in evaluating the usefulness of the motor program concept is that several possibilities exist for the content of a program. The content can be abstract, nearly free of the actual details or motor implementation, or it can be concrete and detailed to the point of specifying the motor units to be recruited. Consider the following three versions of a motor program concept.

(1.) The concept of a motor program might be based on Lashley's (1951) hierarchical solution to the problem of serial order in behavior. Lashley proposed the operation of at least three interrelated mechanisms in controlling a behavior such as speech: *determining tendency, priming of expressive units, schema of order* (or syntax of the act). The determining tendency represents the idea or semantic value to be expressed; the priming mechanism arouses and selects the appropriate linguistic (or production) units, which remain at this stage cotemporal and therefore unordered; and the schema of order accomplishes the actual seriation of the aroused and selected units. Lashley's ideas were used to explain sequencing errors in normal speech production (reviewed by Kent, 1976) and to account for a variety of speech errors in persons with brain damage (LaPointe & Johns, 1975; Lecours & Lhermitte, 1969; Lhermitte, Lecours, & Bertaux, 1969, O'Connell, 1981). The form of programming that derives from this theory is that selected production units are stored in an unordered fashion until a syntagmatic processor operates on them to yield a sequence which is then capable of directing lower level motor operations. Obviously, sequencing errors could occur because of dysfunction of the schema of order. In addition, substitution errors other than sequencing errors (that is, errors other than pre- or post positioning or metathesis) could result from mistakes in priming, such that incorrect production units are selected and aroused, thereby becoming available to the sequencing operation.

(2.) Another way of viewing a motor program is in terms of the phonetic and linguistic requirements that must be expressed in the motor output. An example is Branigan's (1976) speculation on children's acquisition of speech. He proposed that eventually the motor program must be structured to include: a set of articulatory targets (or goals) corresponding to the intended phonemic sequence; assignment of stress to the syllables contained within the sequence; syllable duration sensitivities to stress, segmental composition, and position in utterance; junctural features such as transitions between elements and terminal juncture at the end of a planned unit; and internal ordering of words as it reflects syntactic form to express semantic intentions. In other words, the program must contain a sufficiently complete phonetic representation that all segments, features, and contrasts can be specified for motor implementation. The form of the representation is open to speculation, but there is reason to believe that certain prosodic properties such as stress pattern are stored separately from the set of segmental (articulatory) targets (Fromkin, 1971).

(3.) The motor program also can be considered with respect to the detailed aspects of motor control. Semjen (1977) wrote that a motor program can control long motor sequences without reliance on peripheral feedback if the program contains information on (a) the identity of the effector units (muscles or muscle groups) to be activated, (b) the individual function of the selected units (e.g., agonistic-antagonistic, phasic-tonic), (c) the intensity and duration of activation, and (d) the temporal order and the temporal structure that control the timing of the selected units. The amount of detail that could be contained in such a motor program is considerable. There is evidence that movements are programmed directionally at the level of the motor unit: Romeny, ter Haar, van der Gon, Denier, and Gielen (1982) reported that changes in the order of recruitment of motor units apparently result from changes in the direction of exerted forces. This finding is of special interest to the multifunctional muscles of speech insofar as, "The hypothesis of the size principle (of the recruitment threshold of motor units) may still hold, but due to the nonhomogeneous innervation a specification of the exact task of the muscle will be necessary" (p. 367). The directionality requirement is only one complication among many. Another factor is that activation of motoneuron pools may be highly task dependent, such that the activation may extend over the boundaries of several pools. Romeny et al. (1982) cite evidence that activity of single cells of the monkey motor cortex is associated with the coactivation of as many as four arm muscles. Thus, a single cell may have a "motor field" defined across muscles.

Sternberg's Programming Model

Objections to the extreme version of the motor program concept (viz., the claim that a preplanned movement sequence is executed without influences of peripheral feedback; Keele, 1968) do not deny the utility of some form of preprogramming in the regulation of movement sequences. Sternberg, Monsell, Knoll, and Wright (1978) proposed that sequence control can involve both advanced planning and feedback. They suggested that possible roles of feedback would be as a cue to trigger onsets of subunits in a sequence or to provide information for an error-control process. Several possibilities were proposed for scheduling (advanced planning), ranging from the sequential preparation of subunits, to the preparation of some subunits during the execution of other subunits, to the preparation of a whole sequence.

Sternberg et al. proposed that sequence preparation for activities such as speech and typewriting is accomplished by a strategy of subprogram retrieval in which an entire program may be constructed in advance but the subprogram for the first unit is retrieved only when the sequence is to be executed. They obtained experimental data on latencies and durations in rapid movement sequences for speech and typewriting and inferred from these results that sequence control could be conceptualized in terms of a three-stage model. In the first stage, retrieval is accomplished by a self-terminating sequential search through a nonshrinking buffer (that is, the search for a unit stops when the unit is found, but the preplanned units remain in the buffer). The retrieval stage is followed by an unpacking stage and a command stage. Unpacking refers to the separation of the constituents of a retrieved unit. After the constituents are unpacked, an appropriate sequence of commands is issued.

The idea of a motor buffer is helpful in conceptualizing sequencing and coordination errors in apraxia of speech. One hypothesis is that when a large amount of information is contained in the buffer (as in the case of a complex multisyllabic utterance), the apraxic speaker cannot effectively manage the processing demands. Consequently, sequencing errors are committed. If we follow Sternberg et al. (1978) in considering as well the stages of unpacking and commands, then we can predict that other types of errors, in addition to sequencing errors, may occur. Unpacking errors conceivably could result in feature errors or coordination errors, that is, errors affecting certain constituents of a retrieved unit. If mechanisms of markedness (naturalness) come into play when information is lost in the unpacking stage, then it would be expected that feature errors would show patterns consistent with markedness theory. Impairment of the command stage could result in other abnormalities, such as initiation difficulties, slowing of transitions between target positions, or various timing errors affecting individual movements.

In evaluating the model of Sternberg et al. as a means of understanding apraxia of speech, it may be useful to consider if there is any evidence that the different stages can be independently affected by variables in assessment or management. For example, if a variable affects some types of errors but not others, the selective nature of the improvement (or deterioration) might reflect facilitation (or added impairment) of one stage of processing but not the others. Suppose that a given variable can significantly influence sequencing errors or frank substitution errors but does not alter rate of speech, initiation difficulty, or discoordination. Such an outcome might lend support to a stage conception of the speech processing impairment.

Some limitations to the additive-factor method employed by Sternberg et al. should be noted (Mulder, 1983). This method does not directly show stage durations or stage order. Nor does it yield a substantive interpretation of the stages. Finally, if an experimental variable affects both the duration and output of a stage, then the effect of one stage carries over to the subsequent stages.

Shaffer's Model of Rhythm and Timing

In view of the timing abnormalities that appear to characterize apraxic speech, models of speech timing control may hold promise in understanding this disorder. Shaffer (1982) proposed a theoretical framework for the management of rhythm and timing in skilled behavior. He supposed that the reproducible temporal rhythm of a performance is the realization of a *schedule* in a motor program. He noted that the variable which is specified in the schedule does not have to be time per se, but can be any variable "that has a definite timing concomitant within a mode of computation of the motor system" (p. 112). Thus, candidate variables can include factors such as stress level or movement amplitude — any variable that does not itself vary orthogonally with timing. The importance of a schedule is that it allows a motor system to produce a movement to the next temporal target, using a previous target as a reference point in planning the movement trajectory. Thus, movements become capable of anticipating targets in space and time and also of being coordinated within the dictates of a given schedule. Shaffer assumed that the motor system is computationally equipped to serve as a timekeeper that regulates the time scale of movement trajectories, which in the case of speech allows for considerable flexibility to accommodate variations in speaker rate, stress, and other prosodic and paralinguistic variables. In addition, it is assumed that the motor system can construct trajectories to produce more than a single event. This capability for compound trajectories not only could account for patterns of coarticulation in speech production but also could account for interindividual and intra-individual variability in these patterns.

An interesting property of the motor system envisaged by Shaffer is that it "has to be given a perspective on the output string of the motor program to enable it to anticipate movement requirements" (p. 112). This requirement is fulfilled by an advance scanning of the output string. This scan, or look-ahead, has several benefits to the production of speech. First, it provides for the anticipation of movement targets and yields supplementary background information such as respiratory regulation in support of speech production. Second, the scan creates the capability for the grouping of motor commands, and hence the construction of compound movement trajectories. Third, scanning of the output string is the means by which "expressive information" can be interpreted over a sequence of movements. Shaffer proposed that the scan explains certain properties of speech (sequencing) errors, noting that, "A prior scan of the output string, picking up context information, can confuse this with order information and create an ordering ambiguity in the translation from commands to movement" (p. 115).

This last suggestion is intriguing with respect to apraxia of speech. If indeed the apraxic subject continually confuses order information with context prescription, then errors should show strong context determination, such as errors of pre-positioning, postpositioning, or metathesis. However, the group mean of sequential errors in apraxic utterances was only 7% in the data of LaPointe and Johns (1975), which is perhaps insufficient to register unequivocal support for the hypothesis of order-context confusion. It may be that in the face of such confusion, the impaired motor system demonstrates entropic patterns in which unmarked sounds are selected (Klich et al., 1979; Marquardt et al., 1979).

Roy's Hierarchical Model

A good example of a hierarchically organized programming model of motor skill performance is described by Roy (1978). This model is particularly germane to this volume because it was developed partly on the basis of considerations of (nonspeech) apraxic errors in movement control. The dominant position in Roy's model is occupied by a goal selector, which functions to choose the goal for an action, especially for nonhabitual actions. The possibility that the goal selector may not be needed for habitual or automatic behaviors is an attractive explanation for the preservation of motor control in behaviors that are highly routinized but not in behaviors that require novel formulation. The next highest level of the model is the sequencer, which makes decisions about sequential order by means of both a cognitive and a perceptual component. The first of these makes decisions about the sequential activities of several effectors, whereas the perceptual component provides sensory information required for the decision processes. The goal selector and the subdominant sequencer constitute the *planning component* of the model. The lower levels of the model form the *executive component* consisting of a programmer, movement subroutines, and the individual movements (units) of which the subroutines are composed. The programmer works on specifications from the planning component and determines the combination of movement subroutines that will accomplish the desired movement result.

Roy describes how damage to different regions of the brain is associated with different apraxic syndromes and with presumed functional impairment at different levels of his hierarchical model. Disorders of planning and sequencing of motor acts (ideational and ideomotor apraxia) result from damage to frontal and parietal-occipital areas of cortex. Damage to premotor cortex impairs the ability to execute movement sequences (premotor apraxia) even though planning of the motor activity may be intact. Finally, lesions of the primary areas of the motor cortex disrupt individual movements within a sequence (limb-kinetic apraxia).

Hierarchical models like Roy's lead to two important statements about apraxic syndromes. First, as just summarized, different apraxic syndromes can be associated with impairment at different levels of the model. Thus, the model can be the basis for syndrome delineation. Second, the model can show us that a given apraxic error can be explained at two (or possibly more) levels of processing. For example, substitution errors in apraxia of speech can arise either from dysfunction of the planning component (and within this component from dysfunction of either the goal selector or the sequencer) or from dysfunction of the executive component. Itoh and Sasanuma (this volume, Chap. 5) remark similarly about explanatory ambiguity, noting that "so-called substitution errors" may have three different origins: (1) errors occuring at the level of phoneme selection; (2) errors in articulatory programming; or (3) errors resulting from a combination of (1) and (2) which are likely to manifest themselves as multiple-feature errors.

Motor Schema

Still another theoretical alternative is one in terms of a spatiotemporal (motor) schema (Schmidt, 1975). The schema is a generalization that encompasses various factors such as current conditions, past experience, and desired outcomes to formulate response specifications for a particular, even novel, motor performance. In discussing this theory with respect to apraxia of speech, Kent and Rosenbek (1983) note that a subject might retain effective control over nonverbal movements and perhaps even some automatic utterances but lose effective control for voluntary, purposive speech production because of a deterioration of the spatiotemporal schemata that subserve phonetic performance. In a similar vein, Paillard (1960) commented that the disintegration of schemata can contribute to apraxic disorders in which the subject cannot plan an ordered motor sequence.

Kent and Rosenbek discuss several aspects of schema theory that might be useful in explaining error patterns in apraxia of speech. For instance, the observation that initial consonants are more often in error than consonants in other positions may reflect a more complex motor encoding for this position, insofar as the articulation of an initial consonant usually is modified by the articulatory requirements for the following segments (cf. Klich et al., 1979). Therefore, the motor schema must deal with a greater amount of information for initial position consonants than for consonants in other positions. That is, the schema must contend with (1) information on the current state of the vocal tract, not only as it pertains to the initial consonant but for following sounds as well; (2) preparation of motor commands that are suitable for the first consonant but also efficiently anticipate upcoming articulations; and (3) generation of the predicted feedback by which the actual motor outcome is evaluated to ensure satisfaction of the target and by which any modifications of the schema can be made to improve successive attempts. Schema theory also can account for variations in error frequency with changes in place of production. It would be expected that schemata for alveolar sounds (the most frequently occurring sounds in the language) would be strongly established through motor experience and therefore less likely to deteriorate. As a final example, schema theory may help to explain why apraxic patients cannot always immediately correct their errors even though they appear to be aware of them (Deal & Darley, 1972). Schema theory proposes that a motor performance is evaluated by comparing the actual performance with the intended action (ie., predicted feedback). Accordingly, deterioration of a motor schema in apraxia of speech would impair the generation of response specifications to perform a sequence, *but also* would impair the derivation of error information by which the response specifications could be revised for future attempts.

DEVELOPMENTAL APRAXIA OF SPEECH

This essay is primarily about acquired *apraxia* of speech, but it would be incomplete without at least a mention of *developmental* apraxia of speech. Diagnosing apraxia of speech in children seems to be increasingly popular. There are problems, however, and it is the problems we want to mention. The term, apraxia, appeared first in the adult literature and the earliest discussions were of limb movements and constructional activities rather than of speech. Apraxia for oral, nonverbal movements emerged next, followed by apraxia for speech movements as it appeared in adults with acquired lesions of the nervous system. Much of the early research on developmental apraxia used adult models because no other ones existed. Unfortuntely, adults who lose speech because of apraxia-causing lesions are different from children who fail to develop speech normally because of an impaired ability to develop skilled speech movements as rapidly as their normal speaking peers.

The literature on apraxic limb movements in adults has not worked all that well even as a guide for defining and researching adult apraxia of speech. Differences between development and acquired problems further dilute that literature's usefulness to the study of children. And some writers are reluctant even to allow apraxia to refer to any but a *loss* of skill, making it impossible conceptually for a *developmental* apraxia to exist. But while admitting to these and other problems, researchers have nevertheless set about trying to identify and describe a group of children with developmental apraxia of speech. Furthermore, clinicians apparently remain convinced that some portion of their caseload, made up primarily of children with multiple articulation errors who are painfully slow to respond in treatment, are appropriately classified as developmentally apraxic. Yoss and Darley (1974) describe a group of such children, and readers may want to look at that report. Williams, Ingham, and Rosenthal (1981) could not replicate Yoss and Darley's findings. Guyette and Diedrich (1981) review the extant literature and find no pathognomonic symptoms of the condition. Perhaps there are none, although if the term is to survive, some distinctive cluster of speech and perhaps nonspeech symptoms will have to emerge.

The label, despite its tenuous status and perhaps short life expectancy, seems to be guiding clinicians to a set of helpful management procedures, borrowed in part, like the nomenclature itself, from the adult literature. The apraxic child's reputation for resistance to treatment might well have turned into notoriety if it were not for such methods. Besides making better talkers of such children, response to treatment may eventually have the additional benefit of helping to define this population more exactly. Diagnosis ex juvantibus works in the diagnosis of myasthenia gravis, certain kinds of dementia, and in a host of other conditions. The method can work for speech disorders too if clinicians are careful to use specific, focused, and controlled interventions and to combine perceptual with instrumental measurement of treatment effects. Using instrumental measures in combination with perceptual ones to diagnose suspected apraxic children may help also.

CLINICAL EVALUATION

The "clinical" in clinical evaluation is crucial, because the days when clinical and experimental evaluation both relied on broad phonetic transcription are gone. Experimental evaluation has become increasingly sophisticated (cf. Fromm, Abbs, McNeil, & Rosenbek, 1982), and broad phonetic transcription, while enduring as a clinical tool, is increasingly unacceptable in experimentation. This is not to indict the early perceptual research nor to discourage certain forms of it in the future. Broad phonetic transcription helped. It produced data that illuminated apraxia of speech's boundaries—or at least some of them. The data it produced, however, also created problems of definition and description almost from the beginning, problems that endure even today, especially for those who may have failed to stay abreast of recent research. Scholars reluctant to permit any but aphasic disorders to arise from cortical damage seized upon the high proportion of substitutions which broad phonetic description identified as the cardinal symptoms of apraxia of speech and said they were evidence that apraxia of speech was really aphasia. They apparently forgot Shankweiler and Harris' (1966) warning that broad phonetic transcription could not provide data adequate to an understanding of a disorder's underlying neuropathophysiology. Considerable energy was wasted feuding about whether apraxia is aphasia, but signs suggest that most of the combatants have now moved on, either to new issues or new data. Meanwhile, patients with apraxia of speech continue to appear in clinics and clinicians continue to diagnose them. A few words on how that is done and how it is being influenced by modern research make up the next section of this essay.

A Clinical, Diagnostic Battery

Apraxia of speech needs to be distinguished from aphasia, cognitive deficit, the dysarthrias, and from normal speech; and perhaps types of apraxia of speech need to be distinguished from each other. These needs dictate the clinical battery. Foremost in the battery are language measures that sample performance in reading, writing, listening, and oral language. Some clinicians use only a single test; others use a variety. The object is to rule out aphasia. To rule out cognitive deficits, clinicians rely on their neuropsychology colleagues; on the history; on a few selected tests of cognitive function, uncluding memory; and on the types of speech-language symptoms that differentiate aphasia, dementia, and apraxia of speech (Halpern, Darley, & Brown, 1973; Obler & Albert, 1981). Dysarthria and apraxia of speech and perhaps subtypes of apraxia of speech are distinguishable by responses to a variety of nonspeech and speech tasks. Nonspeech tasks include such activities as blowing, biting one's lip, puckering one's lips, chewing, and swallowing. Speech tasks such as syllable repetition (diadochokinesis), word and sentence imitation, picture description, and reading complete the battery. Clinicians look for evidence of weakness, ataxia, abnormal tone, and for those clusters of speech symptoms that have come to be associated with the various dysarthrias and apraxia of speech. These same nonspeech and speech tasks may also help differentiate types of speech apraxia, although a more fine grained analysis than characterizes the broad phonetic transcription presently in vogue will probably have to become standard if types are to be reliably differentiated.

Special Tests

Tests promising to diagnose a certain condition whistle a siren's song. Clinicians understandably want tests that tell them what each of their patients has. Treatment is easier when we know what we are treating. Several informal and at least one formal test for diagnosing apraxia of speech in adults have emerged. The validity of even the published one is only now being established, but it warrants description.

The Apraxia Battery For Adults. The Apraxia Battery for Adults (ABA) published by Dabul (1979) is a compilation of many tasks familiar from scattered earlier writings. It draws heavily from work on the descriptive nature of apraxia of speech in the 1960s and 1970s, especially from that of researchers with a Mayo Clinic orientation to the disorder. The purpose of the ABA, as stated in the manual, is to verify the presence of apraxia in the adult patient and "to gain a rough estimate of the severity of the disorder." (Dabul, 1979, p. 1).

The test is comprised of six subtests including Diadochokinetic Rate; Increasing Word Length; Limb Apraxia and Oral Apraxia; Latency and Utterance Time for polysyllabic Words; Repeated Trials Test; and Inventory of Articulation Characteristics of Apraxia. The ABA can be administered in approximately 20 min and requires only the test manual, response forms, a stopwatch, and tape recorder.

The test is a laudable attempt to organize tasks that elicit apraxic behavior. The ABA is somewhat thin on suggestions for interpretation and as stated in the manual, "minimal normative data are available, and the battery has not yet been standardized" (Dabul, 1979, p. 16). In order to fulfill its stated purposes, the ABA is badly in need of psychometric studies of reliability and particularly content and concurrent validity. In the meantime it can serve as a useful source of tasks to supplement the traditional clinical evaluation of the apraxic individual.

Influence of Contemporary Research On Clinical Evaluation

While modern research has had scant influence on diagnostic stimuli, it has influenced what clinicians listen and look for. As a result of acoustic (Kent & Rosenbek, 1983) and physiologic (Fromm et al., 1982) research, it is now commonplace to admit a high proportion of distortions into the symptomatology of apraxia of speech. Previously it was assumed that dysarthric speakers made primarily distortions and apraxic ones made primarily substitutions. Recent studies, including some recorded in this volume, are confirming timing and coordination errors resulting in varying amounts of distortion. Fromm et al. (1982) identified a variety of movement abnormalities that were not perceived by a listener either as substitutions or distortions. Such findings do not erase the differences between dysarthric and apraxic speech: Apraxia and dysarthria do not sound identical or even similar. Even with the most fine grained analysis, substitutions that are different from and more numerous than those seen in the dysarthrias will continue to be identified. What recent data have done is provide evidence that a combination of distortions and substitutions does not necessarily mean a combination of dysarthria and apraxia. Our clinical rule is that dysarthria is the most likely diagnosis if a patient has a high proportion of relatively consistent distortions. Apraxia of speech is the likely diagnosis if distortions are mixed with what sound like substitutions, especially if such errors are relatively inconsistent.

Recent research has also begun quantifying a variety of prosodic abnormalities previously reported anecdotally to be present in apraxia of speech. These have been discussed at length previously, and the difficulty in determining the degree to which they are primary or secondary symptoms has been confirmed. Despite the controversy over their nature, clinicians continue to consider that apraxic talkers sound labored and dysprosodic, and that this feature helps to separate them from their aphasic brethren. They are justified in doing so. Researchers and clinicians may eventually discover that the amount and type of prosodic abnormalities also help define various apraxic subtypes. One of us is convinced that at least two subgroups exist, and that they are distinguishable in part by the absence of significant prosodic disturbance in one and the presence of significant prosodic disturbance in the other. Another distinguishing characteristic may be the relative number of substitutions compared to distortion errors, the number being higher in the group with less prosodic disturbance.

A Clinical Profile of the Apraxic Talker

The apraxic talker is relatively easy to identify clinically, although diagnosis is harder the closer to onset a patient is. Thc difficulty at onset is created by the other residuals of brain damage such as confusion and fear rather than because apraxia necessarily undergoes changes with time (although it certainly does change with time). During both the acute and chronic stages, the clinician should consider apraxia of speech as the appropriate diagnosis if the speaker follows one- and occasional two-step written and oral commands despite being speechless, if the speaker shows evidence of trying to talk and of being frustrated by failure, and if dysphagia, dysphasia, and dementia can be ruled out by the history and testing. Writing is usually of little help to the diagnosis, especially during the acute stage, because it is often as involved as the speech. In the chronic stage, however, and sometimes even in the acute, writing, if it is more intact than speaking, can be used to support a diagnosis. Speech, when the patient is not mute, may or may not be helpful. We have seen two groups of apraxic speakers during the acute stage: One group was fluent and produced jargon, although in limited amounts; the other was nonfluent and nearly speechless.

Sometimes clinicians begin treatment with no more than a hypothesis — often weak — about whether a speaker is apraxic. The hypothesis gets a rigorous test from skillful treatment, however. Apraxic talkers understand what clinicians are doing and saying once treatment begins. They respond to speech drills. Indeed, with one possible exception, apraxic talkers improve with and without treatment. The possible exception is a group of speakers who remain speechless or nearly so for life, but who are clearly not globally aphasic because their understanding, writing, reading, and gesturing are too good, albeit far from normal. The majority of apraxic people begin learning, and as they learn they begin to show the classical characteristics accompanied by a few idiosyncracies imposed by treatment's procedures and their own quirks. The classical characteristics were described previously. To those one can add the following clinical features: awareness of errors, variability, willingness and ability to work independently; and reasonably rapid grasping of the compensations that are necessary for improved speech.

TREATING APRAXIA OF SPEECH

Treatments for apraxia of speech seemingly have gone along largely uninfluenced by all but the major turmoil over apraxia of speech. That turmoil is whether apraxia is more usefully classified as a neuromotor speech disorder distinct from the aphasias, and requiring speech therapy, or whether it is symptomatic of language disturbance, and requires language therapy. And even this issue, important as it is, has had only slight influence on specific treatments, because good clinicians almost reflexively respond differently to different patients regardless of what the literature advises. But is it not only the naturalness of responding differently to different symptoms that has muted the issue's influence. Also important is the generally accepted notion that treating apraxic symptomatology requires more than articulation therapy and good will. It requires speech-language therapy — an emphasis on both movement and meaning. Because it does, the methodologies for apraxia of speech and aphasia share a number of features.

Commonalities exist for other reasons as well. Both apraxic and aphasic people suffer similar sequelae of brain damage such as fatiguability and poor set-to-attend which must either be accommodated or modified. Shared features have evolved also because apraxia of speech therapy, like its older cousin, aphasia therapy, has been influenced as much by nonlinguistic, general therapeutic principles as by linguistic and phonetic ones. Even experimental treatments such as vibrotactile stimulation (Rubow, Rosenbek, Collins, & Longstreth, 1982) seem to be motivated less by characteristics of apraxia of speech than by general rehabilitation principles such as intersystemic reorganization (Luria,

1970). Finally, the requirements of single-case design research have begun to influence both aphasia and apraxia of speech treatment (LaPointe, this volume, Chap. 10) by dictating some common structural features such as the ordering of stimuli, the focusing and limiting of treatment, and the type and timing of testing.

But apraxia of speech is not aphasia and treatments of the two are not the same. In apraxia of speech treatment, meaning is made to serve movement. Movement is often incidental in aphasia rehabilitation. Suggestions for disorder-specific methods and stimulus selection have also begun appearing in the literature. Rosenbek (1978) described a program of gestural reorganization for apraxic speakers and showed why it is inappropriate to the aphasic speaker. Kearns (1980) recommended that clinicians experiment with the relative efficacy of treating distinctive features rather than individual sounds when dealing with apraxic speakers. Sands, Freeman, and Harris in a series of papers (Sands, Freeman, & Harris, 1978; Freeman, Sands, & Harris, 1978) have added to the accumulating documentation of voice onset time abnormalties in apraxia of speech and have suggested treatments to alter them. In the future, an increasingly sophisticated and specific set of measurements, research designs, treatment procedures, and targets may be created from the kind of linguistic and acoustic research reported elsewhere and in this volume, by the kind of physiological data reported elsewhere (Fromm, Abbs, McNeil, & Rosenbek, 1982), and by the simultaneous perceptual, acoustic, and physiologic research advocated in this essay. A beginning has been made by Duffy and Gawle (this volume, Chap. 6), and we will review those beginnings as well as suggest some others. Before we do, however, we want to review more traditional approaches to apraxia of speech treatment.

Shewan's Summary

Shewan (1980) wrote a reasonable summary of apraxia of speech treatment's goals and organization as the 1980s began. She said the major goal was to help each patient "imprint the correct patterns" of articulatory movements and "have the client remember those patterns by using tactile, proprioceptive, visual or other imagery" (p. 5). She also said drill and repetition established the imprints. To help each patient toward the best, functional communication of which their systems are capable, she emphasized hierarchies of stimuli and cues and a variety of facilitators such as altered rate and finger tapping so that each speaker moved successfully from easy to more difficult responses. As a way of helping clinicians think about what they had to do to make treatment work she organized a "therapy content network" consisting of "stimulation presentation method, stimuli, responses, facilitating response variables, and response criteria" (p. 6). She made recommendations about each component of her network which clinicians eager to check their own practice against the literature's recommendations may want to read.

Treating with Hierarchies

Much of the early treatment literature described treatment hierarchies. Most of these resulted from approximately equal parts of intuition and wishful thinking seasoned with a bit of data. We will review the hierarchies first and the data that will help lead to their revision second.

An eight-step task continuum. Rosenbek, Lemme, Ahern, Harris, and Wertz (1973) assembled an eight-step task continuum to move patients "from limited, automatic-reactive speech to appropriate, volitional-purposive communication" (p. 463). Stimulus selection was based on a series of principles that included attention to the speech sound make-up and length of meaningful stimuli.
Their eight steps are:

(1) integral stimulation with patient and clinician saying each utterance simultaneously;
(2) repetition after a delay with simultaneous cues provided by the clinician only as necessary to save the patient from too many errors;
(3) repetition after a delay with no simultaneous cues by the clinician;
(4) consecutive repetitions by the patient without intervening or simultaneous cues from the clinician;
(5) reading response aloud while looking at the written stimulus;
(6) saying what was written but only after the writing has been taken away;
(7) using treated responses in answer to questions;
(8) using appropriate responses in role playing.

Movement from one step to another depended upon the patient's correctly saying 80% of 20 consecutive responses. The authors were reasonably happy with their continuum because three study patients generally required progressively fewer repetitions to reach criteron as they moved from Step 1 to Step 8 in the course of learning five unique responses each. The one exception was Step 4 which all patients found to be difficult. Rosenbek et al. say they should have dropped the step altogether or remained longer at previous steps. They admit to adorning the basic continuum with a variety of facilitators such as slowed rate and exaggerated stress and that these facilitators were the continuum's flesh, if not its blood and skeleton. They did not write the facilitators into the continuum for fear of complicating it and of imposing a garroting structure on activities that are spontaneous and dynamic in actual practice. And although they liked the continuum and facilitators with the exception of Step 4, they also say "It would be folly to expect that this approach can improve the speech of all severely apraxic adults" (p. 471). Theirs is a truism, but we are glad they said it.

Revisionism. Deal and Florance (1978) revised the Rosenbek et al. (1973) eight-step task continuum. They tried first to replicate the earlier studies' findings with four patients and found they could. This is especially impressive because three of the four were more than 1 year post onset. They also looked for ways of modifying the continuum and found them. One patient, for example, had only to drill at Steps 1 and 4; and one had only to drill Steps 1 through 4. Furthermore, none of Deal and Florance's patients had the difficulty at Step 4 reported by Rosenbek et al. (1973). Deal and Florance reasoned that this step may have been made easier by their more rigid criteria for moving from one step to another. Instead of using a criterion of 80% correct on 20 trials as had Rosenbek et al. they used a cumulative 80% criterion. This more rigid criterion required patients to remain longer at previous steps, especially Step 1. Finally, Deal and Florance used portions of the continuum as home programs for three of the four patients. Establishing a home program for one of the patients "was not feasible." They think the home programs worked.

A continuum emphasizing the stimuli. Dabul and Bollier (1976) published a different kind of hierarchy. They emphasized the ordering of stimuli rather than of stimulus conditions. They make the controversial observation that typical apraxic errors are anticipation, transposition, and addition. They follow this with a less controversial one: "Therapeutic attention must be paid to the process of sequencing speech sounds" (p. 269). They then describe a program. It begins with teaching sounds in isolation, "much as one would learn in alphabet of letters before attempting to read or write a language" (p. 269). Once an individual sound is learned to criterion (18 of 20 correct productions) it is combined with /a/ and practiced until it reaches a speed of 60 repetitions in 15 sec. The next step is to learn rapid CVCV and CVC productions. They defend their purposeful use of nonsense syllables in part by saying "automatic repetition of a familiar, meaningful syllable or word is not generalizable" (p. 270). Their program's last step is called "Word Attack by Phone and Syllable" (p. 270). They suggest three facilitators for those patients who fail to learn: presenting sounds visually rather than auditorily, using placement techniques, and using written words.

Studying Components of the Therapy Content Network

A number of studies have evaluated components of what Shewan called the therapy content network. A review of selected studies among these may point the way to new task continua, and by their influence on speech accuracy by apraxic talkers may reveal additional information about what apraxia of speech is.

Modality of stimulation. Clinicians like to have apraxic speakers begin by watching. Visible sounds are highly touted first-treatment stimuli, and the visual modality, either alone or in combination with the auditory, figures prominently in the task continua already reviewed. Predictably the literature confirms that the matter is more complex. In an early study, Johns and Darley (1970) compared reading single words, repeating single words heard through earphones, and repetition of words subjects saw and heard an experimenter produce. The live voice presentation elicited significantly better speech than did the response to taped stimuli. It was not better than reading, however, nor were reading and taped stimuli significantly different. LaPointe and Horner (1976) compared four conditions: auditory (A), in which patients repeated each of 10 words after hearing them, but not through earphones; auditory and visual (AV_1), in which patients both heard and watched the clinician's model; reading (V_2); and auditory plus reading (AV_2). Differences by mode were not striking, but response adequacy was significantly better for auditory than for the other three, which did not differ significantly from each other.

Our clinical impression, and one not altogether challenged by the literature, is that the way stimuli are presented may not have potent clinical significance depending on the clinician's acumen and choice of stimuli. We also recognize from our practice that patients differ in what they like. Simmons (1980) offers the obvious clinical solution. She urged testing individual patients and following their lead. To demonstrate her point she used an apraxic blind patient to test whether auditory or auditory-plus-braille presentation was more powerful. Her results demonstrated that auditory-plus-braille stimulation was superior to auditory alone.

She admits that her patient is unique. He was. Her study is useful, nevertheless. It shows how single-case design can be used to exploit variance rather than bury it in statistical analysis as is done in group research.

We have two suggestions about the modality of stimulation. *Do what works.* That means testing each patient. *Keep it simple.* Telling the speaker what to say is quick and easy. If it works as well as other things, use it.

Response conditions. Johns and Darley (1970) report the relative potency of three response conditions: consecutive, distributed, and successive. Differences were not significant, but the authors seemed to have felt that the successive condition in which the speaker had three uninterrupted chances to reproduce a single word in imitation of the clinician was the most facilitating of correct articulation. Having read Johns and Darley (1970) and treated a number of patients both clinically and experimentally, LaPointe and Horner (1976) studied the speech of seven apraxic talkers in two response conditions and under four modes of stimulus presentation. The modes were discussed previously. The two conditions were: (1) 1:10, 1 stimulus and 10 consecutive responses; and (2) 1:1, 10 responses, each preceded by the clinician's stimulus. No differences in these two emerged from their first analysis. Prompted to analyze the data further (understandable since they scored 5600 responses) they looked for deterioration in the 1:10 condition by comparing performance in the first five trials with that in the second five. They described "a strong trend toward deterioration," that was nonetheless not statistically significant. This trend is not surprising. Many patients, especially during treatment's early days, need frequent restimulation if they are to stay on target. Inadequate memory, attention, or motor control may explain this tendency.

Delay. Because clinicians want to leave apraxic patients as independent and as successful as possible, they make liberal use of delay. Usually the clinician provides the target and then directs the patient to delay for varying intervals before responding. Deal and Darley (1972) were among the first to study delay's influence on apraxic articulation. They compared articulatory accuracy for single words after 0, 3, and 6 sec of delay. No differences emerged. This is good news for the clinician. It means that responses do not necessarily degenerate if an apraxic talker is allowed or forced to wait: Clinician and patient do not necessarily need to speak simultaneously or bunch closely together in a clinical game of follow the leader.

Wilson (1977) developed an additional rationale for studying delay in apraxia, and she expanded the design for its study. Her research was governed by selected of learning psychology's findings about stimulus discrimination and response differentiation. She underlines the common sense observation that responses are increasingly less likely as time elapses between stimulation and response. To test this observation with apraxic speakers, she compared the ability of three severely apraxic-aphasic people to imitate 10 one-syllable words in four conditions: 0 delay; 5-sec delay; 10-sec delay; and 15-sec delay. During the 15-sec delay each patient was required to imitate a series of nonspeech gestures. Responses deteriorated as a function of the length of delay, and response was apparently impossible in the 15 sec, interpolated activity condition. These results combined with what she considers the salutary effect of rehearsal lead her to recommend a hierarchy of temporal manipulations. She recommends beginning with no delay; moving to several consecutive responses with no delay and no clinician cuing between them; advancing to consecutive, uncued responses with steadily increasing delay; and ending with delays in which the patient does something during the delays. This hierarchy, she says, is to be used with inconsistent responses and when responses degenerate with time. She was one of the first to consider the influence of what one does during the pause. Others have followed suit.

Delay and rehearsal. Bugbee and Nichols (1980) studied a group of 10 apraxic speaker's articulatory accuracy in five conditions. In the *control* condition, each patient merely repeated each of 30 words after they were presented by the clinician. In two experimental conditions each patient was either allowed to determine the amount of delay before repeating or the number of spoken rehearsals before repeating. In the final two experimental conditions, the clinician controlled the delay (3 sec) or the number of spoken rehearsals (four). The apraxic speakers as a group were significantly more accurate when they controlled the number of rehearsals than when they repeated immediately, after a clinician imposed number of rehearsals, and after a clinician imposed delay. Patients seldom rehearsed more than three times on their way to this significantly superior performance. Unfortunately, the delay interval they imposed on themselves is not reported nor is what they might have been allowed or observed to do during that interval. Nevertheless the potency of self-control is suggested in this study and self-control should probably appear more frequently in treatment programs.

Immediate imitation versus silent rehearsal. Warren (1977) tested the relative efficacy of immediate imitation and silent rehearsal on the ability of five apraxic speakers to name pictures. The study is well-designed, making it easy to recommend for more details. In *imitation*, the patient was provided with the picture to be named and then the clinician said the word up to 20 times per minute and the patient imitated each. In the *rehearsal condition* the patient was shown the picture, told its name, and instructed to say it over and over silently. In this condition each patient was also to say each target aloud immediately after the clinician and at the 5-, 15-, 30-, and 60-sec marks. Each patient's productions immediately after a condition's completion and at 3-, 5-, and 7-day follow-up sessions were tape recorded and evaluated.

Warren found that all five subjects profited from both conditions but that they profited differently. Two profited about equally from both conditions. One did best with rehearsal, and two did best with imitation. At the 7th day follow-up, performance for all five had sagged; and the difference between repetition and rehearsal had disappeared for all but one patient whose performance continued to favor the imitation condition. Warren says his "result questions the usefulness of response delays as a separate procedure in paradigms for apraxia of speech" (p. 89). We agree. He also says it is important how patients use delay. We agree again. Unfortunately the proper uses of delay are still to be discovered, although Wilson's (1977) finding is powerful support for not having patients perform nonspeech activities during long intervals. Also to be discovered is whether any delay regardless of how exotically and efficiently the apraxic speaker uses it is time well spent. Perhaps better than delay is systematic aloud rehearsal.

Rehearsal as a way of classifying patients. Collins, Cariski, Longstreth, and Rosenbek (1980) were less concerned about silent and audible rehearsal's specific influences on speech than they were about the differential diagnostic possibilities of these conditions. They selected one classically apraxic speaker, one apraxic speaker with significant aphasia, and one patient with apraxic features but who best fit the diagnosis of conduction aphasia. They compared the three under four conditions: aloud rehearsal, whispered rehearsal, silent rehearsal while looking at the stimulus written on a card, and silent rehearsal during binaural masking. The two apraxic speakers did best in Condition 3, a silent condition in which they looked at the stimulus for 10 sec before saying it. The conduction aphasic speaker did best with aloud rehearsal. These results were not treated statistically and should be replicated.

Implications. Existing continua are probably all right; but a host of questions exist and clinical researchers can answer them. One of the most crucial is: How appropriate is imitation? Neurocontrol over imitation may be different enough from control over spontaneous speech so that therapeutic gains from imitation generalize only slowly and incompletely to spontaneous speech. It is possible that imitative steps in existing paradigms may be ineffective, or at best, inefficient. While research is being done, clinicians should be chary in their use of published programs. They should evaluate for themselves and for each patient the influence of particular continua.

Treating Apraxic Speech Without Treating The Speech

A variety of authors have recognized that apraxic symptoms result not only from brain damage but from a variety of internal and external forces. Therefore, both stress and environment have been manipulated and the speech effects noted.

Electromyography-assisted biofeedback. McNeil, Prescott, and Lemme (1976) created a case for treating tension in a group of four aphasic patients, three with coexisting apraxia of speech. That case is based primarily on a brief review of the interaction of anxiety and a variety of normal and abnormal behaviors. Their four patients, in addition to a set of speech-language abnormalities, also gave evidence of being upset by errors and of performing less well following an error — typical findings among apraxic speakers.

To effect relaxation, surface electrodes were placed over the frontalis muscle, and then a traditional biofeedback regime to teach relaxation was completed. Visual feedback, in the form of three lights, and auditory feedback, in the form of clicks, were provided in the beginning; and a short experiment was conducted to see which was preferable. Once that was completed, each patient had 15 sessions of biofeedback training using auditory feedback. A treatment effect was looked for in both feedback and no feedback conditions using the Porch Index of Communicative Ability (PICA; Porch, 1967), the Revised Token Test (McNeil & Prescott, 1978), and a standard speech sample (Wertz & Rosenbek, 1971).

The data indicate that all four patients learned to relax. Adequacy of performance increased on PICA verbal and gestural subtests and on the Revised Token Test. Patients varied across tasks, but the patient's families all reported improved communication overall. And as the authors say, "Subjectively, subjects appeared to perform the therapeutic tasks better . . . when receiving feedback" (p. 158).

The authors wanted their data to be seen as preliminary. Unfortunately, subsequent research has been slow to appear. This slowness is especially discouraging because this study is one of the few to consider that apraxia of speech is more than a speech or even a communication disorder. A variety of influences determine how the apraxic speaker does. Stress is one such influence. Stress management may be therapeutic. McNeil, Prescott, and Lemme's (1976) findings suggest it. Future research may confirm it.

Changing the Environment. Florance, Rabidoux, and McCauslin (1980) moved apraxia of speech treatment from the clinic into patients' homes and built a program emphasizing enhanced communication skills rather than motor speech skills to improve communication and guarantee carryover. They report on three patients, two of whom had endured egregious previous treatments. Talking by two of the three improved after the patients and family or friends were taught to change the way they communicated. Family and friends were taught, for example, to "engage in clinical interviewing tactics" (p. 288), such as open ended questions and paraphrasing of what they thought the speaker had said. The third patient received training in what the authors call self-regulation and pseudoconversation, among other things. In other words, he was taught to confront his apraxia, generate cues to help himself, and score his own successes. All three patients apparently thrived.

We applaud such efforts for all patients having neurogenic communicative disorders. Patients and families are, like the rest of us, ill prepared to cope with brain damage's sequelae. The ways they try to communicate are not always the best. Clinicians can help. Part of the clinical art is predicting how much improvement can be expected from environmental manipulation and how much work will be required to improve specific motor control.

An Emphasis on Sounds and Syllables

In the midst of discussion about units of speech and how speech is programmed, clinicians continue to struggle with selecting drill material for apraxic speakers. Unless an individual patient is very mild, such struggle usually includes attempts to select and order single sounds and syllables. This is not to say that apraxia of speech therapy inevitably begins with sounds or syllables. It does not. Clinicians, with few exceptions, want their patients to say something when they talk, so meaningful stimuli appear early in most treatment programs. But even programs that emphasize meaning often begin with drills of individual sounds and syllables. Most general discussions of treatment (cf. Rosenbek, 1978; Shewan, 1980) review guidelines for selecting and ordering these, and some treatment programs are very specific.

Multiphonemic articulation therapy. Holtzapple and Marshall (1977) report on using multiphonemic articulation therapy with one apraxic person. This program, which was apparently first described by Bradley and McCabe (1975), was created for cleft palate children. The program teaches 24 speech sounds first in isolation and progresses by systematically moving them to spontaneous speech. As described by Holtzapple and Marshall (1977), presentation of stimuli comes in three parts: visual only, in which the patient reads the stimuli; auditory and visual where the clinician says the stimulus while the patient reads it; and visual and auditory combined with phonetic placement. The program also comes with a sound production sheet for noting how a speaker responds to each mode of stimulation. Apparently one begins with the most elaborate stimulus presentation (presumably the third) and then moves toward less cuing when "80% accuracy is achieved" (p. 47). As originally described the program had three phases: establishment, transfer, and maintenance.

Alternative activities, what the authors call "Branching steps" (p. 49), are also available for patients who fail to reach certain criteria after a certain number of sessions.

Holtzapple & Marshall's apraxic patient improved. He improved more quickly in his production of voiceless than voiced sounds. The authors admit that the specific effects of multiphonemic articulation therapy on the patient's improvement are hard to ferret out because it was but one-tenth of the total treatment. We mention the approach because it is typical of those programs for apraxic people which emphasize articulation. Holtzapple and Marshall realize the inadequacy of such an articulation approach; they made it a small portion of the patient's total treatment. Our recommendation is that simple articulation training always be but a soupcon of a total speech-language therapy.

Treating with Special Methods

The Metronome. Shane and Darley (1978) were among the first to study the influence of the metronome on apraxic speech. Unfortunately, no palliative emerged in their data, perhaps because patients were not taught to use the device (were not taught, for example, to time their speech so that a syllable or word accompanied each click). It may have failed also because speech rhythms are not a metronome's rhythm.

Delayed auditory feedback. Considerable research has been done with delayed auditory feedback (DAF) and "Broca's aphasic" people. Inevitably some patients are better under the delay. Presumably some of these people had apraxia of speech as a prominent symptom. We are not surprised that DAF is sometimes salutary. An important theoretical question is why apraxic speech is improved under DAF's influence — when it is. A parsimonious, but not necessarily correct, explanation is that improvement results from the conscious control and slowed rate that speakers use under the influence of the machine. They are more careful, and they give their articulators more time to get where they want them to go. An alternative explanation is that the DAF reduces apraxic variability by imposing artificial restraints on sensorimotor systems. To speak under delay, one has to settle into a mode of stereotyped rate, rhythm, stress, and intonation. Reducing the prosodic variability may leave the speaker free to concentrate on specific movements and may even make the movements easier.

Vibrotactile stimulation. Rubow, Rosenbek, Collins, and Longstreth (1982) demonstrated that a vibrotactile program was more successful than a simple imitative program in helping an apraxic talker produce more accurate single, polysyllabic words. The imitative program was traditional: The patient first watched and listened while the clinician provided the stimulus and then tried to duplicate it. In the vibrotactile condition, the patient rested his hand against a vibrator. The clinician not only said each word but simultaneously provided a vibrotactile cue to each syllable's length and relative intensity. Also the patient was taught to respond in accompaniment to a repetition of the vibrotactile cues. Relative progress with the two conditions was measured by having the speaker imitate randon presentations of all treated words. All words improved, but those treated in the vibrotactile condition were significantly better than those treated in the simple imitative condition.

The authors speculate that the vibrotactile stimulation may have acted as an intersystemic reorganizer (Luria, 1970; Rosenbek, 1978). Another way to think about the vibrotactile treatment's influence is as a pacer of motor activity. Like the metronome and DAF, vibrotactile stimulation applied simultaneously with efforts to talk may reduce variability by imposing a definite rhythm on the speech responses. Or the vibrotactile condition may merely enhance a speaker's concentration. Only a series of studies such as that outlined by Rubow et al. (1982) will allow us to sort through the number of possible explanations.

Gestures in apraxia of speech treatment. Meaningful gestures have been used as alternative and augmentative communication with apraxic patients (Dowden, Marshall, & Tompkins, 1981) and to improve apraxic speech (Rosenbek, 1978; Rosenbek, Collins, & Wertz, 1976; Skelly, Schinsky, Smith, & Fust, 1974). Any set of meaningful gestures can be used to replace speech or to augment it. Skelly's (1979) system based on American Indian sign language is one of the more popular of such systems. When paired systematically with speaking, gestures augment and may even be the basis for improved speech (Skelly et al., 1974). The augmenting effect of meaningful gestures is easily demonstrated, but researchers have had difficulty demonstrating that improved gestures can be the basis for improved speech. Anecdotes abound. Unfortunately anecdotes are not proof.

Nonmeaningful gestures, which Ekman and Friesen (1972) call illustrators, also have therapeutic potential, and that potential has been studied. Among the illustrators is a class of gestures called batons which are simple, repetitive gestures that accompany speech. They are the rhythmical but variable "timing" gestures common to most of us we talk, especially during animated discussion. A program with the goal of pairing the two — batons and oral gesturing (or speech) — so that speech is improved was described by Wertz, LaPointe, and Rosenbek (1984). Unlike American Indian sign, batons do not replace speech. They may, however, help selected speakers pace the speech they already have.

WHEN TO TREAT

The clinical litany is that treatment for aphasic and apraxic people should begin as early as possible. The issue is more complex. Acutely ill patients may be emotionally and physically unfit for treatment. Certainly they are sometimes unresponsive to our specific drills, but even then they and their families may be bolstered by our advice, support, prognostication, and promise to help when appropriate and needed.

Coping with Patient Compensations and Physiological Change

One of the concerns about early treatment even for apraxic talkers who are well enough to want to get better is that they may be variable, because, as one of several influences, they begin immediately doing what they think is best to cope with the disability. Good clinicians can guide these coping efforts.

Because most changes, even by those who may unwittingly be getting in their own way, are positive, the clinician has mostly to be a protean creature and try to keep pace with the patient's progress. Even a quick journey toward recovery can be a frightening one, and the good clinician can illuminate the dark places and be a companion along the way.

Somewhat inexplicably, the clinician sometimes seems reluctant to begin early treatments because proving they have done good, that they have contributed to a patient's recovery, is difficult or impossible. Often it is, but that does not make speech disorders or speech treatments unique. Any number of conditions are self-limiting and recovery from them is in the natural process of things. Besides, physiological recovery need not victimize the clinician. Some apraxic patients can be treated in ways that allow for documenting a clinician's contribution even within the first few days or weeks. Rosenbek, Becher, Shaughnessy, and Collins (1979) documented a contribution to the recovery of one 62-year-old apraxic-aphasic man whose treatment began 1 week following a thromboembolic stroke involving the left hemisphere. Even though that patient got considerable help from physiological change, the data showed that treatment helped as well. In addition, that speaker continued to use the gestural accompaniment to speech he had learned in therapy until the end of his days. He was convinced once he left the clinic and without any coaxing from us that gestures were essential when outside pressures against his speech were great.

Aphasiologists are fond of proclaiming that recovery with treatment is greater than physiological change alone could have caused. Perhaps. Our feeling, however, is that physiological recovery is the nonpareil clinician. Speech pathologists improve patients faster; they do not need to claim they can take them higher, unless data yet to be published document it.

PROGNOSIS

With few exceptions, data on the apraxic speaker's prognosis is buried in data on aphasia. This contamination coupled with the ubiquitous problem created by the lack of a standard label and description that makes it impossible to know just what kind of patients are being described in the literature make firm conclusions impossible. A summary of the literature appears in Wertz, LaPointe, and Rosenbek (1984) and by Wertz in this volume (Chap. 9) and will not be repeated here. A few highlights, however, are appropriate.

Little Broca's Aphasia

Mohr, Pessing, Finkelstein, Funkenstein, Duncan, and Davis, (1978) report convincing recovery and localization data on what they call little Broca's aphasia, an articulation disorder accompanied by an oral apraxia. They distinguish this syndrome from a big Broca's aphasia, a language deficit manifest as agrammatism. Little Broca's aphasia, which follows a circumscribed Broca's area lesion, begins with speechlessness and language impairment. Soon thereafter language returns without agrammatism, and the patient's motor speech function also returns except that it is marred by varying degrees of apraxia of speech. The apraxia, too, improves relatively quickly—within weeks or months. We suspect that speech pathologists have encountered and reported this phenomenon less often than have neurologists because such patients may well not be referred. Rapidly improving patients often are not. We have sometimes seen little Broca's aphasic speakers. They are what we call apraxic. Often recovery is rapid and complete so that only a trained listener can hear the residual dysprosody. Sometimes recovery is less complete, but functional speech emerges nevertheless. The amount of residual may well be as much a function of the coexisting aphasia as of the apraxia of speech.

Speechless Patients

And what of the patient who begins and stays speechless but who does not have a profound dysarthria or aphasia? Can that happen to an apraxic person? Can you be so apraxic as to remain speechless? We need data on the speechless: on their language, limb control, site of lesion; and ability to learn, generalize, and retain in the various modalities. By contrasting the chronically speechless with the traditional apraxic who regains functional spech and the global aphasic who remains severely handicapped, we may eventually identify signs that will improve our ability to make early prognostic judgments. To reply, "Well we don't really know. We'll see him twice a day this month and maybe we'll know more in a few weeks'' when asked by a concerned family for a prediction is of no help and probably even very little succor. We can eventually do better. We need to try.

Prognosis with Treatment

Except for the speechless person who fails to learn even a few sounds predictably and whose failure can be predicted after only a few controlled sessions, typical apraxic speakers thrive in treatment. Their gains and carry over are limited only by their cognition, language, or need (and occasionally by their clinician's skills). Extensive treatment data are reported by Wertz, LaPointe, and Rosenbek, 1984. These data confirm that improvements can be expected from even severely apraxic patients (not to be confused with severe Broca's or globally aphasic people). In this present volume (Chap. 9), Wertz also reports on treatment effects. The Veterans Administration Cooperative Study on aphasia (Wertz, Collins, Weiss, Brookshire, Friden, Kurtzke, & Pierce, 1981) from which those data are selected was not designed to provide information on apraxia of speech. Wertz (Chap. 9), in this volume therefore, is appropriately cautious with his statements.

Data on recovery by individual treated patients have also been reported. Sands, Freeman, and Harris (1978) compared the speech of one of Shankweiler and Harris' original patients (1966) at the time of the original study in 1965 with his performance in 1975 after 10 years of therapy, presumably done for free. The treatment is only described as being traditional and emphasizing imitation. The authors are not concerned with proving that treatment worked but they did want to discover how the patient's speech errors changed. Fortunately for the speaker and anyone having to justify such protracted treatment, the patient made fewer errors in 1975 than in 1965. Changes were most obvious in initial and final position singleton consonants and in initial but not final position clusters. Place, manner, and omission errors were substantially reduced. Voicing errors changed only 3%, and addition errors, most of which resulted from the speaker's adding what listeners thought was an /s/ at the beginning of many utterances, were unchanged.

What the authors make of these changes (Freeman, Sands, & Harris, 1978), coupled with the conclusion from their earlier report (Sands, Freeman, & Harris, 1978) is of greatest clinical interest. They say the voicing and addition errors result from ''poor temporal coordination of airflow, phonation, and articulation'' (p. 103). That such errors persist, they hypothesize, may result from the extreme difficulty of such coordination, from the inability of traditional treatments to manage this condition, from the clinician's failure to recognize the errors (especially of voicing), or from some combination of these.

Theirs is a stimulating cluster of testable hypotheses typical of contemporary research reports. To test them, one might first attempt to alter voicing errors with traditional methods and use both perceptual and acoustic (maybe even movement and EMG) measures of progress. If voicing errors persist, instrumental methods for their eradication can be tried. For example, the patient can be fed back information, perhaps in the form of a visual display, on his voice onset time. Or behavioral and biofeedback methods can be contrasted in an alternating treatment design. The combination of careful perceptual, acoustic, and physiologic observation with equally careful and focused treatment may well characterize future apraxia research. Sands, Freeman, and Harris (1978) are among those pointing the way.

A POSSIBLE FUTURE FOR CLINICAL MANAGEMENT

Our review of apraxia treatment has been tendentious. Thousands of clinicians have contributed to their patient's well-being, if not to the literature, and certainly there are more treatment contributions than we have mentioned. We have tried to discuss what is typical. Yet to be discussed is how contemporary research is altering treatment's face. Alterations are this section's topic.

Contemporary research is providing clinicians with fine-grained analyses of apraxic errors and more insight about why those errors appear. Already this research has confirmed the traditional practice of treating apraxic speakers as if they need structured drill.

If we think of apraxia of speech as a movement disorder rather than as an articulation or even a speech disorder, and if we think of even perceived substitutions as when /d/ becomes /n/, as resulting from distortions of the temporal sequence of component movements, then our attitudes about apraxic errors and our treatment approaches are altered. We begin to think of substitutions (assimilitive errors probably should be excluded from the analysis) as only extreme degrees of distortion resulting from significant movement impairment. In treatment, speech targets are replaced by movement targets. In this revised view, the speech sounds one selects are merely facilitators of movement on a par with other facilitators such as rate, rhythm, and stress. Talk about speech sound adequacy and how to achieve it by careful selection of stimulus length and frequency, stimulus mode, response mode, facilitators, and reinforcements is replaced by talk about the timing and coordination of movement sequences. The "sounds" we choose to have patients say are as important — but no more so — than other dimensions of the speech signal.

Thinking of the apraxic talker as motorically rather than linguistically involved and of apraxic errors as frequently being distortions rather than substitutions changes therapy in other ways. In combination those two attitudes make legitimate an evaluation of what apraxic speakers do to make themselves as intelligible as they are. In other words, clinicians can winnow apraxic speech for evidence of rules that individual patients are capable of following and how they compensate for rules they can barely or not follow at all. Studies like that by Duffy and Gawle in this volume (Chap. 6) are exemplary. Some of their apraxic patients produced voicing differences despite having durations of the preceding vowel that were all within the range of the durations that normal speakers use when the following consonant is voiceless. That listeners hear voice-voiceless distinctions means apraxic speakers are compensating, perhaps by exaggerating other cues to the voiced-voiceless distinction. Treatment eventually may be enhanced as additional acoustic and yet-to-be-completed physiologic studies show us how successful apraxic speakers compensate.

More than one type of apraxia is predicted by models of motor performance. Careful diagnosis may reveal them. Deutsch (this volume Chap. 4) is among those making a start. If types are identified, differential treatments may follow. Differential treatments for different apraxic types may also make the neuropathophysiology of the different types clearer. In this way models can be influenced by treatment data.

Clinicians train their patients to slow down, to change posture, to increase effort, to concentrate, to heighten prosodic profiles; and some patients seem to improve. Often it is unclear what has changed, however. By combining the rigor of alternating treatment designs with the precision of acoustic and physiologic measures, clinicians may begin finding out what changes, how much, and why. Do rate changing or pacing treatments work because they influence rate, or attention, or overall effort, or for some other reason? Answers will make the next generation of clinicians better than the present one, because only in a laissez faire world can people be content to say, "I don't care why it works, I'm just glad it does."

SUMMARY AND CONCLUSIONS

Charge to the Clinical Researcher

Itoh and Sasanuma (this volume, Chap. 5) draw our attention to an immediate and practical question: What can be done in a clinical setting to resolve the many persistent questions about the nature of apraxia of speech? They recommend that we start by becoming more keenly aware of the "core symptom" of apraxia of speech (viz., articulatory distortions) and by training our ears to discern these often subtle articulatory variations. But our ears may need help, if not from techniques for the direct observation of articulatory movements, then at least from acoustic analysis. Real-time acoustic analysis can be particularly helpful by supplementing the ear with visual displays which may be frozen for careful inspection of spectral or temporal characteristics of a sound pattern. Frequently, sound distortions that are difficult to identify in the fleeting auditory event of speech can be determined from an acoustic analysis. Acoustic analysis is additionally helpful in the quantification of various dimensions of speech production (e.g., the ever popular voice onset time, formant structure for vocalic sounds, noise spectra for stops and fricatives, durations of phonetic segments, intonation contours, and a host of measures of the short-term spectrum or the waveform of speech).

When instrumental methods are not available, it is particularly important that speech patterns be described with narrow phonetic transcription. Narrow transcription is being used increasingly in studies of children's speech development, and the lessons learned in descriptions of early phonetic development might be applied to studies of aphasia and apraxia. Only infrequently has narrow transcription been reported in studies of apraxia of speech. Much more frequent use has been made of broad (phonemic) transcription, perhaps because investigators assumed from earlier studies that substitutions would be the predominant error category. The papers of Itoh and Sasanuma and of Kent and Rosenbek (1983) suggest that this assumption be reevaluated. From the standpoint of articulation scoring, it is not particularly informative if perceived distortions are indicated simply by an abbreviatory device such as "*D*", "*X*", or whatever. If narrow transcription is used, then information about patterns of deviance can be obtained. It can be the case that many errors perceived as substitutions and many errors perceived as distortions share the same dimension or feature of articulatory variation, for example, errors in control of voicing can be perceived as distortions (such as a partially voiced /s/) or as substitutions (z/ for /s/). Because systems of diacritic marks used for narrow transcription in traditional linguistic phonetics are not always suitable for clinical transcription, it seems appropriate to develop phonetic coding systems more suited to the clinical need (Shriberg & Kent, 1982).

Substitutions And Distortions

Given first of all that greater care must be taken in distinguishing errors of substitution from errors of distortion, it is likely that apraxia of speech will be characterized phonetically as a mix of these two types of errors. Whether one type of error predominates over the other may not be as important as identification of dimensions of dysfunction that are common to both types of errors.

Even with stringent critera for identification of substitution errors, we believe that flurries of substitutions will continue to be a major pathognomic feature of the disorder. The origin of these errors is obscure. However, assuming that the fundamental impairment lies in either paradigmatic or sequential/hierarchical structure of motor output, substitutions can result from (a) confusions of context information with specifications for the current target or trajectory, or (b) entropic selection in which the most probable or natural targets are retrieved. The first of these alternatives is expected to yield sequencing errors (postpositionings, pre-positionings, and metathesis). The second would generate substitutions accountable largely by markedness or naturalness considerations. It is logical to expect that errors would be more likely for sounds that occur less frequently, because paradigmatic and syntagmatic mechanisms would be less easily accessed for these targets. Thus, this framework accounts for three major properties of apraxic speech errors: (1) errors are more likely to occur for less frequently occurring sounds in the language; (2) many substitution errors are sequencing errors, or confusions of elements in an output string; and (3) substitution errors show a general preference for unmarked (natural) items.

What then can be said about the relationship between substitutions and distortions? Are they causally independent? First, let us consider the possibility that substitution errors (in the strict sense of actual phoneme target replacements) are secondary to impairments in the programming or specification of movements. The rationale here is that uncertainty or failure in the implementation of an action or motor goal leads to a deterioration in the representation of that action or goal (and perhaps other partially activated goals as well). That is, difficulty in motor implementation may cause a loss of goal information or a confusion of the information associated with several sequential goals. Attempts at recovery of the lost information or at resolving the confusion lead to altered goals, that is, phoneme substitutions. As explained above, these substitutions would follow two general patterns — a pattern of sequential error and a pattern of entropic deterioration.

On the other hand, it is conceivable that substitutions arise as a primary impairment, particularly one that causes a deterioration of the goal itself (a kind of phonetic aphasia) or one that disturbs the retriveal of correct representations. Distortions and other accompanying abnormalities presumably would be the result of another level of impairment, one that affects programming or control of movement.

Methods of Study

What is the best method for studying apraxia of speech? In the final analysis, there probably will not be a single best method, but rather a synthesis of the results obtained from a variety of methods. Thus, we agree with Itoh and Sasanuma (this volume, Chap. 5) that each of the approaches to the study of apraxia of speech is valuable in complementing other approaches, so that ultimately the disorder will be understood through an integration of the various types of data. However, there is one problem that should not be overlooked or dismissed too quickly. Granted that each method has its own strengths and weaknesses, one should take care to avoid overinterpretation of the data from any one approach or set of results. For example, Kent and Rosenbek (1983) cautioned against motoric level interpretations of perceptually derived data, such as phonetic-feature or distinctive-feature characterization of apraxic utterances. All too often perceptually derived data are the result of processes of abstraction that partially or totally obscure some underlying articulatory events. On the other side of the coin, physiologic data often are severely limited with respect to the parameters or articulators under observation and present inferential difficulties of their own. Unfortunately, few studies have been conducted that offer various levels of analysis on the same set of apraxic utterances. It would be extremely helpful to have correlated information on perceptual deviance, acoustic structure, and associated physiologic patterns (articulator movements, air pressures and flows, or EMG signals). Of course, the total amount of information to be collected an analyzed is huge, which brings up another problem for both clinical and research purposes.

Crystal (1982) compared the current demands on speech-language pathologists as being similar to those placed on medical doctors at the turn of the century. The doctors themselves performed their own pathological analysis "in their back rooms" and voiced complaints (that should sound familiar) about the pressure of time. Speech-language clinicians are faced with tasks of analysis that are challenging if not overwhelming. Thus, we all might join with Crystal in looking forward to the day when this burden of mechanical analysis "will be taken off the speech therapist's back by the provision of automatic analytic techniques — techniques of analysis using word-processors, techniques of remediation using interactive instrumentation" (p. 18). The papers in the volume point up the need for extensive analyses of apraxia of speech — analyses at several levels, from perceptual to acoustic to physiologic. In addition, several levels of linguistic analysis are required, from phonetic (narrow transcription) to syntactic and semantic levels.

Summary by Allegory

The study of apraxia of speech might be likened to the proverbial story of the six blind men describing their perception of an elephant (one examining the tail, another the trunk, another the massive body, etc.), A more contemporary analogy is Kety's (1975) imaginary example of scientists from a future society, sophisticated but illiterate, who seek to understand a peculiar archeological discovery — a book. The chemist among them might burn the book to discover its chemical constituents; a microscopist might examine the fine structure (cytoarchitectionics?) of each page, and perhaps a biologist would be intrigued by evidence of organic compounds showing that the book is a residue (perhaps waste product) of a living organism. Although the linguist, the neurologist, the speech physiologist, the psychologist, and the speech pathologist may not be as far apart as the scientists in our hypothetical example, they each carry a particular kind of sophistication and often a corresponding blindness or ignorance. And, as Wexler (1980) reminds us from work on general system theory, "certain phenomena are inaccessible at each level of analysis," so that some basic phenomena cannot be detected at a high level of analysis and some complex phenomena simply do not exist at lower levels of analysis.

Wexler also warned of the "imperial paradigm" of psychology, which appropriates other perspectives to impose its own concepts on the organization of data. He cites Pavlov's (1963) warning that because psychological conceptions are not essentially spatial conceptions, they cannot penetrate into the mechanism of mutual connections between brain centers. Some attempts at clinicoanatomic studies may shatter on the same rocks, particularly so as they seek to map psychological dysfunction on neural tissue.

NOTES

[1]The concept of entropy has been applied to diverse fields, including economics, geology, city planning, art, and psychotherapy. The generalization of the concept to such different fields is made by associating entropy with disorder or chaos. In equilibrium thermodynamics the degree of disorder can be gauged by reference to the positions and velocities of the molecules in a thermal system. Katakis and Katakis (1982) suggest that disorder becomes higher in biopsychosocial systems "if there are many phases having comparable probabilities of occurring, and if these phases interact with the environment in nonselective ways" (p. 122). The notion of linguistic entropy based on markedness theory is similar to this concept, except that probabilities are defined with respect to natural outcomes (i.e., not all linguistic changes are equally probable). This idea of linguistic entropy assumes an underlying order, that of a functional mode of language expression, or else there would be nothing linguistic to characterize.

[2]As Brown (1979, p. 140) put it, "This theory (disconnection), which is an outgrowth of nineteenth century sensory psychology, at least of the version that contaminated the early days of neurological study, is open to all of the criticisms of area localization previously discussed, since it presupposed a localization of function in precise brain areas."Brown finds the disconnection hypothesis unsatisfactory because it "says nothing about the organization of the disturbed psychological process."

REFERENCES

Bailey, C.-J. N. The garden path that historical linguistics went astray on. *Language and Communication,* 1982, *2,* 151–160.

Basso, A., Salvolini, U., & Vignolo, L. A. Localization of aphasic symptoms: Preliminary observations with C.T. scanner (Italian). *Rivista di Patologia Nervosa E Mentale,* 1979, *100,* 94–102.

Blumstein, S. *A phonological investigation of aphasic speech.* The Hague: Mouton, 1973.

Blumstein, S. Review of "generative phonology—Evidence from aphasia" by M. Schnitzer. *Cortex,* 1974, *10,* 206.

Blunk, R., DeBlesser, Willmes, K., & Zeumer, H. A refined method to relate morphological and functional aspects of aphasia. *European Neurology,* 1981, *20,* 69–79.

Bradley, D., & McCabe, R. Systematic multiple phonemic approach to articulation therapy. *Acta Symbolia,* 1975, *1,* 1–18.

Branigan, G. Syllable structure and the acquisition of consonants: The great conspiracy in word formation. *Journal of Psycholinguistic Research,* 1976, *5,* 117–113

Brown, J. W. On the neural organization of language: thalamic and cortical relationships. *Brain and Language,* 1975, *2,* 18–30.

Brown, J. W. Language representation in the brain. In H. D. Steklis & M. J. Raleigh (Eds.), *Neurobiology of social communication in primates: An evolutionary perspective.* New York: Academic Press, 1979.

Buckingham, H. W., Jr. Explanation in apraxia with consequences for the concept of apraxia of speech. *Brain and Language,* 1979, *8,* 202–226.

Buckingham, H. W., Jr. Explanations for the concept of apraxia of speech. In M. T. Sarno (Ed.), *Acquired aphasia.* New York: Academic Press, 1981, pp. 271-301.

Bugbee, J. K., & Nichols, A. C. Rehearsal as a self-correction strategy for patients with apraxia of speech. In R. H. Brookshire (Ed.), *Clinical aphasiology: Conference proceedings 1980.* Minneapolis: BRK, 1980, pp. 277–284.

Butterworth, B. Hesitation and the production of verbal paraphasias and neologisms in jargon aphasia. *Brain and Language,* 1979, *8,* 133–161.

Cappa, S., Cavalotti, C., & Vignolo, L. A. Phonemic and lexical errors in fluent aphasia: Correlation with lesion site. *Neuropsychologia,* 1981 *19,* 171–177.

Cohen, A., Collier, R., and 't Hart, J. Declination: Construct or intrinsic feature of speech pitch? *Phonetica,* 1982 *39,* 254–273.

Collins, M., Cariski, D., Longstreth, D., & Rosenbek, J. Patterns of articulatory behavior in selected motor speech programming disorders. In R. H. Brookshire (Ed.), *Clinical aphasiology: Conference proceedings 1980.* Minneapolis, BRK, 1980, pp.196–208.

Cooper, W. E., & Sorenson, J. M. *Fundamental frequency contours at syntactic boundaries. Journal of the Acoustical Society of America,* 1977, *62,* 683–692.

Cooper, W. E., & Sorenson, J. M. *Fundamental frequency in sentence production.* New York: Springer, 1981.

Crichton-Browne, J. On the weight of the brain and its component parts in the insane. *Brain,* 1880, *2,* 42-67

Critchley, M. Articulatory defects in aphasia. *Journal of Laryngology and Otology,* 1952, *66,* 1-17.

Critchley, M. *Aphasiology.* London: Arnold, 1970.

Crystal, D. Terms, time and teeth. *British Journal of Disorders of Communication,* 1982, *17,* 3-19.

Dabul, B., *Apraxia Battery for Adults.* Tigard, Oregon: C. C. Publications, 1979.

Dabul, B. L., & Bollier, B. Therapeutic approaches to apraxia. *Journal of Speech Hearing Disorders,* 1976, *41,* 268-276.

Damasio, A. R., Damasio, H., Rizzo, M., Varney, N., & Gersh, F. Aphasia with nonhemorrhagic lesions in the basal ganglia and internal capsule. *Archives of Neurology,* 1982, *39,*15-20.

Darley, F. L. Lacunae and research approaches to them, IV. In C. H. Millikan & F. L. Darley (Eds.), *Brain mechanisms underlying speech and language.* New York: Grune & Stratton, 1967, 236-290.

Darley, F. L. *The classification of output disturbance in neurologic communication disorders.* Paper presented at the American Speech and Hearing Association Convention, Chicago, 1969.

Darley, F., Aronson, A., & Brown, J. *Motor speech disorders.* Philadelphia: Saunders, 1975.

Darley, F. L. *Aphasia.* New York: Saunders, 1982.

Deal, J. L., & Darley, F. L. The influence of linguistic and situational variables on phonemic accuracy in apraxia of speech. *Journal of Speech and Hearing Research,* 1972, *15,* 639-653.

Deal, J., & Florance, C. L. Modification of the eight-step continum for treatment of apraxia of speech in adults. *Journal of Speech Hearing Disorder,* 1978, *43,* 89-95.

Divenyi, P. L., & Efron, R. Spectral versus temporal features in dichotic listening. *Brain and Language,* 1979, *7,* 375-386.

Dowden, P. A., Marshall, R. C., & Tompkins, C. A. Amer-Ind sign as a communicative facilitator for aphasic and apractic patients. In Robert H. Brookshire (Ed.), *Clinical aphasiology: Conference proceedings 1981.* Minneapolis: BRK, 1981. pp.133-140.

Eccles, J. C. The initiation of voluntary movement by the SMA. *Archiv für Psychiatrie und Nervenkrankheiten,* 1982, *231,* 423-441.

Eguchi, S., & Hirsh I. J. Development of speech sounds in children. *Acta Otolaryngologica,* 1969, Supplement 257.

Ekman, P., & Friesen, W.V. Hand movements. *Journal of Communication,* 1972, *22,* 353-374

Falzi, G., Perrone, P., & Vignolo, L.A. Right-left asymmetry in anterior speech region. *Archives of Neurology,* 1982, *39,* 239-241.

Florance, C. L., Rabidoux, P. C., & McCauslin, L. S. An environmental manipulation approach to treating apraxia of speech. In R.H. Brookshire (Ed.), *Clinical aphasiology: Conference Proceedings 1980.* Minneapolis: BRK, 1980. pp. 285-293.

Fowler, C.A. Coarticulation and theories of extrinsic timing. *Journal of Phonetics,* 1980, *8,* 113–133.

Freeman, F. J., Sands, E. S., & Harris, K. S. Temporal coordination of phonation and articulation in a case of verbal apraxia: A voice onset time study. *Brain and Language,* 1978, *6,* 106–111.

Fromkin, V. A. The non-anomalous nature of anomalous utterances. *Language,* 1971, *47,* 27–52.

Fromm, D., Abbs, J., McNeil, M., & Rosenbek, J. Simultaneous perceptual-physiological method for studying apraxia of speech. In R.H. Brookshire (Ed.), *Clinical aphasiology: Conference proceedings 1982.* Minneapolis: BRK, 1982. pp. 251–262.

Fry, D.B. Phonemic substitutions in an aphasic patient. *Language and Speech,* 1959, *2,* 52–60.

Galaburda, A. M., Sanides, F., & Geschwind, N. Human brain. Cytoarchitectonic left-right asymmetries in the temporal region. *Archives of Neurology,* 1978, *35,* 812–817.

Geschwind, N. The apraxias: Neural mechanisms of disorders of learned movement. *American Scientist,* 1975, *63,* 188–195.

Geschwind, N., & Levitsky, W. Human brain: Left-right asymmetries in temporal speech region. *Science,* 1968, *161,* 186–188.

Goodglass, H. Phonological factors in aphasia. In R.H. Brookshire (Ed.), *Clinical aphasiology: Conference proceedings.* Minneapolis. BRK, 1975. pp. 28–44.

Grimm, R.J., & Nashner, L.M. Long loop dyscontrol. In J.E. Desmedt (Ed.), *Cerebral motor control in man: Long loop mechanisms.* Basel: Karger, 1978. pp. 70–84.

Grossman, M. A central processor for hierarchically-structured material: Evidence from Broca's aphasia. *Neuropsychologia,* 1980, *18,* 299–308.

Guyette, T. W., & Diedrich, W. M., A critical review of developmental apraxia of speech. In N. Lass (Ed.), *Speech and language: Advances in basic research and practice* (Vol. 5). New York: Academic Press. 1981. pp. 1–49.

Halpern, H., Darley, F. L., & Brown, J. R. Differential language and neurological characteristics in cerebral involvement. *Journal of Speech and Hearing Disorders,* 1973, *38,* 162–173.

Hammond, G. R. Hemispheric differences in temporal resolution. *Brain and Cognition,* 1982, *1,* 95–118.

Heilman, K. M. Apraxia. In K.M. Heilman & E. Valenstein, (Eds.), *Clinical Neuropsychology.* New York; Oxford University Press, 1979. pp. 159–183.

Holtzapple, P., & Marshall, N. The application of multiphonemic articulation therapy with apraxic patients. In R.H. Brookshire (Ed.), *Clinical aphasiology conference proceedings 1977.* Minneapolis: BRK, 1977, 46–58.

Itoh, M., Sasanuma, S., Hirose, H., Yoshioka, H., & Ushijima, T. Articulatory dynamics in a patient with apraxia of speech: X-ray microbeam observation. *Annual Bulletin of the Research Institute of Logopedics and Phoniatrics,* University of Tokyo, 1978, *12,* 87–96.

Itoh, M., Sasanuma, S., Tatsumi, I. F., Murakami, S., Fukusaki, Y., & Suzuki, T. Voice onset time characteristics in apraxia of speech. *Brain and Language,* 1982, *17,* 193–210.

Itoh, M., Sasanuma, S., & Ushijima, T. Velar movements during speech in a patient with apraxia of speech. *Brain and Language,* 1979, *7,* 227–239.

Jackson, H. Notes on the physiology and pathology of language: Remarks on those cases of disease of the nervous system in which defect of expression is the most striking symptom. *Brain,* 1915, *38,* 40–58.

Johns, D. F. A systematic study of phonemic variability in apraxia of speech. Ph.D. dissertation, Florida State Univ., 1968.

Johns, D. F., & LaPointe, L. L. Neurogenic disorders of output processing: Apraxia of speech. In H. Whitaker & H.A. Whitaker (Eds.), *Studies in neurolinguistics* (Vol. I). New York: Academic Press, 1976. pp. 161-200.

Johns, D., & Darley, F. Phonemic variability in apraxia of speech. *Journal of Speech and Hearing Research,* 1970, *13,* 556–583.

Jonas, S. The thalamus and aphasia, including transcortical aphasia: A review. *Journal of Communication Disorders,* 1981, *14,* 349-373.

Joynt, R. *Reading, perception and language,* Baltimore: York Press, 1975.

Katakis, D. F., & Katakis, C. D. Teleonomic entropy in biopsychosocial systems. *Behavioral Science,* 1982, *27,* 118–124.

Kearns, K. P., The application of phonological process analysis to adult neuropathologies. In R.H. Brookshire (Ed.), *Clinical aphasiology: Conference proceedings 1980.* Minneapolis: BRK, 1980. pp. 187–195.

Keele, S. W. Movement control in skilled motor performance. *Psychological Bulletin,* 1968, *70,* 387-403.

Kelso, J. A. S., & Tuller, B. Toward a theory of apractic syndromes. *Brain and Language,* 1981, *12,* 224–245.

Kent, R. D. Models of speech production. In N.J. Lass (Ed.), *Contemporary issues in experimental phonetics.* New York: Academic Press, 1976.

Kent. R. D. Sensorimotor aspects of speech development. In R.N. Aslin, J.R. Alberts, & M.R. Peterson (Eds.), *Development of perception: Psychobiological perspectives (Vol. 1).* New York: Academic Press, 1981. pp. 161-189.

Kent, R. D. Segmental organization of speech. In P.F. MacNeilage (Ed.), *The production of speech.* New York: Springer-Verlag, 1983. pp. 57–89.

Kent, R. D. Brain mechanisms of speech and language: With special reference to emotional interactions. In R. Naremore (Ed.), *Recent advances: Language science.* San Diego, CA: College-Hill Press, in press. (a.)

Kent, R. D. Windows to the brain: Functional impairment and the surgical field (Commentary on George Ojemann's paper). *Brain and Behavioral Sciences,* in press. (b.)

Kent, R. D., Carney, P. J., & Severeid, L. R. Velar movement and timing evaluation of a model for binary control. *Journal of Speech and Hearing Research,* 1974, *17,* 470–488.

Kent, R. D., & Forner, L. L. Speech segment durations in sentence recitations by children and adults. *Journal of Phonetics,* 1980, *8,* 157–168.

Kent, R. D., Netsell, R., & Abbs, J. H. Acoustic characteristics of dysarthria associated with cerebellar disease. *Journal of Speech and Hearing Research,* 1979, *22,* 627–648.

Kent, R. D., & Rosenbek, J. C. Acoustic patterns of apraxia of speech. *Journal of Speech and Hearing Research,* 1983, *26,* 231–249.

Kertesz, A. *Aphasia and associated disorders. Taxonomy, localization and recovery.* New York: Grune & Stratton, 1979.

Kety, S. S. A biologist examines the mind and behavior. In T. Millon (Ed.), *Medical behavioral science.* Philadelphia: Saunders, 1975.

Kirzinger, A., & Jurgens, U. Cortical lesion effect and vocalization in the squirrel monkey. *Brain Research,* 1982, *233,* 299–315.

Klich, R. J., Ireland, J. V., & Weidner, W. E. Articulatory and phonological aspects of consonant substitutions in apraxia of speech. *Cortex,* 1979, *15,* 451–470.

Kolb, B., Sutherland, R. J., Nonneman, A. J., & Wishaw, I. Q. Asymmetry in the cerebral hemispheres of the rat, mouse, rabbit, and cat: The right hemisphere is larger. *Experimental Neurology,* 1982, *78,* 348–359.

Kornhuber, H. H. Introduction. In H. H. Kornhuber & L. Deecke (Eds.), *Motivation, motor and sensory processes of the brain: Electrical potentials, behaviour and clinical use. Progress in brain research* (Vol. 54). Amsterdam: Elsevier/North Holland, 1980.

LaPointe, L. L. An investigation of isolated oral movements, oral motor sequencing abilities and articulation of brain injured adults. Ph.D. dissertation, University of Colorado, 1969.

LaPointe, L. L. & Horner, J. Repeated trials of words by patients with neurogenic phonological selection-sequencing impairment (apraxia of speech). In R.H. Brookshire (Ed.), *Clinical aphasiology conference proceedings 1976.* Minneapolis: BRK, 1976. pp. 261–277.

LaPointe, L. L., & Johns, D. F. Some phonemic characteristics in apraxia of speech. *Journal of Communication Disorders,* 1975, *8,* 259–269.

Larimore, H. W. Some verbal and nonverbal factors associated with apraxia of speech. Ph.D. dissertation, University of Denver, 1970.

Lashley, K. S. The problem of serial order in behavior. In L.S. Jeffress (Ed.), *Cerebral mechanisms in behavior.* New York: Wiley, 1951.

Lecours, A. R., Dordain, G., & Lhermitte, F. Recherches sur le langage des aphasiques: I. Terminologie neurolinguistique. *Encephale,* 1970, *59,* 520–546.

Lecours, A. R., & Lhermitte, F. Phonemic paraphasias: Linguistic structures and tentative hypotheses. *Cortex,* 1969, *5,* 193–228.

Lecours, A. R., Lhermitte, F. The "pure form" of the phonetic disintegration syndrome (pure anarthria); anatomo-clinical report of a historical case. *Brain and Language,* 1976, *3,* 88–113.

Lehmkuhl, G., & Poeck, K. A disturbance in the conceptual organization of actions in patients with ideational apraxia. *Cortex,* 1981, *17,* 153–158.

Lesser, R. *Linguistic investigations of aphasia.* London: Arnold, 1978.

Lhermitte, F., Lecours, A. R., & Bertaux, D. Activation and seviation of linguistic units in aphasic transformations. In L.D. Proctor (Ed.), *Biocybernetics of the central nervous system.* Boston: Little, Brown, 1969.

Locke, S. Motor programming and language behavior. In G.A. Miller & E. Lenneberg (Eds.), *Psychology and biology of language and thought.* New York: Academic Press, 1978.

Luria, A. R. *Traumatic aphasia: Its syndromes, psychology and treatment.* The Hague: Mouton, 1970.

Marquardt, T. P., Reinhart, J. B., & Peterson, H. A. Markedness analysis of phonemic substitution errors in apraxia of speech. *Journal of Communication Disorders,* 1979, *12,* 481–494.

Martin, A. D. Some objections to the term apraxia of speech. *Journal of Speech and Hearing Disorders,* 1974, *39,* 53–64.

Martin, A. D., & Rigrodsky, S. An investigation of phonological impairment in aphasia, Part 1. *Cortex*, 1974, *10*, 317–328.

Marx, O. Aphasia studies and language theory in the 19th century, *Bulletin of the History of Medicine*, 1966, *40*, 328–341.

Mazzucchi, F., & Vignolo, L.A. Localization of lesions in aphasia: Clinical C.T. scan correlations in stroke patients. *Cortex*, 1979, *15*, 627–654.

McNeil, M. R., & Prescott, T.E. Revised Token Test. Baltimore: University Park Press, 1978.

McNeil, M.R., Prescott, T.E., & Lemme, M. L. An application of electromyographic biofeedback to aphasia/apraxia treatment. In R.H. Brookshire (Ed.), *Clinical aphasiology: Conference proceedings 1976*. Minneapolis: BRK, 1976. pp. 151–171.

Merzenich, M. *Rules underlying use-dependent alteration of cortical maps in adult primates*. Paper presented at Waisman Center, University of Wisconsin, Madison, February 8, 1983.

Metter, E. J., Wasterlain, C. G., Kuhl, D. E., Hanson, W. R., & Phelps, M. E. FDG positron emission computed tomography in a study of aphasia. *Annals of Neurology*, 1981, *10*, 173–183.

Millikan, C. H., & Darley, F. L. *Brain mechanisms underlying speech and language*. New York: Grune & Stratton, 1967.

Mills, L., & Rollman, G. B. Left hemisphere selectivity for processing duration in normal subjects. *Brain and Language*, 1979, *7*, 320–335.

Mlcoch, A. G., & Noll, J. D. Speech production models as related to the concept of apraxia of speech. In N.J. Lass (Ed.), *Speech and language: Advances in basic research and practice*. New York: Academic Press, 1980.

Mohr, J. P., Pessing, M. S., Finkelstein, S., Funkenstein, H. H., Duncan, G. W. & Davis, K. R. Broca aphasia: Pathologic and clinical. *Neurology*, 1978, *28*, 311–324.

Morley, M. *The development and disorders of speech in children*. Edinburgh: Churchill Livingstone, 1972. 3rd ed.

Mulder, G. The information processing paradigm: Concepts, methods and limitations. *Journal of Child Psychology and Psychiatry*, 1983, *24*, 19–35.

Naeser, M. A. Language behavior in stroke patients. *Trends in neurosciences*, 1982, *43*, 53–59.

Naeser, M. A., Alexander, M. P., Helm-Estabrooks, N., Levins, H. L., Laughlin, S. A., & Geschwind, N. Aphasia with predominantly subcortical lesion sites: Description of three capsular/putaminal aphasia syndromes. *Archives of Neurology*, 1982, *39*, 2–14.

Noel, G., Bain, H., Collard, M., & Huvelle, R. Clinico-pathological correlations in aphasiology by means of computerized axial tomography: Interest of using printout and prospective considerations. *Neuropsychobiology*, 1980, *6*, 190–200.

Obler, L. K., & Albert, M. L. Language in the elderly aphasic and in the dementing patient. In M.T. Sarno (Ed.), *Acquired aphasia*. New York: Academic Press, 1981. pp. 385–398.

O'Connell, P.R. Neologistic jargon aphasia: A case report. *Brain and Language*, 1981, *12*, 292–302.

Ojemann, G. A. Subcortical language mechanisms. In H. Whitaker & H.A. Whitaker (Eds.), *Studies in neurolinguistics* (Vol 1). New York: Academic Press, 1976. pp. 103–138.

Ojemann, G., & Mateer, C. Human language cortex: Localization of memory, syntax, and sequential motor-phoneme identification systems. *Science*, 1979, *205*, 1401–1403.

Paillard, J. The patterning of skilled movements. In J. Field, H.W. Magoun, & V.E. Nall (Eds.), *Handbook of physiology. Section I. Neurophysiology* (Vol. 3). Washington, D.C.: American Physiological Society, 1960.

Pavlov, I. P. *Lectures on conditioned reflexes.* New York: International Publishers, 1963.

Pierrehumbert, J. The perception of fundamental frequency declination. *Journal of the Acoustical Society of America*, 1979, *66*, 363-369.

Poeck, K., Lehmkuhl, G., & Willmes, K. Axial movements in ideomotor apraxia. *Journal of Neurology, Neurosurgery and Psychiatry*, 1982, *45*, 1125-1129.

Poncet, M., Degos, C., & Deloche, G. Phonetic and phonemic transformations in aphasia. *International Journal of Mental Health*, 1972, *1*, 45-54.

Porch, B. E. *Porch Index of Communicative Ability.* Palo Alto, CA: Consulting Psychologists Press, 1967.

Reed, E. S. An outline of a theory of action systems. *Journal of Motor Behavior*, 1982, *14*, 98-134.

Requin, J. Toward a psychobiology of preparation for action. In G.E. Stelmach & J. Requin (Eds.), *Tutorials in motor behavior.* Amsterdam: North-Holland, 1980.

Riese, W. The early history of aphasia. *Bulletin of the History of Medicine*, 1947, *23*, 322-334.

Roland, P. E., Larsen, B., Lassen, N. A., & Skinhoj, E. Supplementary motor area and other cortical areas in organization of voluntary movements in man. *Journal of Neurophysiology*, 1980, *43*, 118-130.

Romeny, B.M., ter Haar, van der Gon, J. J., Denier, & Gielen, C.C.A.M. Changes in recruitment order of motor units in the human biceps muscle. *Experimental Neurology*, 1982, *78*, 360-368.

Rosenbek, J. C., Treating apraxia of speech. In D.F. Johns (Ed.), *Clinical management of neurogenic communicative disorders.* Boston: Little, Brown, 1978. pp. 191-241.

Rosenbek, J. C., Becher, B., Shaughnessy, A., & Collins, M. Other uses of single-case designs. In R.H. Brookshire. (Ed.), *Clinical aphasiology conference proceedings 1979.* Minneapolis: BRK, 1979. pp. 311-316.

Rosenbek, J. C., Collins, M. J., & Wertz, R. T. Intersystemic reorganization for apraxia of speech. In R.H. Brookshire (Ed.), *Clinical aphasiology: conference proceedings 1976.* Minneapolis: BRK, 1976. pp. 255-260.

Rosenbek, J. C., Lemme, M.L., Ahern, M.B., Harris, E. H., & Wertz, R. T. A treatment for apraxia of speech in adults. *Journal of Speech and Hearing Disorders*, 1973, *38*, 462-472.

Rottenberg, D., & Hochberg, F. *Neurological classics in modern translation.* New York: Hafner, 1977.

Roy, E. A. Apraxia: A new look at an old syndrome. *Journal of Human Movement Studies*, 1978, *4*, 191-210.

Rubow, R., Rosenbek, J. C., Collins, M. J., & Longstreth, D. Vibrotactile stimulation for intersystemic reorganization in the treatment of apraxia of speech. *Archives of Physical Medicine and Rehabilitation*, 1982, *63*, 150-153.

Ryalls, J. H. Motor aphasia: Acoustic correlates of phonetic disintegration in vowels. *Neuropsychologia*, 1981, *19*, 365-374.

Sands, E., Freeman, F., & Harris, K. Progressive changes in articulatory patterns in verbal apraxia: A longitudinal case study. *Brain and Language*, 1978, *6*, 97-105.

Schmidt, R. A., A schema theory of discrete motor learning. *Psychological Review*, 1975, *82*, 225–240.

Schnitzer, M. L. Generative phonology: Evidence from aphasia. Ph.D. dissertation, University of Rochester, 1971.

Seldon, H. L. Structure of human auditory cortex I. Cytoarchitectonics and dendritic distributions. *Brain Research*, 1981, *229*, 277–294. (a)

Seldon, H. L. Structure of human auditory cortex II. Axon distributions and morphological correlates of speech perception. *Brain Research*, 1981, *229*, 295–310. (b)

Semjen, A. From motor learning to sensorimotor skill acquisition. *Journal of Human Movement Studies*, 1977, *3*, 182–191.

Shaffer, L. H. Rhythm and timing in skill. *Psychological Review*, 1982, *89*, 109–122.

Shane, H. C., & Darley, F. L. The effect of auditory rhythmic stimulation on articulatory accuracy in apraxia of speech. *Cortex*, 1978, *14*, 444–450.

Shankweiler, D., & Harris, K. S. An experimental approach to the problem of articulation in aphasia. *Cortex*, 1966, *2*, 277–287.

Shewan, C. M. Verbal dyspraxia and its treatment. *Human Communication*, 1980, *5*, 3–12.

Shriberg, L. D., & Kent, R. D. *Clinical phonetics*, New York: Wiley, 1982.

Simmons, N. N. Choice of stimulus modes in treating apraxia of speech: A case study. In R.H. Brookshire (Ed.), *Clinical aphasiology: conference proceedings 1980*. Minneapolis: BRK, 1980. pp. 302–307.

Skelly, M. *Ameri-Ind gestural code based on Universal American Indian Hand Talk*. New York: Elsevier, 1979.

Skelly, M., Schinsky, L., Smith, R. W., & Fust, R. S. American Indian Sign (Amerind) as a facilitation of verbalization for the oral verbal apraxic. *Journal of Speech and Hearing Disorders*, 1974, *39*, 445-456.

Sorenson, J. M., & Cooper, W. E. Syntactic coding of fundamental frequency in speech production. In R.A. Cole (Ed.), *Perception and production of fluent speech*. Hillsdale, NJ: Erlbaum, 1980.

Sternberg, S., Monsell, S., Knoll, R. L., & Wright, C. E. The latency and duration of rapid movement sequences: Comparisons of speech and typewriting. In G. E. Stelmach (Ed.), *Information processing in motor control and learning* New York: Academic Press, 1978.

Thach, W. T. Timing of activity in cerebellar dentate nucleus and cerebral motor cortex during prompt volitional movement. *Brain Research*, 1975, *88*, 233-241.

Thomas, L. *The medusa and the snail*. New York: Bantam, 1979.

Thorsen, N. A study of the perception of sentence intonation—Evidence from Danish. *Journal of the Acoustical Society of America*, 1980, *67*, 1014-1030.

Tognola, G. R., & Vignolo, L.A. Brain lesions associated with oral apraxia in stroke patients: A clinic-neuro-radiological investigation with the C.T. scan. *Neuropsychologia*, 1980, *18*, 257–272.

Tonkonogy, J., & Goodglass, H. Language function, foot of the third frontal gyrus, and rolandic operculum. *Archives of Neurology*, 1981, *38*, 486–490.

Trost, J. E. Patterns of articulatory deficts in patients with Broca's aphasia. Ph.D. dissertation, Northwestern University, 1970.

Walker, S. F. Lateralization of functions in the vertebrate brain: A review. *British Journal of Psychology*, 1980, *71*, 329–367.

Warren, R. Rehearsal for naming in apraxia of speech, In R.H. Brookshire (Ed.), *Clinical aphasiology: conference proceedings 1977*. Minneapolis: BRK, 1977. pp. 80–90.

Wertz, R. T., Collins, M. J., Weiss, D., Kurtzke, J. F., Friden, T., Brookshire, R. H. Pierce, J., Holtzapple, P., Hubbard, D. J., Porch, B. E., West, J. A., Davis, L., Matovitch, V., Morley, G. K., & Resurreccion, E. Veterans Administration cooperative study on aphasia: A comparison of individual and group treatment. *Journal of Speech and Hearing Research,* 1981, *24,* 580–594.

Wertz, R. T., LaPointe, L. L., Rosenbek, J. C. *Apraxia of Speech: The disorder and its treatment*. New York: Grune & Stratton, 1984.

Wertz, R. T., & Rosenbek, J. C. Appraising apraxia of speech. *Journal of the Colorado Speech and Hearing Association*, 1971, *5*, 18–36.

Wexler, B. E. Cerebral laterality and psychiatry: A review of the literature. *American Journal of Psychiatry*, 1980, *137*, 279–291.

Williams, R.,Ingham, R. J., & Rosenthal, J. A further analysis for developmental apraxia of speech in children with defective articulation. *Journal of Speech and Hearing Research,* 1981, *24,* 496-505.

Wilson, P. Temporal relationships in therapy for apraxia. In R.H. Brookshire (Ed.), *Clinical aphasiology: conference proceedings, 1977*. Minneapolis: BRK, 1977. pp. 119–123.

Yoss, K., & Darley, F. Developmental apraxia of speech in children with defective articulation. *Journal of Speech and Hearing Research*, 1974, *17*, 399–416.

2

Subcortical Lesions and Verbal Apraxia

Andrew Kertesz

INTRODUCTION

The role of subcortical structures in language is incompletely understood although their contribution to motor function is a subject of much research. Observations connected with stereotaxic surgery for Parkinson's disease directed attention to the role of the thalamus in language, and the dysarthria and word-finding difficulty following thalamotomies have been known for some time. "Dysarthria" and confusion are common features and interfere with language testing. Aphasia was noted in 42 percent of thalamotomies by Selby (1967). He described the disturbance as hesitant speech but preserved repetition. Bell (1968) considered the deficit to be similar to the aphasias of the frontal regions. Darley, Brown, and Swenson (1975) also reported cases of language changes after neurosurgery for Parkinsonism. One hundred one thalamotomy patients were reviewed. Language change occurred twice as often after left as opposed to right thalamotomy. Eighty-eight percent of the subjects had reduced accuracy and completeness, 65% reduced fluency, and 50% a reduction in auditory comprehension.

Smyth and Stern (1938) reported speech disturbances with tumors especially of the medial and anterior but not the ventral nuclear group of the thalamus. Only two cases of the 24 thalamic tumors reported by McKissock and Paine (1958) had aphasia. Thalamic hemorrhage, diagnosed on computerized tomographic (CT) scans or at autopsy, can produce an unusual aphasic syndrome with anomia, perseveration, and occasional neologisms with intact comprehension and repetition (Mohr, Watters, & Duncan, 1975). Some of these features such as the good repetition and fluent paraphasic speech, are also characteristic of transcortical sensory aphasia (Cappa & Vignolo, 1979), but the good comprehension and aspontaneity are more characteristic of transcortical motor aphasia. Thus, thalamic lesions produce a complex and variable picture which occasionally has been noted to be alternating and fluctuating within a single case. Perhaps the extent and the locus of the lesion will eventually be identified as the determiners of the consistency and degree of aspontaneity, the neologisms, and the level of comprehension.

CT scanning makes it possible to look at other subcortical lesions. The striatum consists of the putaminal portion of the lenticular nucleus connected through strips (striatum) of fibers across the internal capsule to the caudate nucleus. Naeser, Alexander, Helm-Estabrooks, Levine, Laughlin, and Geschwind (1982) reported a number of aphasic patients with lesions in the putamen and internal capsule. The predominant aphasia pattern for lesions with putaminal-capsular involvement and anterior-superior extension was that of good comprehension and syntax but slow, dysarthric speech. With posterior extension, comprehension was poor with rapid, paraphasic speech and jargon. Repetition was also impaired. When extension was both anterior-superior and posterior, lasting global aphasia resulted. These subcortical global aphasias were due, according to Naeser et al. (1982), to isolation of Broca's area both from afferent and efferent pathways. Damasio, Damasio, Rizzo, Varney and Gersh (1982), reported on atypical aphasia associated with small nonhemorrrhagic lesions of the anterior limb of the internal capsule and the striatum in the dominant hemisphere. Some of the patients had fluent speech as judged from phrase length, but decreased verbal agility.

It is the purpose of this chapter to present cases with subcortical stroke lesions and features of so-called verbal apraxia. The association of relatively isolated verbal apraxia in the acute patient with subcortical lesions is of diagnostic and pragmatic value to the clinician and has important implications for psychological models of language processing and motor physiology of speech.

METHODS

Assessment

We studied the speech production and articulation on a corpus of elicited speech and repetition tasks from the Western Aphasia Battery

(WAB) (Kertesz, 1982). That test was also used to provide data for establishing the severity of impairment or aphasia quotient (AQ), content of communication, and the fluency of spontaneous speech including a combined paraphasia and grammaticality rating (Kertesz, 1979). Comprehension was measured by yes-no tasks requiring no speech output, auditory word discrimination, and sentence comprehension utilizing sequential commands with preposition and relational words. A repetition task of words of increasing length and articulatory difficulty, number, word-number combinations, and high- and low-probability sentences; a naming task of 20 common objects presented visually and haptically; a comprehensive test of limb and oral praxis, drawing, block design, line bisection, calculation; and the Raven's Progressive Matrices completed the assessment.

Rating of Speech

The rating scale for speech production is specified in Table 2-1.

TABLE 2–1
Rating scale of speech output

Volume

0 No speech
1 Mostly unintelligible
2 Very low, barely intelligible
3 Moderately low
4 Slightly decreased
5 Normal

Phonemic Paraphasias

0 Not enough speech to judge
1 Severe (more than 2 per sentence or per 4 words)
2 Moderate (1–2 per sentence or per 4 words)
3 Mild (3–4 per interview)
4 Only occasional (1–2 per interview)
5 None (normal)

Semantic Paraphasias

0 Not enough speech to judge
1 Severe (more than 2 per sentence or per 4 words)
2 Moderate (1–2 per sentence or per 4 words)
3 Mild (3–4 per interview)
4 Only occasional (1–2 per interview)
5 None (normal)

Phonemic Perseverations (includes conduit d'approche)

0 Not enough speech to judge
1 Severe (more than 2 per sentence or per 4 words)
2 Moderate (1–2 per sentence or per 4 words)
3 Mild (3–4 per interview)
4 Only occasional (1–2 per interview)
5 None (normal)

Neologistic Jargon

0 Not enough speech to judge
1 More than 50% unintelligible utterances
2 Moderate (2 per sentence or 25%)
3 Mild (3–4 per interview)
4 Occasional (1–2 per interview)
5 None (normal)

Rate of Speech

0 No speech
1 Very hesitant (few utterances)
2 Nonfluent hesitation
3 Slowing and mild hesitation
4 Occasional hesitation
5 Normal

Dysarthria

0 Not enough speech to judge
1 Severe slurring of most words
2 Moderate (1–2 per sentence)
3 Mild (3–4 per interview)
4 Occasional (1–2 per interview)
5 None (normal)

Phonemic substitutions or paraphasias were defined as clearly articulated, recognizable alterations of a target phoneme, while neologistic utterances were defined as unintelligible transformations of lexical units. Phonemic perseveration, characterized by groping or repetitive approximations (the conduit d'approche), was rated separately. Volume and rate alterations were judged according to their deviation from normal. The dysarthria rating considered slurring, straining, wetness, and nasality that consistently distorted rather than altered phonemes. Three independent judges listened to the tape of each patient. The final scores used to document the characteristics of speech output were arrived at by using two of the concordant judgments or, if a range was obtained, the median value. In 94.3% of the scores, two-thirds or complete agreement was achieved. Broken down into subtests, the agreement was 91.3% for volume of speech, 91.3% for phonemic paraphasias, 89.8% for semantic paraphasias, 91.3% for phonemic perseverations, 100% for neologistic jargon, 97.8% for rate of speech, and 97.8% for dysarthria.

Experimental and Control Subjects

The target population consisted of a group of patients identified as having subcortical lesions with speech-language impairment (N = 15). Three patients did not have tapes, two patients were excluded because the speech production was so severely affected that most of the parameters could not be judged, and one patient for a significant foreign accent. The remaining 10 patients are the subjects of this study, in addition to a control population of aphasics with cortical lesions only (N = 12) and another group with combined cortical-subcortical lesions (N = 10).

CASE REPORTS

(1.) M.J., a 50-year-old, right-handed woman, developed a sudden dense right hemiplegia; she could only produce effortful, unintelligible sounds. A CT scan (Figure 2-1) revealed a 1.5-cm hemorrhage in the posterior limb of the left internal capsule, putamen, and globus pallidus. Two weeks poststroke she was formally tested with the WAB. Spontaneous, conversational speech was slightly slow with word-finding difficulty and some slurring. Occasional phonemic paraphasias were noted. Syntax and comprehension for all auditory material was normal although she had mild difficulty comprehending long written phrases. Writing was mildly impaired. No oral or limb apraxia was detected.

Three months later she had improved but still exhibited mild hesitancy and phonemic errors. Mild reading and writing deficits persisted. She was scored as a recovered aphasic with mild agraphia.

(2.) R.H., a 34-year-old man, became hemiplegic and mute for a week, but by the time he was formally tested 3 weeks poststroke he had low volume, nonfluent speech with dysarthria, anomia, and phonemic substitutions. His writing was impaired and he had some oral apraxia but not limb apraxia. The CT scan showed a lesion in the putamen, anterior limb of the internal capsule, and the caudate (Figure 2-2).

(3.) R.W., a 63-year-old man, developed moderately severe right hemiplegia and low volume, hesitant speech with a moderate number of phonemic substitutions, and some perseveration and dysarthria. On testing 2 weeks poststroke, he showed word-finding difficulty and severe agraphia. He also had moderate oral apraxia. At 3 months retest he still had some phonemic substitutions, but his fluency was improved. At 6 months he was still agraphic and anomic.

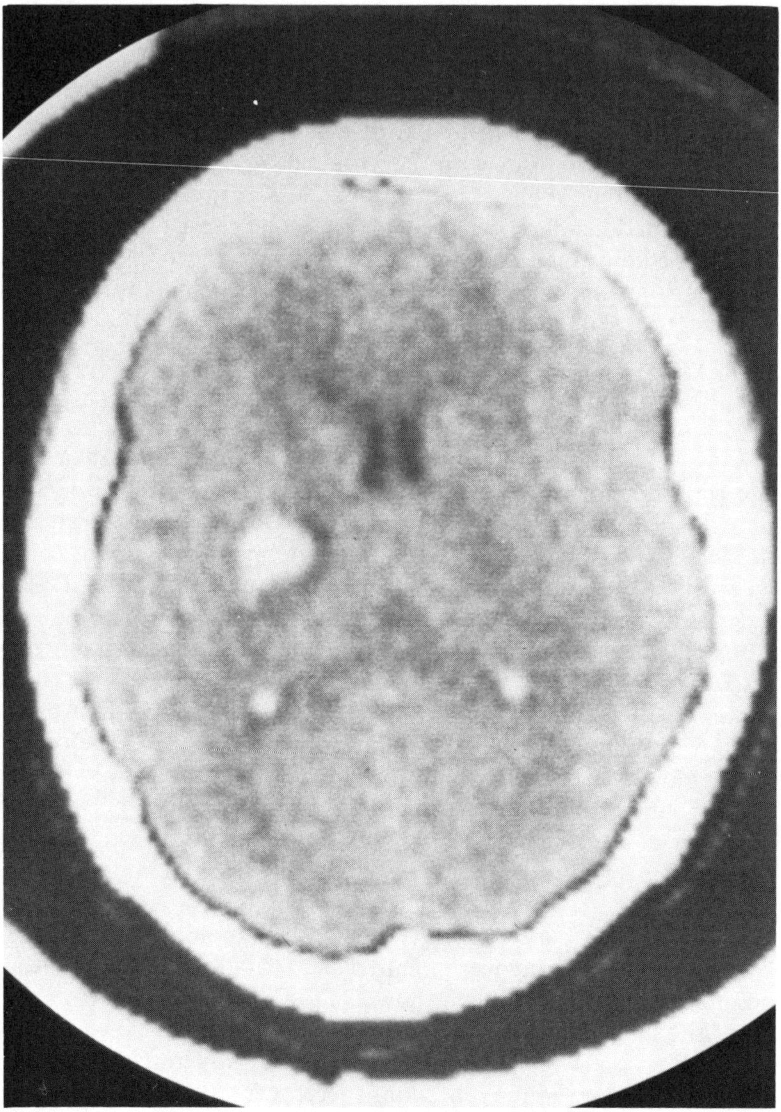

FIGURE 2–1
C.T. scan of Case 1. A small putaminal hemorrhage with a slight halo of edema involving the globus pallidus and internal capsule.

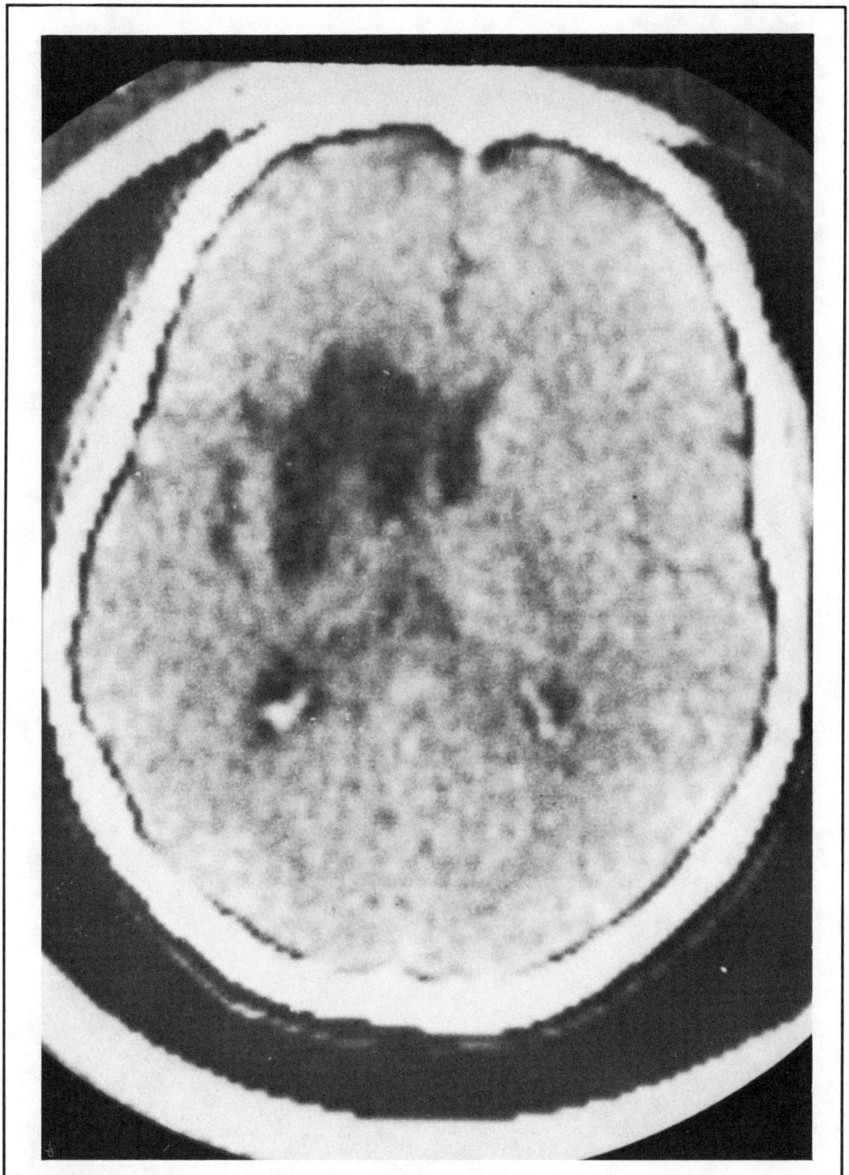

FIGURE 2–2
C.T. scan of Case 2. A moderately large striatal lesion destroying the putamen, the head of the caudate and some of the anterior limb of the internal capsule. The left ventricle is enlarged.

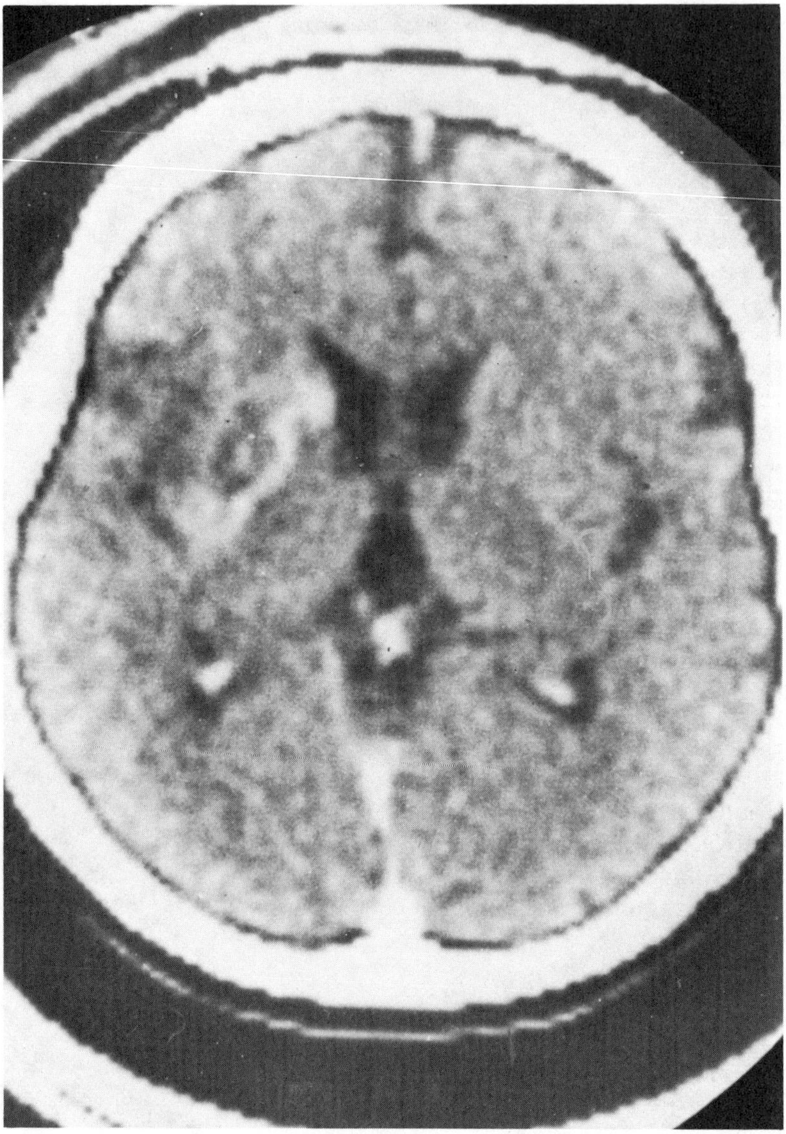

FIGURE 2–3
C.T. scan of Case 3. The lesion is similar to that in Case 2 but intravenous contrast was injected giving the whitish halo around it. The anterior insular region may also be involved.

The CT scan showed a relatively large size, striatal lesion, involving the putamen, caudate, and the anterior limb of the internal capsule (Figure 2-3).

(4.) J.H., a 64-year-old man, suddenly became hemiplegic and aphasic. His speech was low in volume, at times unintelligible, with hesitation and anomia, a large number of phonemic substitutions, and even some neologistic utterances. Comprehension and repetition were good but he still had anomia and agraphia a year later.

His lesion was in the putamen, caudate, and anterior portion of the internal capsule. The ventricles were enlarged.

(5.) B.M., a 67-year-old woman, developed slightly hesitant, anomic speech. Her reading and writing were poor. She had a few phonemic substitutions, perseveration, and a slightly slowed rate of speech. Her verbal apraxia was considered very mild at the time of testing 2 weeks poststroke. Her agraphia persisted.

The CT scan showed a striatal lesion involving the caudate, putamen, and the anterior limb of the internal capsule.

(6.) P.V., a 62-year-old man, was seen 2 weeks poststroke with slurred, slow, hesitant speech of mostly single words. Occasional phonemic perseveration, paraphasias, and word-finding difficulty but better confrontation naming and repetition were also noted. His comprehension was impaired for complex material. He also had alexia and severe agraphia; he could not write his name or letters of the alphabet. He was considered to have Broca's aphasia. A year later his speech was fluent with occasional phonemic substitutions but his hemiplegia persisted.

His CT scan, 1 year poststroke, showed a lesion involving the putamen and internal capsule, with enlargement of the left anterior horn of the lateral ventricle.

(7.) E.W., a 71-year-old woman, developed right hemiplegia and a mild speech disturbance with hesitation, phonemic substitutions, anomia, and severe agraphia. She was only able to print a few single letters in addition to her name. She did not have oral or limb apraxia.

A CT scan showed a small hemorrhage deep in the left lenticular nucleus at the border of the putamen and the globus pallidus.

(8.) A.B., a 70-year-old woman, had an acute onset of anomic aphasia, without hemiplegia. She had phonemic substitutions and slow speech, but her oral praxis was not impaired. She had significant agraphia, which improved at 3 months.

A CT scan showed a left anterior internal capsule and striatal lesion that involved some of the putamen and caudate.

(9.) F.T., a 71-year-old man, had a stroke in evolution with emotional lability initially that cleared, and when he was tested 2 weeks poststroke he had a nonfluent aphasia with mild right hemiplegia. His speech was telegraphic and halting with phonemic substitutions and groping. He had agraphia and apraxia for oral and complex movements.

A CT scan showed a deep infarct of the anterior capsular and caudate region.

(10.) V.E., a 66-year-old woman, developed right facial weakness and at times unintelligible speech. She made paraphasic errors and perseverated. On formal testing 3 weeks poststroke, she had only a few phonemic and semantic substitutions. Mild agraphia but no oral or limb apraxia was seen.

The CT scan showed a deep infarct in the left anterior internal capsule, and lenticular and caudate nuclei.

SUMMARY OF FINDINGS

The results of the speech output, aphasia, and apraxia ratings are summarized in Table 2-2. All 10 patients were aphasic, 6 of them very mildly, 4 moderately, according to the Aphasia Quotient of the WAB. Most of our patients with subcortical lesions are only mildly aphasic. Two exceptions with severe aphasia were included in this group. One patient (P.V.) had Broca'a aphasia with low fluency and dysarthria in addition to verbal apraxia. The patient with conduction aphasia (F.T.) had an Aphasia Quotient similar to the Broca's aphasic but with better fluency and poorer repetition. Phonemic groping was the most marked in this patient. This conduit d'approche or phonemic approximation is so often seen in conduction aphasics that it is virtually diagnostic of this type. It usually carries a good prognosis (Kertesz, 1979). The rest of the patients had anomic aphasia.

The rating of spontaneous speech for verbal apraxia revealed that all patients had some phonemic substitutions, usually of initial consonants. In four out of ten these were mild, in three moderate, and in one quite frequent. The most severely affected patient was also the one whose utterances were considered unintelligible the most often, therefore the score for neologistic utterances was significant. His dysarthria and low volume also undoubtedly contributed to the low intelligibility rating. Yet his speech was fluent enough to categorize him as anomic aphasic and to allow his frequent phonemic substitutions to be rated.

The rating scales for the ten patients show that while phonemic substitutions are uniformly present, semantic substitutions are absent or usually very mild, and jargon is absent. The rate of speech is usually decreased, although the patient's speech is still considered fluent in most instances. Voice volume is variable, and while some of this may reflect

TABLE 2–2
Output rating and language in subcortical lesions

		Score									
	Range	*MJ*	*RH*	*RW*	*JH*	*BM*	*PV*	*EW*	*AB*	*FT*	*VE*
Volume	0–5	4	5	3	2	5	5	4	4	3	4
Rate of Speech	0–5	3	4	3	4	4	3	4	3	3	4
Dysarthria	0–5	2	5	4	3	5	2	5	5	4	5
Phonemic Substitutions	0–5	3	4	3	1	4	4	3	3	3	4
Groping (Perseverations)	0–5	5	4	4	5	4	4	4	4	3	5
Neologistic Utterances	0–5	5	5	5	2	5	5	5	5	5	5
Semantic Paraphasias	0–5	5	4	4	5	4	5	4	4	4	4
Fluency	0–10	9	9	5	5	9	2	9	9	5	9
Content	0–10	9	9	7	5	9	5	9	8	6	8
Comprehension	0–10	9.9	9.5	9.2	8.9	9.9	8.6	8.5	9.6	7.6	8.9
Repetition	0–10	9.0	9.9	7.2	9.3	9.9	6.6	9.7	9.3	5.5	9.8
Naming	0–10	8.8	7.4	7.6	6.7	7.7	6.7	8.6	8.1	4.7	8.2
Reading	0–100	84	87	52	40	80	67	83	76	35	64
Writing	0–100	74	42	13	18	82	20	8	34	22	80
Oral Praxis	0–15	14	11	12	13	14	14	15	14	11	15
Limb Praxis	0–15	15	15	14	12	15	15	14	14	10	12
AQ (Severity)	0–100	92	90	72	70	91	58	90	88	58	88
Aphasic Type		A	A	A	A	A	B	A	A	C	A

normal variation, at least in three of the ten cases there was a significant decrease. Dysarthria was prominent in three cases and mild in two others.

Oral (buccofacial) apraxia was mild in four cases and not significant in six, although completely absent in only two. The presence of oral apraxia was associated with more marked verbal apraxia in three and mild verbal apraxia in one case. Limb praxis was affected in three cases. In two cases it cccurred in conjunction with oral apraxia and with agraphia in one case.

Writing was significantly impaired in all cases, in five cases quite severely; in two others, prominent; and in three cases, mildly. The severity of limb apraxia did not correlate with severity of agraphia.

Comprehension of verbal and written material was good except for three patients who were significantly alexic on the reading portion of the WAB. Three others were less severely affected, and the rest of the patients had only mild reading problems. Naming was affected universally, albeit mildly. Repetition was only impaired in three of the patients, most severely in the patient with conduction aphasia.

DISCUSSION

Although verbal apraxia is often seen in cortical or combined cortical and subcortical lesions of the posterior frontal lobe, especially in recovering stroke patients or patients with head injuries, the subcortical lesions of the striatum are specifically associated with prominent verbal apraxia without many other features of aphasia in the more acute stages of stroke. The comparison of these subcortical cases with a similarly examined cortical group (Kertesz, Bub, & Crook, 1982) indicates that the cortical syndrome tends to be more severe but is otherwise indistinguishable from the subcortical syndrome in many cases. The comparison is made difficult by the significant differences in lesion size which tend to be larger in cortical lesions. Occasionally, however, some signs emerge which do distinguish the two groups. The subcortical group shows more phonemic substitutions, perseverations, and approximations; and the rate and volume tends to be lower, some of which are features of verbal apraxia. The overall fluency is lower in the subcortical group and they also have more dysarthria. The cortical group, on the other hand, has more semantic paraphasias.

Verbal apraxia is difficult to define in an objective fashion, but the term enjoyed recent popularity because clinicians agree that there is an articulatory disturbance that is distinct from dsyarthria and that is not a necessary feature of aphasia. Darley, Aronson, and Brown's, (1975) description of verbal apraxia can be summarized as follows:

(1.) Effortful groping for correct articulatory postures, at times with facial grimacing;
(2.) Consonants more involved than vowels, and clusters more involved than singletons (Shankweiler & Harris, 1966);
(3.) Inconsistent articulatory errors;
(4.) Substitutions, additions, repetitions primarily; less frequently distortions or omissions (Johns & Darley, 1970);
(5.) Analysis of errors by distinctive features indicates that the majority of errors are close approximations of the target (Trost & Canter, 1974);
(6.) Perseverative, anticipatory, and transposition errors;
(7.) Alteration of prosody and rate.

None of these features has been quantified satisfactorily to provide accurate or exclusive diagnostic criteria for verbal apraxia. Our rating scale emphasizing phonemic substitutions, perseverative groping, rate, and volume and contrasting these to semantic and neologistic paraphasias is an attempt in this direction.

Systematic quantitative studies of verbal apraxia are relatively few. Shankweiler and Harris (1966) studied five recovering Broca's aphasics, 6 months to 7 years postonset. At the time of the testing, the aphasic symptoms were greatly diminished, leaving a major residual deficit in articulation. These patients did not have apraxia of nonverbal, oral movement, although "dexterity and speed" were diminished. Speech sound discrimination was preserved in some of these patients, and when it was impaired it was most impaired for vowels while production was most impaired for consonants. Analysis of the articulatory errors indicated initial consonant clusters and fricatives were most often involved. They are also the most difficult to perceive. The voiced stop consonants were more often substituted than others. Many of the substitutions were unrelated and inconsistent. Vowels were well produced except in one patient who was the poorest in other respects of production also. Fricatives, which were among the most difficult sounds for these five patients, are among the last to be added to a child's vocabulary and they require closer control of the amount and timing of movements than the other consonants.

Further study of verbal apraxia by Johns and Darley (1970) emphasized the inconsistency and unpredictability of errors in the apraxic group — characteristics that are hardly conducive to quantification and reliable classification. They also thought that the disturbed prosody was the result of compensation. They emphasized the difference between volitional (purposive) and spontaneous (reflexive) performance.

Trost and Canter (1974) confirmed that repetition was easier than naming, inadequate responses being made more often in spontaneous production than in repetition. Final consonants were easier than initial ones and vowels were easier than consonants. Single consonants were easier than clusters. Substitutions and additions were the majority of errors made on consonant singletons; omissions, substitutions, and their combination were the most frequent errors on clusters. Subphonemic feature (place, manner, voicing, nasality) analysis of substitution errors showed a majority of errors to be close approximations (one or two feature errors) to target sounds. Frequent inadequate responses were indicators of the severity of the verbal apraxia.

Many of the studies of "verbal apraxia" with a few notable exceptions (Martin & Rigrodsky, 1974; Deal & Darley, 1972; Martin, Wasserman, Gilden, Gerstman, & West, 1975; Hardison, Marquardt, & Peterson, 1977) disregard the linguistic changes, and many studies of agrammatism similarly ignore the articulatory deficit. Yet Broca's aphasia represents a syndrome that is characterized by both phenomena in addition to other interesting linguistic and behavioral symptoms such as literal or phonological (deep) alexia; ideomotor (limb and facial) apraxia; catastrophic reaction (easy frustration); perseveration (at times stereotypies); impaired comprehension of sequential or grammatically ambiguous sentences, relational words, prepositions, etcetera. In most cases of Broca's aphasia the linguistic and articulatory errors are so closely combined that they cannot and perhaps should not be separated.

Liepmann (1900) considered motor aphasia to be apraxia of speech. Marie (1906) was the most influential to regard "anarthria" as distinct from aphasia. Alajouanine, Ombredane, and Durand (1939), on the other hand, described "phonetic disintegration of language" and considered it an element and often a residual disorder of motor aphasia or Broca's aphasia.

In recent times the term verbal apraxia has been used to describe a range of behaviors from the few instances of the "pure" syndrome to the articulatory phonemic difficulty found in many aphasic people. The term is liberally applied to any output problem as long as it is not dysarthria. Many authors simply equate verbal apraxia with Broca's aphasia, yet at the same time insist that verbal apraxia is distinct from aphasia. Martin (1974) objected to the term "apraxia of speech" and argued that motor programming disturbances are inextricably tied to language deficits and cannot be defined except within the framework of aphasia.

It is difficult to draw a line between aphasic and articulatory disturbances. It would be ideal to study the pure phenomenon in isolation. The cases described in this chapter all had a relatively isolated verbal apraxia (some very mildly) from the outset, although all were considered aphasic as well, by virtue of at least some anomia and agraphia.

Verbal apraxia is often elicited with repetition of words or consonant-vowel syllables. Yet the spontaneous speech production of the patients could be quite different from the imitative speech. In some patients, repetition may increase errors (conduction aphasia); in others the errors often improve with repetition (Johns & Darley, 1970). A patient with transcortical motor aphasia, however, may have verbal apraxia on spontaneous speech but not on repetition.

Comprehension, writing, and oral praxis, as well as other language parameters, often remain unreported. This is usually the situation when cases of "pure verbal apraxia" are referred to. The articulatory disturbance may be prominent, but when other language parameters are examined, such as in our study, the patients will be found aphasic on several accounts. Word finding difficulty is often prominent, and semantic paraphasias are undoubtedly linguistic and not articulatory errors.

The severe agraphia was a striking and somewhat surprising finding in the majority of our cases. It is not explained by limb apraxia or a generalized disturbance of written language because reading was usually better preserved. The persisting prominent agraphia in these cases supports the aphasic nature of the output disturbance.The co-occurrence of verbal apraxia and agraphia could be related to the particular location of the lesions, but this particular area has not been described to be associated typically with agraphia. Agraphia associated with alexia occurs characteristically with parietal lesions of the angular gyrus, and occasionally agraphia that is more prominent is described with superior parietal lesions. However, we found that the persistence of agraphia is characteristic of recovery from aphasic stroke from variously located lesions (Kertesz, 1979). Many reports of verbal apraxia are vague or equivocal about agraphia which is not often documented. The degree of agraphia cannnot be explained on the basis of apraxia since these features were not associated.

Buccofacial apraxia and verbal apraxia were not particularly associated in this group of subcortically affected patients. The dissociation of the two phenomena has been frequently observed (Goldstein 1948; DeRenzi, Pieczuro, & Vignolo, 1966). Alajouanine and Lhermitte (1960) thought that nonverbal oral apraxia represented a less complex problem than "phonetic disintegration" and that it could recover more quickly. Mateer and Kimura (1977) found nonfluent aphasics impaired on oral movements and repetition of phonemes and syllables. Fluent aphasics were impaired also on the imitation of multiple nonverbal oral movements, an impairment which was not accounted for by visual memory span deficits. They thought that simple oral movements were controlled by the anterior speech area but multiple movements or sequences were elaborated by the posterior area. The alternative explanation would be that a hierarchy of difficulty between the observed deficits exists, and that the more severe anterior lesions would affect the simpler movements as well as the complex ones.

Verbal apraxia due to trauma has distinctive features when compared to those resulting from stroke. After head injuries the loss of voice is more common than in stroke. Aphonia recovers in a predictable order: vowels are first, and consonants follow (Nathan, 1947). Apraxia seems more severe for the lips and tongue than for the larynx. Nathan's cases showed interesting disturbances rarely seen in stroke cases. One patient omitted all consonants, another spoke in syllables, and another was unwilling to talk at all. Automatic phrases such as "I don't know" were well preserved in one patient, and another could sing before he could talk. The output is improved by emotional content and rhythm, linking a series of items in a familiar sequence. The slowness, excessive pausing, syllabic pacing, and inappropriate segmentation lend a special prosodic quality to the posttraumatic speech deficit that cannot be characterized by the usual descriptions of dysarthria, aphasia, or verbal apraxia associated with vascular cases. Nathan's (1947) overlap of skull defects included the foot of the third frontal convolution, the pre- and postcentral gyri, and the inferior parietal lobule. The subcortical extent of the lesions was not known. Most of Nathan's patients had agraphia as well as anomia.

Johns and Darley (1970) made the point that the distinctiveness of apraxia and dysarthria warrant different therapeutic approaches. They emphasized the substitution and omission errors of apraxia in contrast to the distortion errors of dysarthria. They also noted the superiority of the auditory-visual mode over the purely auditory or visual modes for treating verbal apraxia. Any claims for therapeutic success must be tempered by the frequently observed rapid recovery when verbal apraxia is the presenting feature, such as in our cases. Systematic studies of recovery from verbal apraxia are needed to document the pattern of recovery of motor speech disturbance in stroke as distinct from trauma.

The articulatory-phonemic disturbance in verbal apraxia appears to be linguistic and motoric at the same time. A separation of these two may be an artificial one and even clinically not all that useful. The motor function of subcortical nuclei that were affected in this series of patients with verbal apraxia plays an important role in coordinating skilled motor movement. The putamen and caudate nuclei (together called the striatum) receive their major input from the cortex, especially the frontal lobe, but also from temporal and parietal areas. They also receive innervation from the substantia nigra and centrum medianum of the thalamus. Their output provides the major afferent path to the globus pallidus that in turn supplies the thalamus and from there the cortex with modulated feedback (Purpura, 1976). There is recent evidence that the striatum integrates intention and perception into movement (Hassler,

1978). This major circuitry of the basal ganglia integrates purposeful movement and can be assumed to play a special role in the sequential integration of the complex activity of speech.

The lesions affecting subcortical structures often involve several structures in a variable degree of combination along with the intervening internal capsule that funnels cortical impulses to the thalamus and pontine nuclei, thereby providing the essential pathways for speech output. Partial or complete involvement of the capsule or thalamus would add to the variations in the resulting speech deficit.

Verbal apraxia, although superficially a "motor deficit," is likely an impairment of the complex interaction of communicative intention translated into programmed motor function and perceptual feedback from the executory organs of speech as well as cortical areas responsible for phonemic selection and syntactic programming. The integrated functions of language transcend mere descriptive levels such as articulation or phonemic selection or parsing. It is unlikely therefore that central lesions that result in verbal apraxia will affect motor function alone.

REFERENCES

Alajouanine, T., & Lhermitte, F. Les troubles des activités expressives du langage dans l'aphasie leurs relations avec apraxies. *Revue Neurologique,* 1960, *102,* 604–629.

Alajouanine, T., Ombredane, A., & Durand, M. *Le syndrome de la desintegration phonetiques dans l'aphasie.* Paris: Masson, 1939.

Bell, D. S. Speech functions of the thalamus inferred from the effects of thalamotomy. *Brain,* 1968 *91,* 619–638.

Cappa, S. F., & Vignolo, L. A. Transcortical features of aphasia following left thalamic hemorrhage. *Cortex* 1979, *15,* 121–130.

Damasio, A. R., Damasio, H., Rizzo, M., Varney, N., & Gersh, F. Aphasia with nonhemorrhagic lesions in the basal ganglia and internal capsule. *Archives of Neurology,* 1982, *39,* 15–20.

Darley, F. L., Aronson, A. E., & Brown, J. R. *Motor speech disorders.* Saunders: Philadelphia, 1975.

Darley, F. L., Brown, J. R., & Swenson, W. M. Language changes after neurosurgery for Parkinsonism. *Brain and Language,* 1975, *2,* 65–69.

Deal, J. L., & Darley, F. L. The influence of linguistic and situational variables on phonemic accuracy in apraxia of speech. *Journal of Speech and Hearing Research,* 1972, *15,* 639–653.

DeRenzi, E., Pieczuro, A., & Vignolo, L. A. 1966. Oral apraxia and aphasia. *Cortex,* 1966, *2,* 50–73.

Goldstein, K. *Language and language disturbances.* New York: Grune & Stratton, 1948.

Hardison, D., Marquardt, T. P., & Peterson, H. A. Effects of selected linguistic variables on apraxia of speech. *Speech and Hearing Research,* 1977, *20,* 334–343.

Hassler, R. Striatal control of locomotion, intentional actions and of integrative and perceptive activity. *Journal of Neurological Science,* 1978, *36,* 187–224.

Johns, D. F., & Darley, F. L. 1970. Phonemic variability in apraxia of speech. *Journal of Speech and Hearing Research,* 1970, *14,* 141–143.

Kertesz, A. *Aphasia and associated disorders.* New York: Grune & Stratton, 1979.

Kertesz, A. *The Western Aphasia Battery.* New York: Grune & Stratton, 1982.

Kertesz, A., Bub, D., & Crook, S. *Subcortical aphasia.* Paper presented at the International Neuropsychological Society European Conference, Deauville, 1982.

Liepmann, H. Das Krankheitsbild der Apraxie (''motorischen asymbolie''). *Monatsschr Psychiatr Neurol,* Bd VIII, Berlin: Monographie, 1900.

Marie, P. Revision de la question de l'aphasie: l'aphasie de 1861 a 1866: essai de critique historique sur la genere de la doctrine de Broca. *Sem Med Paris,* 1906, *26,* 565–571.

Martin, A. D. Some objections to the term ''apraxia of speech''. *Journal of Speech and Hearing Disorders,* 1974, *39,* 53–64.

Martin, A. D., & Rigrodsky, S. An investigation of phonological impairment in aphasia, Part 1 and 2. *Cortex,* 1974, *10,* 317–346.

Martin, A. D., Wasserman, N. H., Gilden, L., Gerstman, L, & West, J. A. A process model of repetition in aphasia: An investigation of phonological and morphological interactions in aphasic error performance. *Brain and Language,* 1975, *2,* 434–450.

Mateer, C., & Kimura, D. Impairment of nonverbal oral movements in aphasia. *Brain and Language,* 1977, *4,* 262–276.

McKissock, W., & Paine, K. W. E. Primary tumors of the thalamus. *Brain,* 1958, *81,* 41–63.

Mohr, J. P., Watters, W. C., & Duncan, G. W. Thalamic hemorrhage and aphasia. *Brain and Language*, 1975, 2, 3–17.

Naeser, M. A., Alexander, M. P., Helm-Estabrooks, N., Levine, H. L., Laughlin, S.A., & Geschwind, N. Aphasia with predominantly subcortical lesion sites. *Archives of Neurology*, 1982, *39*, 2–14.

Nathan, P. W. Facial apraxia and apraxic dysarthia. *Brain*, 1947, 70, 449–478.

Purpura, D. P. Physiological organization of the basal ganglia. In M.D. Yahr, (Ed.), The basal ganglia, New York: Raven Press, 1976.

Selby, G. Stereotaxic surgery for the relief of Parkinson's disease. II. An analysis of the results of a series of 303 patients (413 operations). *Journal of Neurological Sciences*, 1967, *5*, 343–375.

Shankweiler, D., & Harris, K. S. An experimental approach to the problem of articulation in aphasics. *Cortex*, 1966, *2*, 277–292.

Smyth, G. E., & Stern, K. Tumors of the thalamus — A clinicopathological study. *Brain,* 1938, *61*, 339–374.

Trost, J. E., & Canter, G. J. Apraxia of speech in patients with Broca's aphasia: A study of phoneme production accuracy and error patterns. *Brain and Language*, 1974, *1*, 63–79.

ACKNOWLEDGMENTS

I am grateful for the assistance of Sharon Crook, Daniel Bub, and Kim Kassa. The study was supported by Ontario Ministry of Health Grant PR 969. Some of the data were collected with the aid of Ontario Ministry of Health Grant DM 324 to Dr. C. Shewan and Dr. A. Kertesz.

3

The Elusive Lesion—Apraxia of Speech Link in Broca's Aphasia

Thomas P. Marquardt
Harvey Sussman

INTRODUCTION

Perhaps the overriding goal of aphasiology is to understand the relationship between clinical syndrome and site/extent of focal brain damage within the language dominant left hemisphere. With the advent of computerized axial tomography (Hounsfield, Ambrose, & Bridges, 1973) it is now possible to examine this elusive clinical-neurological relationship. The idealisitic hope in this endeavor is to find some commonality across patients in terms of specific brain areas undergoing damage and concomitant motoric and/or cognitive language impairment. In this chapter we address the issue of whether or not such a commonality exists in a group of nonfluent Broca's aphasic patients. Using a battery of diagnostic tests of verbal, oral, and limb apraxia, we attempted to correlate lesion data to these clinical measurements.

The only study known to us that has previously undertaken this type of comparison is that of Tognola and Vignolo (1980) who examined oral apraxia in relation to size and loci of brain lesions. Forty-four patients were studied during the time interval 21 to 60 days poststroke. Oral apraxia (OA) was assessed by an imitation 10-item test with a maximum score of 20. Patients scoring 15 or less were classified as having oral apraxia; those scoring below 10 were classified as severely orally apraxic. Composite contour maps showing maximum areas of cortical lesion overlap were derived from CT scan sections following a graphical procedure outlined in Mazzocchi and Vignolo (1978). Lesion areas were measured from a standard lateral diagram by use of a planimeter. There were three categories of lesion size: large (greater than 36 cm^2), medium (20–36 cm^2), and small (less than 20 cm^2). In addition to the lateral overlays showing cortical involvement, Tognola and Vignolo also included descriptions of frequency of involvement of deep structures such as the insular cortex, lenticular nucleus, and internal capsule. The format of their data was descriptive and no numerical analyses were undertaken.

In the large lesion group ($n = 6$) with patients having both OA and aphasia, the entire left frontotemporoparietal area of the left hemisphere was involved with added deep involvement of the insula and lenticular nucleus. All patients with large lesions in this area had severe OA ($\bar{X} = 2.5$, range 0–10). The composite contour cortical map for the medium-sized lesion group ($n = 7$) having both OA and aphasia showed greatest overlap near the central operculum and adjacent temporal lobe. All lesions in this group "encroached" (p. 259) upon the insula and five of seven reached the lenticular nucleus. The mean severity score of OA in this group was 8.6 (range 0–15). The small lesion group ($n = 6$) coincided with the medium-sized group in showing the central operculum and adjacent T_1 areas as maximally involved. The mean OA score for this group was 9.6 (range 7–13). All of the small lesions also involved the insula and one third of the cases involved the lenticular nucleus. Seven patients with OA and aphasia had purely deep lesions and in all cases the insula was involved. Six had lenticular involvement and four had internal capsule involvement. The mean OA score was 9.2 (range 0–15) for the deep lesion group.

Sixteen of Tognola and Vignolo's patients did not have OA (12 were aphasic and 4 were not). All lesions of this group were medium to small in size; only four were deep enough to involve the insula, and none reached the lenticular nucleus. The cortical lesion overlays showed the posterior peri-Sylvian cortex as having the maximum overlap in lesion site.

Tognola and Vignolo concluded that "the crucial area for oral gestures comprises approximately the following cerebral structures of the left hemisphere: frontal and central (Rolandic) opercula, the adjacent parts of the first temporal convolution, and the anterior portion of the insula (p. 269)." Patients without OA had only medium or small lesions which were located posteriorly, sparing both frontal and central opercula. Deep lesions in the non-OA group spared the insula or only involved posterior portions of the insula. The lenticular nucleus was always spared in this group. Interestingly, patients with no OA and purely deep lesions often had internal capsule involvement but not insulolenticular involvement.

The study we are reporting expanded upon the Tognola and Vignolo investigation in two important respects. First, verbal apraxia, limb apraxia, and articulator reaction time tasks were administered in addition to measures of oral apraxia. Second, a computer software routine was used to extract three-dimensional lesion centroids and lesion volumes which then were correlated with clinical measures of apraxia. Since our subject pool represented a more homogeneous and neurologically stable sample compared to Tognola and Vignolo's group, we were able to refine our inquiry by examining relationships between motor performance and lesion loci and volume in patients with lesions restricted to more anterior speech and language representation areas.

METHOD

Subjects

Subjects were 15 neurologically stable patients with Broca's aphasia selected on the basis of performance on the Boston Diagnostic Aphasia Examination (Goodglass & Kaplan, 1972). All subjects were at least 3 months postonset of brain damage and premorbidly right-handed. None had positive histories for *precerebral* insult oral-facial anomalies or communicative disorders. Computerized tomography and neurological examination were completed for each patient at the time of testing.

Subject data are shown in Table 3-1. Mean age of the group was 54.1 years. Mean time postonset of brain damage was 35.7 months with a range of 3 to 177 months. Etiology of brain damage was trauma for two subjects, intracerebral hemorrhage for three patients, and occlusive cerebrovascular accident for ten patients.

Lesion Site and Size

A composite of subject brain lesions mapped according to procedures developed by Mazzocchi and Vignolo (1978) is shown in Figure 3-1. The mapping involved several steps. First, the angle of the sections with respect to the orbitomeatal line was determined from identification of skull bone, intracranial calcification, and cerebrospinal fluid space landmarks within the brain scan sections. An atlas of CT scan sections and

TABLE 3–1
Sex, age (in years), etiology of brain damage, postonset time (in months from onset of brain damage to initiation of testing) and CT scan interpretation for aphasic subjects

Subject	*Sex*	*Age*	*Time Postonset (in months)*	*Etiology*	*Brain Scan Interpretation*	*Boston Score*
1	F	35	39	Occlusive CVA	Large area of diminished density in left postfrontal region with compensatory dilation of frontal pole of left lateral ventricle.	506.0
2	M	59	16	Occlusive CVA	Area of diminished attenuation in left temporal area that extends over several cuts, representing infarction that primarily involves the anterior limb of internal capsule and part of lentiform nucleus on the left.	534.0
3	M	42	6	Hemorrhagic CVA	Area of decreased density in left hemisphere in region of internal capsule extending from region adjacent to Sylvian fissure inferiorly up to frontoparietal cortex superiorly.	477.5
4	M	56	152	Trauma	Area of diminished density beginning in left temporal region, ascending superiorly in distribution of left cerebral artery.	547.0
5	M	64	48	Occlusive CVA	Marked tissue loss in entire left internal capsule and thalamic region, with a large area of encephalomalacia over left temporal cortical region.	523.0
6	F	78	12	Occlusive CVA	Infarction in left corpus striatum and periventricular white matter on left side with compensatory atrophy of left anterior horn in body of left lateral ventricle.	396.5
7	F	64	15	Hemorrhagic CVA	Lesion in left posterior frontal lobe lateral to lateral ventricle.	508.0
8	M	23	19	Trauma	Lesion involving anterior left temporal lobe, ascending with considerable involvement of left frontal lobe.	364.0

TABLE 3-1 — Continued

Subject	*Sex*	*Age*	*Time Postonset (in months)*	*Etiology*	*Brain Scan Interpretation*	*Boston Score*
9	M	52	7	Occlusive CVA	Prominent, fairly large low density lesion in the left frontal area extending somewhat into the left parietal lobe.	174.5
10	F	61	4	Occlusive CVA	Area of diminished density involving left caudate nucleus, left anterior limb of internal capsule, left globus pallidus and putamen, anteriomedial portion of left temporal lobe and insula; probable involvement of posterior limb of left internal capsule with sparing of thalamus.	466.5
11	F	55	3	Occlusive CVA	Large area of encephalomalacia involving left posterior frontal area and anterior tip of left temporal lobe.	498.0
12	F	46	8	Hemorrhagic CVA	Area of diminished density involving left anterior temporal lobe and left posterior inferior frontal lobe.	470.5
13	M	62	25	Occlusive CVA	Low density area in left temporal lobe and central area. Appears to be a linear zone lateral to left lateral ventricle.	525.0
14	M	54	4	Occlusive CVA	Elongated area of decreased density in the insular region extending to the cortex in the posterior frontal region (precentral gyrus).	539.0
15	M	60	177	Occlusive CVA	Large low density cystic area in the left hemisphere beginning in the basal ganglia and ascending superiority to involve the corona radiata but apparently sparing the cortex.	189.0
		$\overline{X} = 54.1$	$\overline{X} = 35.7$			$\overline{X} = 447.9$

corresponding anatomical structures (Matsui & Hirano, 1978) was used to aid in this process. Second, the lesion contour on each section was traced to allow identification of damage to the cortex and deep structures. Third, the linear distance between the anterior (a) and posterior (p) extremities of the damaged hemisphere, the anterior (l_1) and posterior (l_2) points of the lesion, and the anterior (A) and posterior (P) points of a standard lateral diagram were determined. The formulas AP/ap $\times$ al_1 and AP/ap $\times$ al_2 then were used to plot the anterior and posterior points of the lesion on the lateral diagram and the points were connected with a smooth line to portray the lesion contour.

Standard brain scan section and lateral diagram composites for the 15 subjects are shown in Figure 3-1. As might be expected, all subjects demonstrated lesions deep to the cortex (Figure 3-1A). However, only nine of the subjects had cortical damage. The lateral diagram (Figure 3-1B) shows a concentration of lesions for these nine subjects extending from the posterior frontal lobe to the anterior parietal lobe and superior temporal lobe including the insular cortex and opercula.

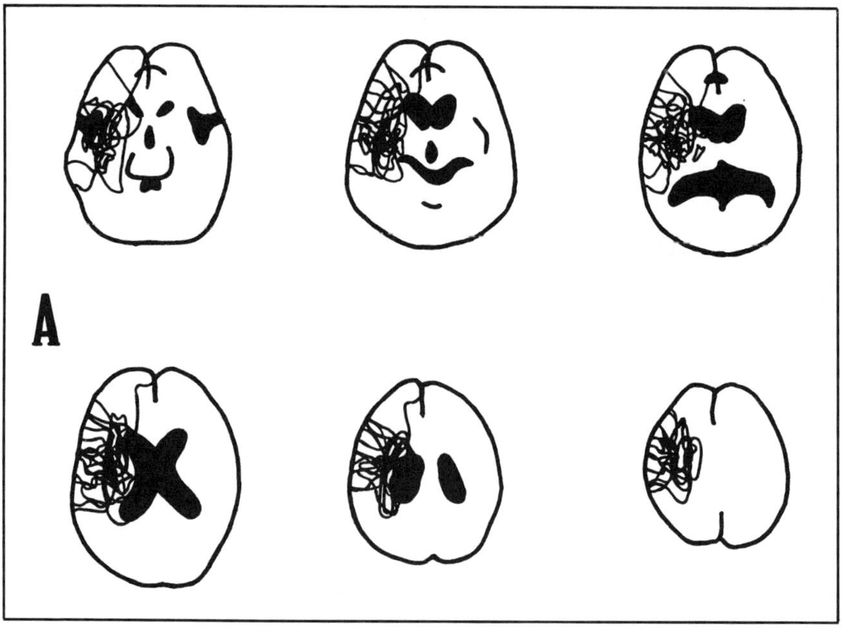

FIGURE 3-1A

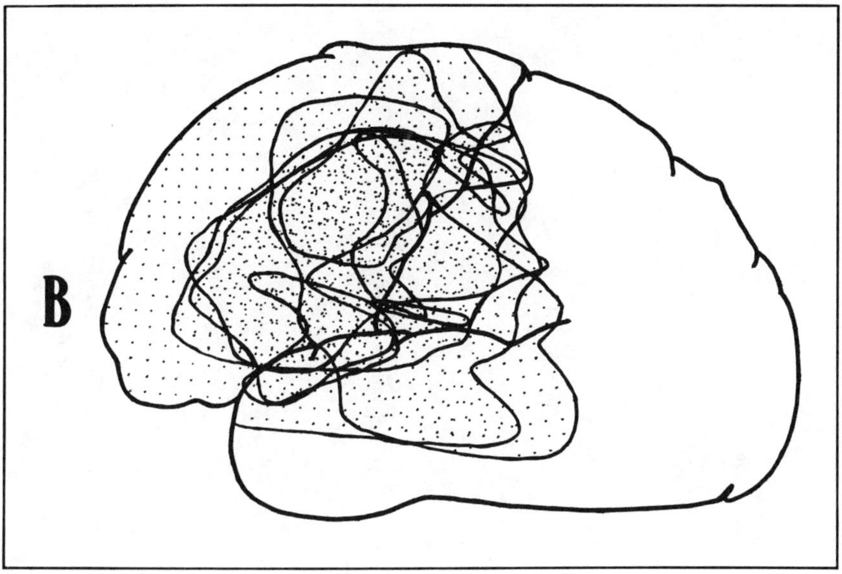

FIGURE 3–1B

Apraxia Measures

A battery of tasks was used to measure the severity of verbal, oral and limb apraxia (Table 3-2). The seven verbal tests included the Boston Verbal Agility measure and subtests from the Madison Veterans Administration Hospital apraxia assessment protocol (Rosenbek & Wertz, 1976). The Boston Oral Agility subtest and tasks that evaluated the subject's ability to produce oral movements in response to commands and in imitation were used to assess oral apraxia. Similarly, intransitive limb, transitive limb, and whole body movements were evaluated in response to commands and in imitation. It should be pointed out that this battery of tests constitutes a substantially larger and more reliable estimate of the degree of apraxia than that employed by Tognola and Vignolo. A four-point scoring system was used for all tasks except the Boston subtests and the sentence imitation. In this system a score of zero was assigned if the patient made no response, an erroneous response was scored 1, a partially adequate response was scored 2, and a correct response was scored 3.

Additional tasks were used to evaluate oral stereognosis, parietal lobe functions, and oral structure reaction times. Oral stereognosis testing included discrimination and matching. On the discrimination task, two 3-dimensional forms were placed in the mouth, one at a time, while the

TABLE 3–2
Apraxia and related assessment tasks

Test Type	*Test*	*Description*	*Total Items*	*Scoring*	*Maximum Score*
Verbal Apraxia	Boston Verbal Agility	Serial repetition of one or two words Example: "Huckleberry"	7	One or two points depending on number of repetitions within a 5-sec interval	14
Verbal Apraxia	Multisyllabic Words	Imitation of multisyllabic words Example: "Impossibility"	6	No points if no response One point if response is attempted but erroneous Two points if response is partially adequate Three points if response is normal	18
Verbal Apraxia	Words of Increasing Length	Imitation of words of increasing length Example: "Zip"–"zipper"–"zippering"	12	Same as above	36
Verbal Apraxia	Identical Initial-Final Consonant Words	Imitation of words with identical initial and final consonants Example: "Church"	10	Same as above	30
Verbal Apraxia	Diadochokinesis	Serial repetition of stop-vowel syllables Example: "Papapa"	4	Same as above	12
Verbal Apraxia	Sentence Imitation	Imitation of five sentences Example: "Arthur was an oozy, oily sneak."	31	One point for each correctly produced word	31

TABLE 3-2 — Continued

Test Type	*Test*	*Description*	*Total Items*	*Scoring*	*Maximum Score*
Oral apraxia	Boston Oral Agility	Production of alternating oral structural movements Example: Protrude and retract tongue	6	One or two points depending on the number of repetitions within a 5-sec interval	12
Oral Apraxia	Oral $Movements_1$	Performance of oral movements in response to commands Example: Open your mouth	22	No points if no response One point if response is attempted but erroneous Two points if response is partially adequate Three points if response is normal	66
Oral Apraxia	Oral $Movements_2$	Imitation of oral movements	22	Same as above	66
Limb Apraxia	Limb $Movements_1$	Performance of intransitive limb, transitive limb, and whole body movements in response to commands Example: Wave goodbye	22	Same as above	66
Limb Apraxia	Limb $Movements_2$	Imitation of intransitive limb, transitive limb, and whole body movements	22	Same as above	66
Auxiliary Test	Oral $Stereognosis_1$	Matching of forms presented orally without visual access	20	No points for incorrect response; one point for correct response	20

Test Type	*Test*	*Description*	*Total Items*	*Scoring*	*Maximum Score*
Auxiliary Test	Oral Stereognosis$_2$	Identification of orally presented three dimensional forms from pictured alternatives	32	Same as above	32
Auxiliary Test	Parietal Lobe Battery	Items used to determine the presence and severity of constructional apraxia, finger agnosia, acalculia, and right-left orientation disorders	—	0–3 depending on task	249
Auxiliary Test	Reaction Time	Reaction time of tongue, lip, and jaw in response to presentation of tone	—	Time in milliseconds	—

patient's eyes were closed. The patient was then required to indicate whether they were the same or different. The matching task required selection of the correct picture of a form from foils after the form had been placed in the mouth and tactually examined. The patient was not allowed to examine the form visually during testing. The Parietal Lobe Battery from the Boston Diagnostic Aphasia Examination included items used to detect the presence and severity of constructional apraxia, finger agnosia, acalculia, and right-left orientation disorders.

Reaction time measures were obtained for each patient from three oral gestures: tongue protrusion, lip protrusion, and mandibular lowering. The patient was instructed to initiate movement of the articulatory structure as fast as possible upon hearing a 100-Hz tone. Attached to the articulator was a thin flexible beam that, when deflected, activated a microswitch which turned off a timer and the tone. Reaction times were obtained to the nearest .1 msec and averaged over 10 trials per articulator. Each patient was given adequate practice trials to ensure understanding of the task.

Digitization of CT Scans

Transaxial sections of CT scans were traced showing the outlines of the brain, ventricles, and lesion (Yeo, Turkheimer, & Bigler, 1983). The tracings were digitized using a Summagraphics "Bit Pad." A manually operated stylus was moved along the outline of each structure giving *x* and *y* coordinates at the rate of 5/sec, not exceeding 200 per in. Areas of each outlined structure (e.g., ventricles) were computed for each CT scan slice using a computational algorithm for area based on the method of directed triangles (Lopshitz, 1963). Volumes were derived using the trapezoidal rule where each volume spanning any two slices equals the mean of the two areas times the distance between them. The reliability of this tracing/digitizing procedure has been previously determined to be .99 (Yeo, Turkheimer, & Bigler, 1983).

Lesion location was summarized by three centroid measures for three spatial coordinates: anterior-posterior (A–P), left-right (L–R), and inferior-superior (I–S). The brain was first divided into four quadrants (left anterior, right anterior, left posterior, right posterior). Left and right halves of the brain were marked by the interhemispheric fissure. Anterior and posterior divisions were derived by first drawing a line connecting the most anterior extensions of the frontal lobes and another doing the same for the farthest posterior extension of the occipital lobes. The interhemispheric fissure line was then extended to intersect these lines anteriorly and posteriorly. The perpendicular bisector of this extended line served as the dividing point for anterior and posterior halves of the brain. A–P and L–R lesion centroid values were expressed in centimeters from dead center of the brain after being converted from CT scan distances to real brain size values. I-S centroid values were expressed as the number of brain scan sections superior or inferior to a dead center horizontal plane.

The centroid values, although a quantitative step in the right direction, are not without definite shortcomings in terms of descriptive accuracy and value. It is entirely conceivable that the same centroid value could be derived from two markedly different lesions. For example, a lesion oriented in the transverse plane, extending a large distance from the cortex to deep subcortical tissue (with very limited anterior-posterior extent) could have the identical left-right centroid value as a lesion oriented in its greatest extent in the anterior-posterior plane and situated deep within the left hemisphere. The two very distinct lesions can be visualized as forming the two parts of a "plus" sign, one horizontally spaced and the other vertically. The centroid would correspond to the common intersection of the two components. In such a situation, little descriptive value would be obtained from the centroid value. A three-dimensional description giving the six farthest extents of the lesion (I–S, A–P, L–R) would be more desirable and we are currently engaged in deriving such values.

Analysis

Apraxia subtest results were converted to ratio values and collapsed to provide mean percentage performance scores for verbal, oral, and limb apraxia. Oral stereognosis and parietal lobe subtest scores were summed and a mean reaction time for the lip, tongue, and jaw was calculated.

Digitization of the brain scans provided four lesion values: A–P, L–R, and I–S centroid locational data and lesion volume. Correlational and multiple regression analyses of the clinical test results and lesion numerical descriptors were used to evaluate the lesion-symptom relationship in our group of Broca's aphasic patients.

RESULTS AND DISCUSSION

Clinical Test and Brain Scan Findings

Apraxia test results expressed as mean ratio scores and measures derived from the digitized CT scan traces — anterior-posterior (A–P), left-right (L–R), and inferior-superior (I–S) centroid values and lesion volumes are shown in Table 3-3. Mean scores for verbal and oral apraxia were very similar (.791 versus .793) while limb apraxia scores were higher (.938). Assuming an approximate equivalence of task difficulty for the three types of apraxia, it appears that Broca's aphasic subjects with ver-

TABLE 3–3
Mean ratio scores for apractic subjects on Boston Examination and Apraxia Subtests and Lesion Centroid Location (cm) and Volume (cm^3)

Subject	*Boston*	*Verbal Apraxia*	*Oral Apraxia*	*Limb Apraxia*	*Mean*	*L–R*	*A–P*	*I–S**	*Volume*
1	506.0	.775	.750	.955	.827	4.242	2.845	−.483	64.270
2	534.0	.612	.777	.992	.794	4.978	1.448	−1.687	7.178
3	477.5	.882	.938	.992	.937	3.200	.660	1.735	26.088
4	547.0	.962	.917	.984	.955	4.521	1.219	.884	86.950
5	523.0	.835	.837	.905	.859	4.826	.991	.302	42.524
6	396.5	.603	.753	.823	.726	1.753	.432	10.447	36.150
7	508.0	.733	.810	.905	.816	3.124	1.270	6.990	51.439
8	364.0	.658	.767	.980	.802	3.302	3.480	−.521	121.592
9	174.5	.662	.513	.725	.633	4.013	2.286	2.205	57.256
10	466.5	.973	.837	.985	.932	3.073	2.311	−.483	42.164
11	498.0	.887	.853	.970	.903	3.835	3.023	1.570	45.376
12	470.5	.843	.867	.960	.890	3.785	1.219	1.844	33.823
13	525.0	.962	.783	.992	.912	3.886	1.676	−.739	4.982
14	539.0	.765	.757	.992	.838	4.724	.635	2.725	7.620
15	189.0	.707	.733	.910	.783	2.946	.762	.800	62.058
Mean	477.9	.791	.793	.938	.840	3.747	1.617	1.706	45.989
SD	119.465	.127	.099	.076	.087	.868	.955	3.175	31.011

*Expressed as number of brain scan sections from a dead center horizontal plane.

bal and oral apraxia do not necessarily demonstrate limb apraxia. If an arbitrary cutoff of less than 95% correct performance is used as an indicator of the presence of significant impairment, 12 subjects demonstrated verbal apraxia and 15 demonstrated oral apraxia but only 5 had limb apraxia.

The A–P (mean = 1.617) and L–R (mean = 3.747) centroid values indicate that all lesions involved the left anterior quadrant of the brain. Negative values for these parameters would reflect a right and posterior lesion location. The negative I–S values for five subjects indicate that the lesion centroid location was below a midpoint horizontal plane. Lesion volumes were extremely heterogenous and ranged from 4.982 to 121.592 cm^3 (mean = 45.989 cm^3).

Results from the reaction time, parietal lobe, and oral stereognosis tasks are shown in Table 3-4. Mean reaction times were greater for the tongue (mean = 414.36) and lip (mean = 413.47) than for the jaw (mean = 386.33). Reaction times for tongue protrusion were not obtained for one subject because he was unable to complete the task. Parietal lobe scores were not available for one subject and stereognosis scores were not obtained for two subjects.

TABLE 3–4

Reaction times (msec) for tongue protrusion, lip protrusion, and jaw lowering and parietal lobe and oral stereognosis scores for Broca's aphasic subjects

Subject	*Tongue*	*Lip*	*Jaw*	*Mean*	*Parietal Lobe*	*Stereognosis*
1	339	310	300	336	228	28
2	369	369	413	384	237	—
3	288	332	214	278	180	—
4	218	217	219	218	229	39
5	252	249	276	259	185	24
6	513	506	531	517	172	35
7	466	249	385	367	216	40
8	274	293	294	287	206	47
9	—	739	818	779	90	19
10	397	352	289	346	177	57
11	477	496	418	464	42	41
12	494	462	287	414	204	35
13	688	781	332	600	189	39
14	259	289	294	281	223	39
15	707	558	725	663	—	34
Mean	414.357	413.467	386.330	412.867	184.143	36.692
SD	154.545	174.329	177.351	162.894	55.076	9.690

Correlational Analyses

Pearson Product–Moment correlation coefficients among the independent measures of verbal, oral, and limb apraxia are shown in Table 3-5. All apraxia scores were significantly and positively correlated. However, none of these measures were significantly correlated with age. The mean reaction time per patient (averaged across articulators) also was used in a correlational analysis with the apraxia measures. Reaction time was found to be significantly correlated with both oral apraxia (r = -.73; $p \leq .01$) and limb apraxia (r = -.66, $p \leq .01$) but not with verbal apraxia (r = -.30). Reaction time was not significantly correlated with any of the CT scan measures. It was slightly encouraging to note that reaction time, a nonlinguistic sensorimotor task, was significantly correlated with only the nonverbal apraxia measures and not the verbal apraxia scores.

TABLE 3–5
Pearson Product-Moment correlation coefficients between indices of verbal apraxia (VA), oral apraxia (OA), and limb apraxia (LA)

	VA	*OA*	*LA*
VA	—	.61**	.51*
OA			.73**

*Significant at P ≤ .05.
**Significant at P ≤ .01.

Lesion centroid and volume data also were correlated with eight clinical measures as shown in Table 3-6. Parietal lobe and oral stereognosis scores were correlated only with the A–P values since these were the only meaningful relationships expected (i.e., low parietal lobe and stereognosis scores should be associated with more posterior lesions). Correlation coefficients were all non-significant except for the relationship between lesion volume and diadochokinetic scores. This significant negative correlation (r = -.57, $p \leq .05$) suggests that the larger the lesion, the lower the diadochokinetic score. The remaining correlations between volume and clinical measures were nonsignificant, but they were, at least, negative since volume was considered the most valid quantitative measure obtained from the CT scan data.

The two centroid measures were weakly related to the clinical results. The interpretation of the correlation between the L–R centroid values and clinical measures is puzzling because the low positive coefficients indicate that the more lateral the center of the lesion, the better the performance on the clinical tests. This interpretation leads to a possible con-

TABLE 3-6
Pearson Product-Moment correlation coefficients between CT-scan parameters (lesion volume, left/right centroid, and anterior/posterior centroid) and various clinical indices

	OA	*VA*	*LA*	*VG*	*DK*	*BDAE*	*PL*	*SG*
Lesion Volume	−.07	−.13	−.12	−.10	−.57*	−.36		
L-R Centroid	.32	.19	.31	.30	.32	.42		
A-P Centroid	.25	.05	.07	.12	.11	.09	−.35	−.22

NOTE. OA = oral apraxia, VA = verbal apraxia, LA = limb apraxia, VG = verbal agility, DK = diadochokinesis, BDAE = Boston Diagnostic Aphasia Exam, PL = parietal lobe battery, SG = stereognosis.
*Significant at $P \leq .05$.

clusion that the closer the lesion is to the lateral cortex (as opposed to subcortical involvement), the better the performance on speech and language tests. As we shall see, this conclusion points out the dangers in quantifying lesion loci and attempting to relate such oversimplified parameters to speech and language functioning. We are as of yet in no position to make such statements.

The correlations between A–P centroids and clinical results are somewhat more meaningful. Positive albeit nonsignificant correlations were found between parietal lobe and stereognosis scores and the A–P centroids which suggest that more anterior lesions are associated with higher scores on these measures, the expected finding.

Multiple Regression Analysis

The three mean apraxia percentages were arcsin transformed to more closely satisfy the underlying assumptions of a normal distribution and homogeneity of variance. The three centroid parameters (A–P, L–R, I–S) and lesion volume were then separately, and in combination, tested as predictor variables for the apraxia scores and the Boston scores. With the exception of one variable, none of the CT scan derived parameters, either singly, or in combination, approached significance in predicting clinical performance. The sole exception was the I–S centroid that significantly predicted the limb apraxia score ($p \leq .05$). Of interest was the surprising finding that the predictive power decreased as two-, three-, and four-variable models were tested against the clinical scores. In other words, the more you "know" about the lesion size and location, the less well you are able to predict the clinical performance of the patient.

The correlation and multiple regression analyses failed to reveal any significant and meaningful relationships between lesion-derived and clinically derived measures. Although the centroid values were a priori recognized as too primitive to serve as reliable quantifiers of lesion loci, the total lesion volume was expected to yield far greater predictive value than was found. Thus, we must conclude that group volume data devoid of accurate loci quantifiers are inadequate for establishing neurological-clinical relationships.

Case Studies

Examination of individual subjects illustrates the inherent difficulty involved in attempting to relate lesion volume/loci to clinical measures of apraxia. Four subjects will be presented. Each suffered an occlusive cerebrovascular accident at least 3 months prior to testing.

Lesion volume and apraxia. Figure 3-2a shows a tracing of a digitized output reflecting a CT scan slice for *Subject 2* corresponding to 3B in our framework and slice SM in the Naeser and Hayward (1978) framework. The area of the lesion in this slice is 2.32 cm^2. Figure 3-2b is a lateral view of the lesion which involved a small area of the parietal and temporal operculum with deep extension to the internal capsule undercutting the sensorimotor face area. While the overall volume was small (7.2 cm^3), this strategically placed lesion produced apraxia percentages of .61, .78, and .99 for verbal, oral, and limb apraxia, respectively. The verbal apraxia percentage was the second-lowest score of all patients studied, while the Boston score (534) was the third highest.

Subject 10 presents an entirely different picture vis-a-vis the relationship between lesion volume and clinical findings. The lesion location of *Subject 10* (see Figures 3-2c and 2d) overlapped that of *Subject 2*. The subcortical area of tissue damage included the insular cortex, putamen, globus pallidus, caudate nucleus, and the anterior limb of the internal capsule. Cortically, the lesion involved the frontal and anterior-superior temporal operculum with a small intrusion into the parietal operculum. Lesion sizes of the two subjects, however, were markedly different. The lesion volume of *Subject 10* (42.2 cm^3) was six times larger than that of *Subject 2* and the lesion area of slice SM (9.70 cm^2) was four times larger (See Figure 3-2c). Despite the more extensive cortical and subcortical involvement, *Subject 10* had superior apraxia scores: .97, .83, and .99 for verbal, oral, and limb apraxia, respectively. Thus, the patient with minimal cortical and subcortical involvement was more severely apractic than the patient with more extensive neural damage in virtually corresponding loci. This diversity was typical of the cases we examined. Obviously, correlational and multiple regression analyses are doomed to failure with such nonlinearity of neurological and clinical data within a relatively homogeneous sample of patients.

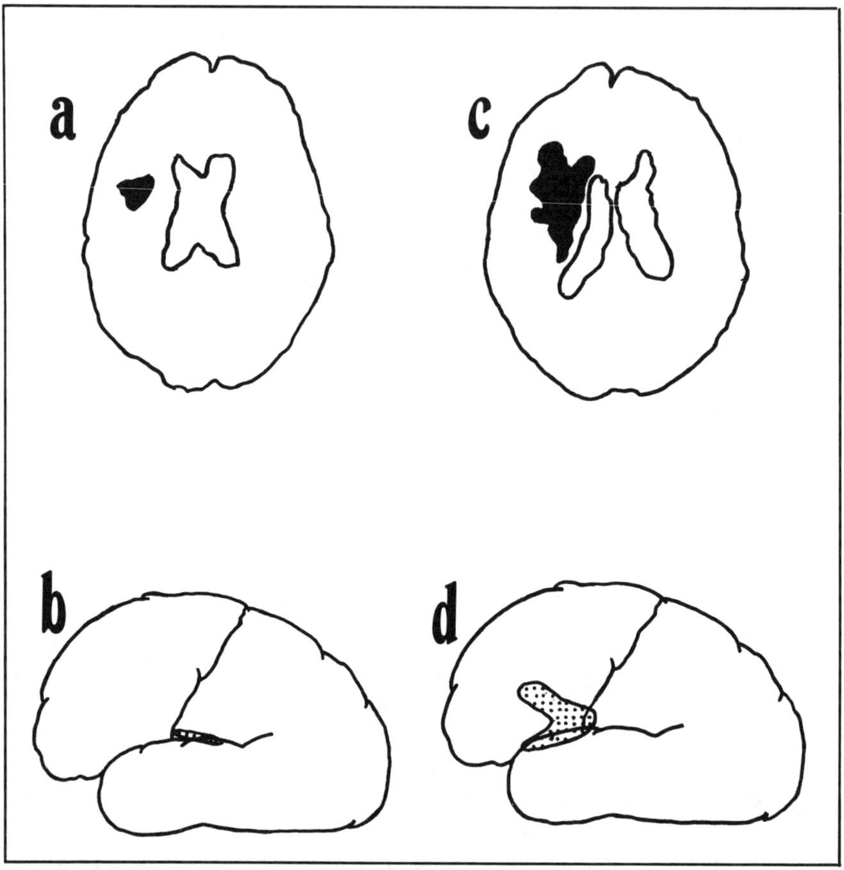

FIGURE 3–2
Subject 2 (a and b), lesion volume 7.2 cm^3; subject 10 (c and d), lesion volume 42.2 cm^3.

Cortical-subcortical involvement and apraxia. The most severely impaired of our patients was *Subject 9* who had a Boston score of 174.5 and a mean apraxia percentage of .63. Figure 3-3a is a sample slice (3B or SM) showing the extent of the damage subcortically, and Figure 3-3b is a lateral view of the lesion. The lesion volume of *Subject 9* (57.3 cm^3) was similar to that of *Subject 10* (42.2 cm^3), but the location was different: *Subject 9* had extensive cortical damage, whereas *Subject 10* had primarily subcortical damage. As can be seen in Table 3-3, *Subject 10* had far superior performance on measures of apraxia (mean = .93) and language performance (Boston = 466.5) compared to *Subject 9*. This comparison would tend to support the overall generalization that the more cortical versus subcortical involvement, the more apractic/aphasic the patient.

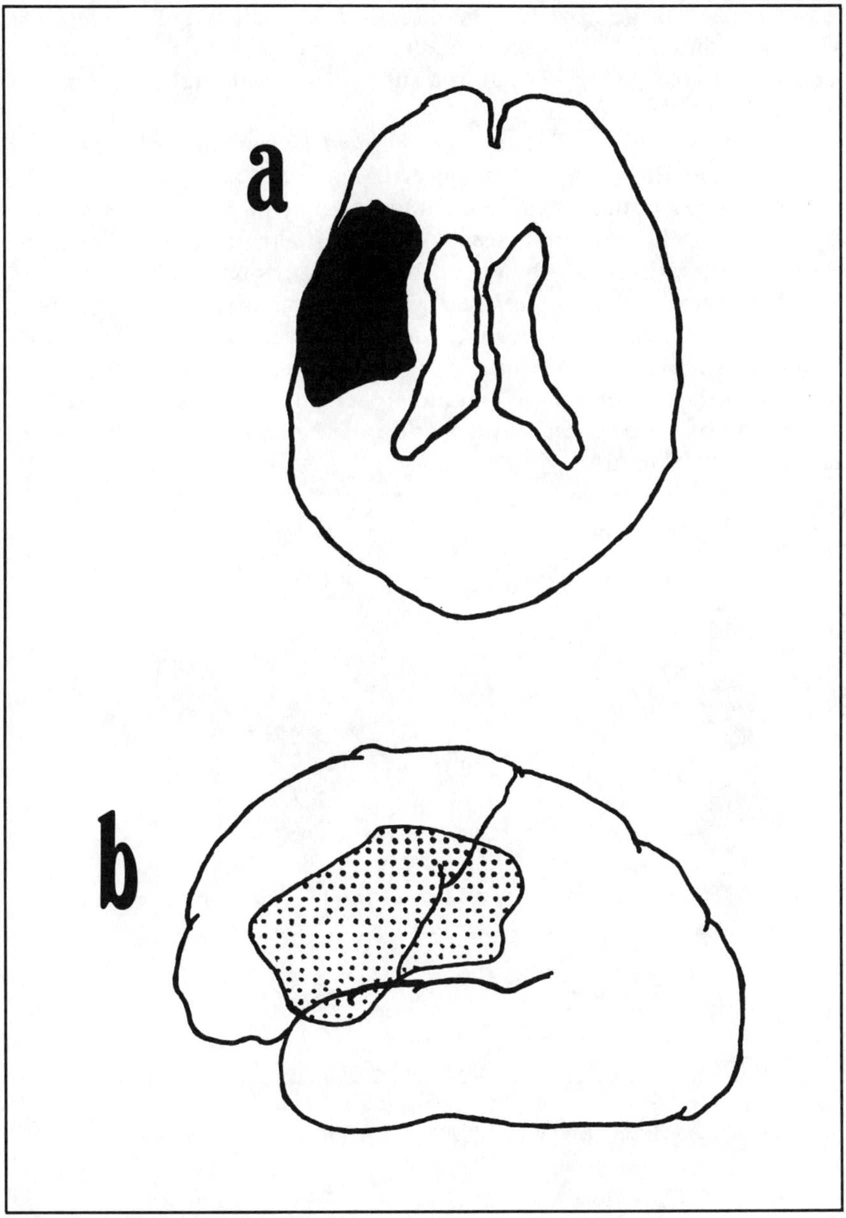

FIGURE 3–3
Subject 9, lesion volume 57.3 cm³.

However, as can be expected, we also studied one patient *(Subject 15)* who had a similar lesion volume (62.06 cm^3) and similar apraxia/aphasia scores compared to *Subject 9*, but a subcortical lesion not involving the lateral cortex at all.

Two representative CT slices from *Subject 15, roughly* corresponding to Naeser and Hayward's (1978) slices BW and SM are shown in Figure 3-4. An extensive subcortical lesion undercutting almost the entire frontal and temporal lobes can be seen. Although the tissue damage was confined almost entirely to subcortical structures, this patient had apraxia/aphasia scores similar to *Subject 9*, who had primarily cortical involvement. Thus, patients with severe cortical compared to subcortical lesions of similar volume may demonstrate similar clinical performances. These case examples are not unique, but merely serve to point out the obstacles in the way of an empirical investigation of the relationship between lesion and clinical data.

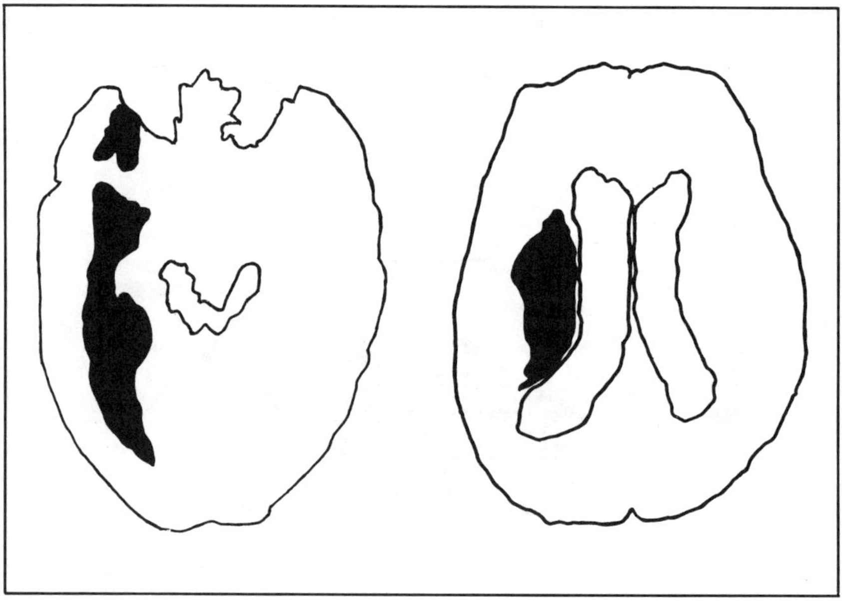

FIGURE 3–4
Subject 15 (left), slice 2A (BW) area: 17.981 cm^2; (right), Slice 3B (SM) area: 9.394 cm^2.

CONCLUSIONS

There are several methodological and neurophysiological reasons for the lack of a direct relationship between brain lesions and clinical symptoms. First, centroid values, as we have noted, do not provide information on the specific lesion configuration or the gyri and deep structures involved. Second, our lesion tracing procedures assumed an equal tissue density reduction within the damaged area revealed by each CT-scan slice, and intact neurons outside of it. Quite obviously, lesions have no such precise demarcation. Third, lesion delimitation does not necessarily reflect the extent of reduced/disrupted neural activity. Diaschisis and associated blood flow and metabolic alterations would be expected to impact on observed symptomotology. Fourth, selection of subjects with lesions restricted to more anterior portions of the left hemisphere may have reduced the variability necessary to demonstrate significant correlations between clinical and lesion measures. Finally, we have no direct knowledge of neural reorganizational changes in areas adjacent or distal to the lesion site or of possible right hemisphere compensation (Sussman & Klingman, 1982).

The negative findings obtained in this study can serve a very positive purpose, however, to future studies of this nature. One such positive outcome is to underscore the need for an adequate model to work from in attempts to understand even the most rudimentary principles of central nervous system cognitive/linguistic functioning. Without such a model or framework, we are limited to making stabs in the dark since the inherent variability of aphasic/apractic performances and lesion sites/sizes makes such an inquiry almost pointless. We tried to study this elusive pairing of lesion and clinical measures, not because we expected crisp relationships to emerge from murky data, but rather because it had not yet been attempted. The shortcomings, as we see them, are more in relation to meaningful CT-scan analyses than in the psychometric integrity of clinical indices. For now, case studies, entirely descriptive, are more fruitful than quantitative group assessments based on neurological parameters that we as of yet do not fully understand.

NOTE

[1]If limb diadochokinesis had been assessed, the incidence of limb apraxia may have been increased for our sample.

REFERENCES

Goodglass, H., & Kaplan, E., *The assessment of aphasia and related disorders.* Philadelphia: Lea and Febiger, 1972.

Hounsfield, G., Ambrose, J., & Bridges, G., Computerized transverse axial scanning. *British Journal of Radiology*, 1973, *46*, 1016–1051.

Lopshitz, M., Computation of the areas of oriented figures. Boston: Health, 1963.

Matsui, Y., & Hirano, A., *An atlas of the human brain for computerized tomography.* Japan: Igaku-Shoin, 1978.

Mazzocchi, F., & Vignolo, L., Computer assisted tomography in neuropsychological research: A simple procedure for lesion mapping. *Cortex,* 1978, *14,* 136-144.

Naeser, M., & Hayward, R., Lesion localization in aphasia with cranial computed tomography and the Boston Diagnostic Aphasia Exam. *Neurology*, 1978, *28*, 545–551.

Rosenbek, J., & Wertz, T., Veterans Administration workshop on speech motor disorders. Madison, Wis., 1976.

Sussman, H., & Klingman, K., *Hemisphericity in aphasic language recovery.* Paper presented at the convention of the American Speech-Language-Hearing Assocation, Toronto, Ontario, 1982.

Tognola, G., & Vignolo, L., Brain lesions associated with oral apraxia in stroke patients: A clinico-neuroradiological investigation with the CT scan. *Neuropsycholigia*, 1980, *18*, 257–272.

Yeo, R., Turkheimer, E., & Bigler, E., Computer analysis of lesion volume: Reliability and utility. *Clinical Neuropsychology*, 1983, *5*, 45.

ACKNOWLEDGMENTS

This research was supported by Grant NS 15336 from the National Institute of Neurological and Communicative Disorders and Stroke. We acknowledge the assistance of Eric Turkheimer, Dennis Nalty, and Alice Richardson in the preparation of this manuscript.

4

Prediction of Site of Lesion from Speech Apraxic Error Patterns

Steven E. Deutsch

In spite of what appears to be a growing recognition of the clinical entity referred to as speech apraxia, there is still considerable controversy regarding the variety of speech production behaviors and the neurophysiologic basis responsible for such output. Most of the contemporary writing that approaches this topic from the frame of reference of localization of brain function reflects the point of view that speech apraxia results from frontal lobe lesions. This now traditional point of view is reflected in studies designed to describe the output of the speech apraxic patient and differentiate it from dysarthria and aphasia (Bay, 1964; Darley, 1964; Darley, 1969; Johns & Darley, 1970; LaPointe, 1969; Shankweiler & Harris, 1966; Trost & Canter, 1974). However, despite the prevailing point of view that verbal or speech apraxia is associated with a frontal lobe lesion, the possibility that a posterior, or temporoparietal lobe lesion may also lead to an apraxic-like disorder exists.

Liepmann, Luria, and Canter have all discussed the possibility that damage to two different cortical areas may produce two dissimilar patterns of disordered speech production. Liepmann (1905, 1913) stated that damage to Broca's area caused labored difficulty in articulation of individual speech sounds, a reduced speech sound repertoire, and problems in articulatory transition. However, if the output problem resulted from a posterior lesion, the speech errors took the form of fluent paraphasic misarticulations and confused speech sound selection. Luria (1966, 1970) believed that pathology of the premotor areas related to speech production may result in: a disruption of the smooth automatic character of the articulatory motor behavior; impairment in the coordination involved in serially organized movements; and, in more severe lesions involving the premotor cortex and its deeper connections to basal ganglia structures, there may be preseveration or fixation on an articulatory motor pattern. He discussed the resultant speech output associated with "afferent kinesthetic apraxia" resulting from a parietal lobe lesion as characterized by inconsistency of error production. The primary defect observed in this disorder is substitution for individual sounds. Canter's (1969) primary verbal apraxia is characterized by a delay in the articulatory transitions between syllables or words and an occasional latency in the initiation of speech. Such patients may exhibit a reduced phoneme repertoire, as well as a pattern of sound substitutions which are generally close in manner and place of articulation to the target. "Secondary verbal apraxia" may take the form of frequently bizarre and erratic substitutions of phonemes. Alteration in the sequencing of phonemes and syllables may be evident, and severe cases may approach neologistic jargon.

These reports suggest that persons referred to as having speech apraxia may represent two populations that differ with respect to site of cortical lesion and the accompanying distinctive pattern of disordered speech production. The present study was designed to explore the possible existence of two identifiable subgroups of patients whose speech production output has been described in the literature as characteristic of speech apraxia. The following specific questions were posed: (1) When subjects exhibiting speech apraxic behavior are selected on the basis of evidence supporting an anterior or posterior site of lesion, do measures of speech errors either singly or combined reliably classify the subjects into two subgroups? (2) Assuming that discrimination of the two subgroups is possible, what single measure or combination of measures best predicts classification of the subgroups? (3) What is the probability of correct and incorrect classification of subjects to an anterior or posterior lesion speech apraxic subgroup on the basis of the measures of interest?

METHOD

Subjects

The subjects selected for this study were 18 left hemisphere brain-injured adults exhibiting a variety of speech production errors, which have been described in the literature as characteristic of speech apraxia. These subjects also exhibited varying degrees of aphasia. They were obtained through the speech pathology divisions of four rehabilitation hospitals in New York City. All were alert, cooperative, and medically stable. Nine of the subjects were classified into a left frontal lobe group (frontal lesions) and nine into a left parietal and/or temporal lesion group (posterior lesions). Subjects were assigned to these groups on the basis of statements and clinical test results in their medical records. These statements and test data permitted classification of the subjects into two groups with confidence that their known sole lesions were either frontal or posterior. Subject classification was also confirmed by a review of available medical evidence by Dr. Arthur Benton, Neurologist, University Hospitals, Iowa City, Iowa.

All subjects were native English speakers with no history of previous speech or language impairment prior to the onset of their disorder. All exhibited a left hemisphere dominance for language (as inferred by premorbid right-handedness and the presence of varying degrees of aphasia), adequate hearing acuity for speech reception and comprehension as measured by pure tone audiometric thresholds, and no evidence of dysarthria either on the basis of medical records or clinical observations by the experimenter. The nine individuals in each subgroup were matched for mean age and duration postonset. Table 4-1 presents a summary of relevent descriptive data.

The diagnostic classification of speech apraxia was determined for all subjects dependent upon the presence of verbal behaviors that have been stated in the literature to be associated with speech apraxia. Specifically, a subject's speech must have presented evidence of two or more of the following: disruptions of smooth articulatory transitions between phonemes, syllables, and words (Luria, 1966; Shankweiler & Harris, 1966); disturbed melodic structure (Luria, 1966; Johns & Darley, 1970); problems in the initiation of speech, including groping and searching for

TABLE 4-1
Summary of apraxic subject data

	Anterior Apraxics (N = 9)					*Posterior Apraxic (N = 9)*				
Measure	*Mean*	*Range*	*CVA*	*Trauma*	*Tumor*	*Mean*	*Range*	*CVA*	*Trauma*	*Tumor*
Age (yr.)	49.67	25–70				51.67	25–73			
Duration (mo.)	22.67	4–38				25.56	8–62			
Severity Score[a]										
Monosyllabic	28.00	4–82				23.00	5–60			
Polysyllabic	93.89	28–173				99.67	15–193			
Etiology			8	1	—			6	2	1

[a]Severity scores were derived from the number of speech apraxic errors produced on a word repetition task.

the correct articulatory position (Canter, 1969; Trost & Canter, 1974); errors in phonemic and syllabic sequencing (Liepmann, 1913; Luria, 1966; Canter, 1969; Darley, Aronson, & Brown, 1975); numerous phonemic errors, including substitutions, omissions, additions, repetitions, and distortions (Johns & Darley, 1970; Trost & Canter, 1974); error inconsistency (Shankweiler & Harris, 1966; LaPointe, 1969; Johns & Darley, 1970); increasing phonemic errors as word length increased (Johns & Darley, 1970; Deal & Darley, 1972). Both the initial interview procedure and a tape recorded, standardized administration of the Boston Diagnostic Aphasia Examination (Goodglass & Kaplan, 1972) provided an opportunity to observe these behaviors.

PROCEDURES

Stimuli

Each subject was required to repeat the examiner's production of individually randomized lists of 64 monosyllabic and 66 polysyllabic words (Appendix A and A-1). The stimuli were selected to elicit a maximum number of speech apraxic errors. That is, the words of both lists contain at least one or more of those consonants and consonant clusters known to be most difficult for apraxic speakers (Trost, 1970). The polysyllabic words were included to provide an opportunity to observe sequencing and syllable omission errors. Each singleton consonant was tested four times in four different stimulus words and each consonant cluster was tested in two different stimulus words. A broad representation of vowels was used in the construction of the stimuli.

Administration and Scoring

The examiner spoke each stimulus word twice before allowing the subject to repeat the word. Each repetition attempt was judged to be adequate or inadequate by the examiner. Inadequate responses were any of the seven types described in Appendix B and B-1. After an inadequate response, the stimulus was presented a maximum of two additional times in an effort to elicit an adequate response. Adequate responses were either judged to be correct or to contain errors that could be described in terms of the six error types used to generate the criterion measures for the study. Appendix C presents a definition and example of each error type. All subject responses were tape recorded by the examiner and assigned an identification code by his assistant.

Five months after the final subject was recorded, the tape recorded responses were transcribed by the examiner using broad phonetic transcription. This delay in transcription and the coding procedure ensured that the examiner had no knowledge of any subjects' identity, medical history, or site of lesion classification. Only the first incorrect, adequate response to each stimulus word was scored. The scorable responses were categorized and tallied according to the six error types: articulation, syllable omission, syllable addition, fluency, sequencing, and complex combination of any of the above. The number of errors tabulated within each error type for both the monosyllabic and polysyllabic stimuli was expressed as a percentage of the total number of errors made by the subject. These percentages generated the 13 criterion measures employed in the data analyses.

Reliability

After all tapes were transcribed and scored, those of the first two subjects were transcribed a second time and rescored for the purpose of obtaining reliability measures. A 98.8% agreement was achieved in the assignment of responses to the adequate and inadequate categories. A 94.3% agreement was achieved in the error classification of the adequate responses. This degree of consistency in classification of responses was considered sufficiently high to permit meaningful interpretation of the data.

RESULTS

The means and standard deviations of the 13 criterion measures for the two subgroups of subjects are presented in Table 4-2. Also presented are the results of one-tailed t tests used to test the significance of the difference between the subgroup means. Only the percent of polysyllabic sequencing errors was significantly higher for the posterior subgroup ($t_{16} = 2.105, p < .05$).

The data were processed through an IBM 360 computer under the direction of Biomedical Computer Program (BMD P7M) designed to compute a stepwise discriminant analysis. The output of this procedure identifies the combination of variables which best divide the two groups of subjects and provides a probability measure of correctly classifying the subjects into their appropriate subgroups on the basis of the selected variables. The "best" prediction of subject subgroup classification was achieved through a combination of 3 of the 13 criterion measures: percent of polysyllabic sequencing errors, percent of monosyllabic articulation errors, and the total number of polysyllabic errors. Table 4-3 lists these variables in the order of their relative strength as discriminating predictors. It can be observed from the probability values reported in Table 4-3 that the linear combination of these three speech production error scores resulted in the maximum strength of accurate subject subgroup classification at the .01 level of confidence.

TABLE 4–2
Comparison of the 13[a] experimental measures obtained from the two subgroups, including t ratios used to test the significance of the difference between means of subgroup performance.

Variable: Percent of Errors	*Frontal Mean*	*SD*	*Posterior Mean*	*SD*	*t*
Monosyllabic					
1. Complex errors	11.4	12.5	12.7	10.2	.228
2. Fluency errors	38.8	24.9	44.6	29.2	.452
3. Articulation errors	57.6	23.7	51.3	25.8	.532
4. Syllable addition errors	1.0	1.8	0.8	1.7	.268
5. Sequencing errors	2.9	4.0	3.4	5.5	.247
6. Total monosyllabic errors	28.0	25.6	23.0	19.4	.467
Polysyllabic					
7. Complex errors	39.1	19.0	49.7	21.8	1.096
8. Fluency errors	35.2	26.0	28.0	15.0	.722
9. Articulation errors	51.2	23.3	51.9	12.4	.078
10. Syllable addition errors	2.7	2.5	3.9	2.9	.780
11. Syllable omission errors	4.0	2.1	4.8	2.1	.959
12. Sequencing errors	6.7	5.3	12.0	5.4	2.105*
13. Total polysyllabic errors	93.9	51.9	99.7	49.6	.241

*$df = 16$; $p < .05$.

[a]Two additional nonspeech variables were employed in the original analysis.

TABLE 4–3
Summary of stepwise discriminant function analysis identifying significant variables which discriminate between frontal and posterior lesion subjects

*Variables(s)**	*Wilkes Lambda*	*Approximate F Statistic*	*Degrees of Freedom*		*P*
1	.7831	4.433	1	16	.05
1 and 2	.6024	4.950	2	15	.025
1, 2, and 3	.4385	5.975	3	14	.01

*Variable 1: percent polysyllabic sequencing errors;
Variable 2: percent monosyllabic articulation errors;
Variable 3: total number of polysyllabic errors.

The number of individuals correctly classified and the percent of correct classification achieved when the best single variable and the best combination of variables were employed in the discriminant analysis are presented in Table 4-4. It can be observed that with the linear combination of three variables, the percent of correct classifications increases over that achieved by the best single measure or best combination of two measures. That is, when the linear combination of three variables was employed in the alanysis, it was found to be sufficient to predict correct subgroup assignment for 16 of the 18 subjects. This is the equivalent of a correct subject classification equal to 88.9%. No additional variables were selected by the program. This indicates that none of the other 10 variables exhibited *F* values sufficiently large to meet entry requirements and provide any improvement in discrimination. Thus, these results indicate that none of the other 10 variables either singly or combined would lead to an equivalent or better prediction of subject assignment than the 3 measures initially identified.

A "leaving one out" procedure was employed to provide a less optimistic, more conservative estimate of the reliability of the predictor variables selected by this analysis. This procedure removes all scores of a single subject from the subject pool and recomputes a new discriminant function. It then attempts to classify the omitted subject on the basis of the newly derived linear function based upon, in this case, the data from the remaining 17 subjects. The procedure continues until all subjects have been reclassified. In each step of this analysis exactly the same number of correct classifications occured as in the original analysis. This result verified the strength of the predictor variables to classify the subjects into their appropriate subgroups.

Intercorrelation

To gain additional information about relationships existing among the 13 criterion measures, a Pearson correlation procedure was employed. Table 4-5 presents the r and p values for each of the seven significant intercorrelations obtained ($p \leqq .005$). The percent of fluency errors was negatively correlated ($p = .0001$) with percent of articulation errors for both the monosyllabic and polysyllabic word repetition tasks. That is, those subjects who exhibited the largest number of fluency errors produced the least number of articulation errors, and inversely, those subjects who were highly fluent committed a large number of articulation errors. Despite the diverse number of specific errors comprising the "fluency error" category, it is notable that the frontal subgroup exhibited more dysfluency on the polysyllabic word task than did the

TABLE 4–4
Number of cases correctly classified and percent of correct classifications employing the best single variable and best combination of variables

	Variable 1		*Variable 1 and 2*		*Variable 1, 2, and 3*	
	Frontal	*Posterior*	*Frontal*	*Posterior*	*Frontal*	*Posterior*
Number of Cases Correctly Classified	6	5	5	8	8	8
Percent Correct Classification	66.7	55.6	55.6	88.9	88.9	88.9
Total Percent Correct Classification	61.1		72.2		88.9	

Note.
Variable 1: percent polysyllabic sequencing errors;
Variable 2: percent monosyllabic articulation errors;
Variable 3: total number of polysyllabic errors.

TABLE 4–5
Significant ($p \leq .005$) Pearson intercorrelations obtained for the 13 experimental variables

	Percent Monosyl. Articulation Errors	*Total Number Monosyl. Errors*	*Percent Polysyl. Articulation Errors*	*Percent Polysyl. Addition Errors*	*Percent Polysyl. Sequencing Errors*	*Total Number Polysyl. Errors*
Percent Monosyl. Complex Errors		.86752 .0001				
Percent Monosyl. Fluency Errors	−.97986 .0001					
Total Number Monosyl. Errors						.75255 .0003
Percent Polysyl. Complex Errors					.64580 .0038	.76539 .0002
Percent Polysyl. Fluency Errors			−.94785 .0001			
Percent Polysyl. Omission Errors				−.63603 .0045		

Note. Top number in each cell is the *r* value, bottom number is the *p* value.

posterior lesion subjects. This observation is consistent with the anticipated result of greater dysfluency exhibited by frontal lesion patients.

The percent of complex errors was significantly correlated ($p \leq .0002$) with the total number of errors on both the polysyllabic ($r = .7653$) and monosyllabic ($r = .8675$) word tasks. This reflects the fact that complex errors constituted a sizable component of the total error score. The complex error category also exhibited a significant correlation ($r = .6458$, $p < .004$) with sequencing errors on the polysyllabic task. This result indicated that sequencing errors were a frequent component of the polysyllabic complex error type.

A significant negative correlation existed between percent of syllable omission errors and percent of sylllable addition errors ($r = -.6360$, $p = .0045$). This relationship represents a tendency for syllabic errors occurring on the polysyllabic word task to be predominantly characterized by either additions or omissions.

Finally, the significant correlation ($r = .7525$, $p = .0003$) between the total number of errors on the polysyllabic and monosyllabic speech tasks suggests that those subjects who produced relatively more errors on the polysyllabic task manifested the same tendency on the monosyllabic task. However, all subjects exhibited significantly more errors on the polysyllabic task than on the monosyllabic speech task ($t = 8.45$, $p < .001$). This result indicates that the subject group as a whole exhibited more speech apraxic difficulties on longer stimuli.

DISCUSSION

The major question of this study was whether a group of subjects exhibiting speech apraxic behaviors could be differentiated into two site of lesion subgroups on the basis of any single measure or combination of 13 speech error measures. The findings indicated that the single best discriminating measure was the percent of polysyllabic sequencing errors. This was also the only error measure upon which the two subgroups' performance differed significantly. That is, the posterior subgroup exhibited significantly more sequencing errors than did the frontal subjects. This outcome agrees with Liepmann (1913), Luria (1966), and Canter's (1969) statements and observations attributing this particular speech error type to a speech apraxic entity resulting from a posterior lesion.

Monosyllabic articulation errors and polysyllabic sequencing errors constituted the best discriminating pair of measures. Beyond the fact that inclusion of articulation errors in the analysis improved classification accuracy, articulation errors by themselves represented the largest portion of the total number of errors made by both subgroups.

Therefore, it may be viewed as the fundamental speech production error feature of both speech apraxic subgroups. This finding also confirms statements by Luria (1966) and Canter (1969) that attribute articulation difficulties to both such subgroups.

It is notable that while articulation difficulty was common to both subgroups the posterior subjects experienced less difficulty on the monosyllabic task. Moreover, all subjects had more difficulty with the polysyllabic words, supporting the findings of Johns and Darley (1970) that accuracy of articulation in apraxic speakers is negatively affected by an increase in stimulus word length. A further indication of greater difficulty associated with polysyllabic stimuli was the selection of the total number of polysyllabic errors as the final constituent of the three best discriminating variables. The posterior subgroup exhibited a larger total number of errors on the polysyllabic repetition task than did the frontal group. This difference appeared to be primarily a reflection of the large number of complex errors produced by the posterior subgroup.

While all error types were not mutually exclusive across subgroups, the posterior lesion patients produced the pattern of more polysyllabic sequencing errors, fewer monosyllabic articulation errors, and a larger total number of polysyllabic errors in comparison to the frontal lesion subjects. Therefore, to the extent that Luria (1966) and Canter (1969) implied that specific types of speech errors result solely from an anterior or posterior lesion, the present results suggest otherwise. Nevertheless, by employing the above pattern of error types, the discriminant function analysis predicted correct subject subgroup assignment for 88.9% of the total subjects.

To determine the factors responsible for the misclassification of one subject from the frontal subgroup into the posterior subgroup (Subject 7), and one subject from the posterior subgroup (Subject 17) into the frontal subgroup, the probability of each individual's subgroup assignment was determined. Specifically, the probability of posterior assignment of Subject 7 was 92%, and the probability of anterior assignment of Subject 17 was 78%. Therefore, it is evident that neither subject was a borderline misclassification. Inspection of the data showed that the performance of Subject 17 was inconsistent. That is, his scores on the monosyllabic speech task were characteristic of subjects classified as having frontal lesion, while on the polysyllabic task his scores were typical of other posterior subjects in this study. The three best predictive criterion measures for frontal Subject 7 were clearly typical of the subjects who had posterior lesions. Several possible explanations are available to account for these two subjects' misclassification. First, in the case of Subject 7, the available clinical information employed in the initial subgroup assignment could be considered potentially ambiguous. It is also possible that each of the two subjects may have actually incurred more extensive and diffuse damage than was reported in their medical records, such that they displayed atypical performance. Finally, it is possible that one or both of these subjects may possess a different neural organization for brain function than is presumed to exist for the majority of individuals.

The present results do provide some suggesions regarding organization of cortical mechanisms involved in speech production. There exists considerable mention of temporoparietal mechanisms participating in some way in motor activity. For example, Ruch and Fulton (1960), states, "a posterior parietal supplementary motor area discharges partly through the pyramidal systems and partly through the extrapyramidal system. The temporal lobe contains two supplementary motor areas" (p. 268). Foerster (in Luria, 1966) studied motor disturbances arising from postcentral lesions. These resulted not only in sensory disturbances but also gross motor defects. He labeled the phenomenon "afferent pareses" and described the disability as resulting from a loss of selectivity and an inability to find the correct destination, resulting in a diffuse contraction of agonists and antagonists. Lesions occurring more posteriorly (Area 5) have been reported by Head (1920) and Denny-Brown (1958) to result in disorganization of spatial integration or the "kinesthetic schemes" of movement which are the foundation for construction of the motor act. Such statements may be interpreted to imply that motor activity is, to some degree, dependent upon the posterior mechanisms or that the information from these regions is in some way supplemental to accurate functioning.

The role of the sensory or afferent mechanism in motor speech activity is somewhat vague. Nevertheless, Luria (1966) states quite succinctly that there is a kinesthetic basis for all voluntary movement that is organized in the parietal lobe. This basis requires the integration of afferent information regarding the position of muscles and joints. To the extent that the temporoparietal regions can be said to integrate the afferent information (e.g., conscious sensation of tough pressure, kinesthesia, and auditory monitoring or unconscious proprioceptive information) and to the extent that a disruption in the formulation and/or transmission of this information to the frontal lobe will result in a disordered speech production output, Luria's statement seems supported by the present findings.

In view of the above, the significant negative correlation observed across both groups between the percent of articulation and fluency errors may be reflective of their self-monitoring ability. That is, the more dysfluent subjects produced fewer articulation errors while those subjects who were highly fluent produced many articulation errors. The highly dysfluent subjects produced phonemic reapproaches at either the syllable or word level; delayed speech initiations; disruptions to the fluency of transitions between phonemic elements; and repetitions of a target phoneme, syllable, or entire word. These behaviors may be interpreted as representing an effort by the subject to maintain control of the speech programming mechanism by attempting to prevent errors with changes in silent articulatory posturing prior to actual verbalization. On the other hand, the posterior group seemingly continued to produce speech fluently without regard to their numerous articulation errors. This disregard may reflect a disruption of the integration of afferent information in the temporoparietal mechanisms which should be forwarded to frontal efferent mechanisms. Also, it may be due to a problem on the part of posterior brain damaged subjects in monitoring, by auditory feedback, their own speech production.

Any interpretation of the results of this study must be considered with certain inherent qualifications and limitations. Perhaps the primary qualification was the potential for subjects to have been initially assigned to the incorrect site of lesion subgroup. While these classifications were based upon the best clinical evidence available, the potential for misclassification must be recognized. This qualification is presented in light of the fact that appropriate diagnostic procedures employed for many patients with closed-skull brain lesions do not permit highly precise identification of the exact location and extent of the lesion. That is, while some clinical procedures may provide adequate information concerning the prime location, they frequently are inadequate to define accurately the peripheral margins of more diffuse lesions.

Generalization of the results should be reserved for persons with mild or moderate speech apraxic involvement as was the case for the present subjects. This restriction was necessitated by the need to exclude extremely severe patients whose performance might have been influenced by comprehension deficits, auditory acuity problems, or dysarthric involvement.

An additional concern relative to the generalizability of these findings relates to the experimenter's inability to control for the exposure of some subjects to prior treatment. It is possible to assume that for some portion of the present subject group, their speech production output may have been influenced by rehabilitative drill procedures similar in format to the experimental tasks. Such a situation would represent an unequally distributed practice effect for those subjects whose therapy programs included similar speech tasks or phonetic drill procedures.

In light of the above considerations, the results of the present study may be interpreted to possess the following important implications for the clinical speech pathologist involved in the diagnosis and rehabilitation of brain injured adults.

Initial assessment procedures to determine the presence and extent of speech apraxia should include a polysyllabic speech task presented imitatively. This recommendation is presented in view of the findings of Johns and Darley (1970) and those of the present study, that a monosyllabic speech task alone failed to reveal the actual extent of speech apraxic-like difficulty for several subjects. Additionally, a corpus of the patient's speech responses should be subjected to a detailed analysis. That is, criteria similar to those employed in the present study to categorically classify verbal output into adequate versus inadequate productions, should be applied to a sample of each patient's speech production. The purpose of such a procedure would be to achieve a more reliable identification of an individual's speech apraxic behaviors as distinguished from aphasic, neologistic productions. Finally, if the negative relationship observed between fluency and articulation accuracy is a valid reflection of attempted self-monitoring or self-correction ability, then remediation procedures for brain damaged persons who show speech behaviors comparable to the posterior group of this study should include efforts to encourage such patients to monitor their speech production output and make the appropriate self-corrections. The outcome of such an approach should be an increased awareness of articulatory accuracy resulting in successively closer target phoneme approximations. For brain damaged persons whose speech efforts are comparable to the present frontal group, their dysfluent behaviors should be analyzed with the goal of extinguishing those which are least productive and maintaining or establishing those behaviors which result in increased self-corrected approximations of the target response.

In conclusion, the findings of the present study tend to support the position that two forms of a speech production problem can be identified and localized to either a frontal or posterior site of brain lesion. These problems are not a result of damage to the neuromotor systems responsible for causing dysarthria, nor do they appear to be related to a language deficit. The two patterns of speech errors exhibited by the subjects of the present study tend to support references by Canter (1969) and Luria (1966) of a primary or efferent kinetic apraxia and a secondary or afferent kinesthetic speech apraxia.

APPENDIX A

List of 64 monosyllabic words presented to the 18 subjects

1. gift
2. jar
3. smile
4. masks
5. wish
6. vail
7. girl
8. square
9. yawn
10. ring
11. tub
12. thick
13. teeth
14. glove
15. squash
16. flute
17. judge
18. hooks
19. slave
20. robe
21. yarn
22. worm
23. swing
24. shoes
25. yolk
26. vase
27. slide
28. frog
29. spring
30. mouth
31. shirt
32. crutch
33. bat
34. wasp
35. yacht
36. string
37. red
38. door
39. clown
40. cage
41. green
42. thread
43. screws
44. watch
45. black
46. think
47. bank
48. dog
49. smoke
50. crown
51. float
52. scrap
53. straw
54. glass
55. blue
56. frame
57. three
58. clasp
59. spruce
60. swan
61. grass
62. tasks
63. raft
64. axe

APPENDIX A–1

List of 66 polysyllabic words ranging from two to four syllables in length

1. jacket
2. gingerbread
3. legislation
4. vaccine
5. vacation
6. advantageous
7. thousand
8. thanksgiving
9. hypothesis
10. Yukon
11. yesterday
12. universal
13. shadow
14. champagne
15. composition
16. critic
17. creation
18. incriminate
19. flapjack
20. flamingo
21. inflammation
22. clothespin
23. clinician
24. inclination
25. donkey
26. document
27. indefinite
28. garlic
29. government
30. mahogany
31. banana
32. bandanna
33. abdication
34. window
35. wastebasket
36. Winnebago
37. stringent
38. strategy
39. instructiveness
40. gravy
41. gravity
42. aggravation
43. scrimmage
44. scrutiny
45. blanket
46. blasphemy
47. blasphemousness
48. fragment
49. frequency
50. fragmentation
51. slingshot
52. slaughterhouse
53. slanderousness
54. threshold
55. thrombosis
56. squeamish
57. squalidness
58. gluten
59. gluttony
60. gluttonousness
61. springboard
62. springiness
63. swallow
64. swastika
65. smokestack
66. smithereens

APPENDIX B

Inadequate response classifications (adapted from Burns, 1975).

1. *No response* was made by the subject after the stimulus word had been presented and a reasonable amount of time had elapsed.

2. *Random phoneme strings* were subject responses which did not yield a word approximation.

3. *Recurrent verbalizations* were repetitious productions that were unrelated to the stimulus word.

4. *Circumlocutions* were defined as responses in which no specific single word production could be isolated, but the utterance was conceptually appropriate.

5. *Commentaries* were responses in which no specific target word could be isolated, but the subject commented on the nature of the required word or related some personal experience in some way associated with the target word.

6. *Semantic or grammatic substitutions* were real, single-word responses consisting of an obvious conceptually related word or a grammatical variant of the target word.

7. *True neologisms* were nonsense phonemic sequences, spoken as a unit with fluency of articulation and no evidence of groping for correct articulatory position. The response did not reasonably approximate the target word or any conceptually related variant. Several arbitrary criteria were devised for distinguishing true neologisms from phonemic paraphasias (adequate responses) which have been attributed to speech apraxic difficulties. These criteria are presented in Appendix B-1.

APPENDIX B–1

Criteria for distinguishing phonemic paraphasias from true neologisms in monosyllabic and polysyllabic words*

Rule	Examples: Phonemic Paraphasias	Examples: Neologisms
CV or VC		
1. The correct target consonant or target vowel must occur in correct positional relation	/tau/toe	/ɔIt/toe
or		
2. The correct target consonant and target vowel must occur in any position	/ot/toe	/od/toe
CVC or CCV or VCC		
1. At least one target consonant must occur in correct positional relation to the correct target vowel	/sIp/ship	/spi/ship
or		
2. The correct target consonants and target vowel must occur in any position	/pIʃ/ship	/pæʃ/ship
or		

*Modified from Burns (1975): Distinguishing polysyllabic phonemic paraphasias from true neologisms required that:

(a) The number of syllables in the response item, equal to one less than the number of syllables in the target word, complied with the above rules; or

(b) more than half the total phonemes produced in the response were not extraneous to the total number of phonemes in the target word, and the response evidenced a loss of fluency of articulation or a groping for the correct articulatory position.

Rule	Examples: Phonemic Paraphasias	Examples: Neologisms
3. The correct target consonants must occur in correct positional relation to any vowel	/ʃɛp/ship	/ʃob/ship
CVCC or CCVC		
1. At least two target consonants must occur in correct positional relation to the correct target vowel	/klæk/black	/klob/black
or		
2. All target consonants and the target vowel must occur in any position	/klæb/black	/plæb/black
or		
3. All target consonants must occur in correct positional relation to any vowel	/blIk/black	/plik/black
CCCVC or CVCCC		
1. At least three target consonants must occur in correct positional relation to the correct target vowel	/triŋ/string	strɔg/string
or		
2. All target consonants and the target vowel must occur in any position	/triŋs/string	trɔŋs/string
or		
3. All target consonants must occur in correct positional relation to any vowel	/stræŋ/string	/stær/string

APPENDIX C

Speech apraxic error types used in scoring responses of the 18 subjects

Error Type	*Definition*	*Example*
Articulation	Conventional phonetic substitution, addition, omission, and distortion errors	/kIf/ for gift
Syllable Omission	Omission of one or more syllables	/dIfɛnt/ for different
Syllable Addition	Addition of one or more syllables other than intrusion of /a/	/græ̆vIdIti/ for gravity
Fluency	*a.* Transitionalization: disruptions to the fluency of smoothly blended articulations in the form of /ə/ or /ʌ/ intrusive vowels between component elements of a consonant cluster, intrusive glottal stop, intrusive pause or hiatus between phonemes or syllables, and prolongations	/kʌrieʃən/ for creation
	b. Delayed speech initiation: interval measured from the end of the investigator's final repetition of the stimulus word to the beginning of a discrete adequate response by the subject. The presence of starter sounds, fillers, recurrent utterances or silent articulatory posturing prior to an audible response was not regarded as the beginning of a discrete response and were scored as a delayed speech initiation. A silent response interval exceeding two seconds was scored as delayed. Timing of delays was determined from the tape recording	
	c. Reapproach: repetition of either a whole word, syllable or a target phoneme during which the target phoneme was changed	/s-j-tri/ for tree
	d. Repetition: an unchanged repeated production of a target phoneme, syllable or whole word	/o-oIk/ for thick

Error Type	*Definition*	*Example*
Sequencing	Transposition of phonemes or substitution of an earlier or later occuring phoneme within and across traditional syllable boundaries and/or transposition of entire syllables	/jɛsdɚte/ for yesterday or /jɛsdetɚ/ for yesterday
Complex	Involves more than one of any of the above error types. Each error type comprising a complex error was recorded in its appropriate error category.	/dIp-dIfɛnt/ for different (scored as a fluency reapproach and a syllable omission)

REFERENCES

Bay, E. Principles of classification and their influence on our concepts of aphasia. In A. deReuck & M. O'Conner (Eds.), *Disorders of language.* Boston: Little, Brown, 1964.

Burns, M. S., *Phonemic behavior of aphasic patients with posterior cerebral lesions.* Ph.D. dissertation, Northwestern University, 1975.

Canter, G. J. *The influence of primary and secondary verbal apraxia upon output disturbances in aphasic syndromes.* Paper presented at the Annual Convention of the American Speech and Hearing Association, Chicago, 1969.

Darley, F. L. *Diagnosis and appraisal of communication disorders.* Englewood Cliffs NJ: Prentice-Hall, 1964.

Darley, F. L. Notes prepared for delivery to American Speech and Hearing Association Convention, Chicago, 1969.

Darley, F. L., Aronson, A. E., & Brown, J. R. *Motor speech disorders.* Philadelphia: Saunders, 1975.

Deal, J. L., & Darley, F. L. The influence of linguistic and situational variables on phonemic accuracy in apraxia of speech. *Journal of Speech and Hearing Research,* 1972, *15*, 639–653.

Denny-Brown, D. The nature of apraxia. *Journal of Nervous and Mental Diseases,* 1958, *126*, 9–32.

Goodglass, H., & Kaplan, E., *The assessment of aphasia and related disorders.* Philadelphia: Lea and Febiger, 1972.

Head, H. *Studies in neurology, Vol. 1.* London: Oxford Medical Pub., 1920.

Johns, D. F., & Darley, F. L. Phonemic variability in apraxia of speech. *Journal of Speech and Hearing Research*, 1970, *13*, 556–583.

LaPointe, L. L. *An investigation of isolated oral movement, oral motor sequencing abilities and articulation of brain injured adults.* Ph.D. dissertation, University of Colorado, 1969.

Liepmann, H. Uber störungen des handelns bei gehirnkranken. Berlin: S. Karger, 1905 (Unpublished translation by Gertrude Eggert, 1969).

Liepmann, H. Motorische, aphasie, und apraxie. *Transaction of the 17th international congress of medicine.* London, Section XI, Part 2, 97-106, 1913.

Luria, A. R. *Higher cortical functions in man.* New York: Basic Books, 1966.

Luria, A. R. *Traumatic aphasia: its syndromes, psychology and treatment.* The Hague: Mouton, 1970.

Ruch, C. T., & Fulton, F. J. (Eds.) *Medical physiology and biophysics.* Philadelphia: Saunders, 1960.

Shankweiler, D., & Harris, K. S. An experimental approach to the problem of articulation in aphasia. *Cortex*, 1966, *2*, 272-292.

Trost, J. E. *A descriptive study of verbal apraxia in patients with Broca's aphasia.* Ph.D. dissertation, Northwestern University, 1970.

Trost, J. E., & Canter, G. Apraxia of speech in patients with Broca's aphasia: A study of phoneme production, accuracy and error pattern. *Brain and Language*, 1974, *1*, 63–79.

ACKNOWLEDGMENT

This article is adapted from a portion of the author's doctoral dissertation conducted at the University of Iowa under the direction of Dr. James A. Hardy. The author thanks Dr. Arthur Benton for his assistance with the project and the staff of Columbia Presbyterian Hospital Speech and Hearing Clinic, as well as many other facilities that must remain nameless, for their contribution to the data collection.

5

Articulatory Movements in Apraxia of Speech

Motonobu Itoh
Sumiko Sasanuma

Clarification of the nature of apraxia of speech is vitally important not only for the differential diagnosis and treatment of the disorder but also for providing crucial information concerning the role of higher cortical functions in speech production. Potentially useful approaches to this goal may include: (1) phonemic/phonetic analyses of speech errors produced by the apraxic patients (e.g., Johns & Darley, 1970; LaPointe & Johns, 1975; Trost & Canter, 1974); (2) investigation of the sensory-perceptual ability of the patients (e.g., Aten, Johns, & Darley, 1971; Rosenbek, Wertz, & Darley, 1973); and (3) direct observations of articulatory gestures in the patients. Each of these approaches with its own strengths and weaknesses can complement the others, providing deeper insight into the problem. Since apraxia of speech, by definition, is a motor speech impairment, however, the last approach appears to yield the most direct and precise information on the impaired articulatory movements per se, the acoustic end products of which are part and parcel of the speech symptoms called apraxia of speech.

A variety of techniques has been developed which permit direct observations of the articulatory gestures. Shankweiler, Harris, and Taylor

(1968) pioneered the use of electromyography (EMG) with two patients who had residual articulatory disorders (presumably what we call "apraxia of speech") following damage to the left cerebral hemisphere from stroke. This research yielded valuable information on the defective articulatory gestures of these patients. Technological advancement in recent years has brought about other new techniques that can, and should, be exploited to gain further information on the articulatory movements in apraxia of speech.

During the past few years we have had the opportunity to conduct a series of experiments which adopted some of the new techniques for direct observations of the articulatory gestures in a patient clinically diagnosed as having a "pure" form of apraxia of speech, and in fluent aphasic patients (Itoh, Sasanuma, & Ushijima, 1979; Itoh, Sasanuma, Hirose, Yoshioka, & Ushijima, 1980; Itoh, Sasanuma, Tatsumi, Murakami, Fukusako, & Suzuki, 1982; Itoh, Sasanuma, Hirose, Yoshioka, & Sawashima, 1983). In this chapter we would like to present some of the essential data obtained from these experiments and to try to interpret these data so as to make the best possible inferences about the nature of apraxia of speech. We hope that such effort might, in turn, enable us to offer some suggestions concerning clinical assessment of this disorder.

Case History

The experimental subject, T.K., was a 55-year-old executive of a large company. He was in his usual state of health until 2 o'clock in the afternoon of March 14, 1970, when he suddenly felt numb in the right arm while golfing and felt dizzy for a while (approximately 30 sec in retrospect). After resting for a few minutes he recovered, went back to his car, and started to drive home. Following a collision he found himself unable to utter a word to an attending policeman and was admitted to a nearby hospital. His phonation returned a week after the day of the accident, but it took more than a month before he was able to produce speech sounds.

According to the medical records, his examination upon admission revealed no gross abnormalities. He had a blood pressure of 140/90 and a regular pulse of 66/min. Upon neurological examination, no cranial nerve involvements were found. Motor and sensory examinations were normal except for a positive Rossolimo on the right side of the lower extremity. The electroencephalogram (EEG) and other special tests were normal. Thus, the findings were inconclusive with regard to the etiology, but it was suspected that T.K. had incurred a transient attack of cerebral infarction due to thrombosis just before the accident. In September 1976, 6 years after the onset, computerized axial tomography (CT scan) revealed an infarct involving the cortical surface near the anterior tip of the Sylvian fissure of the left hemisphere and immediately subjacent subcortical white matter (Figure 5-1).

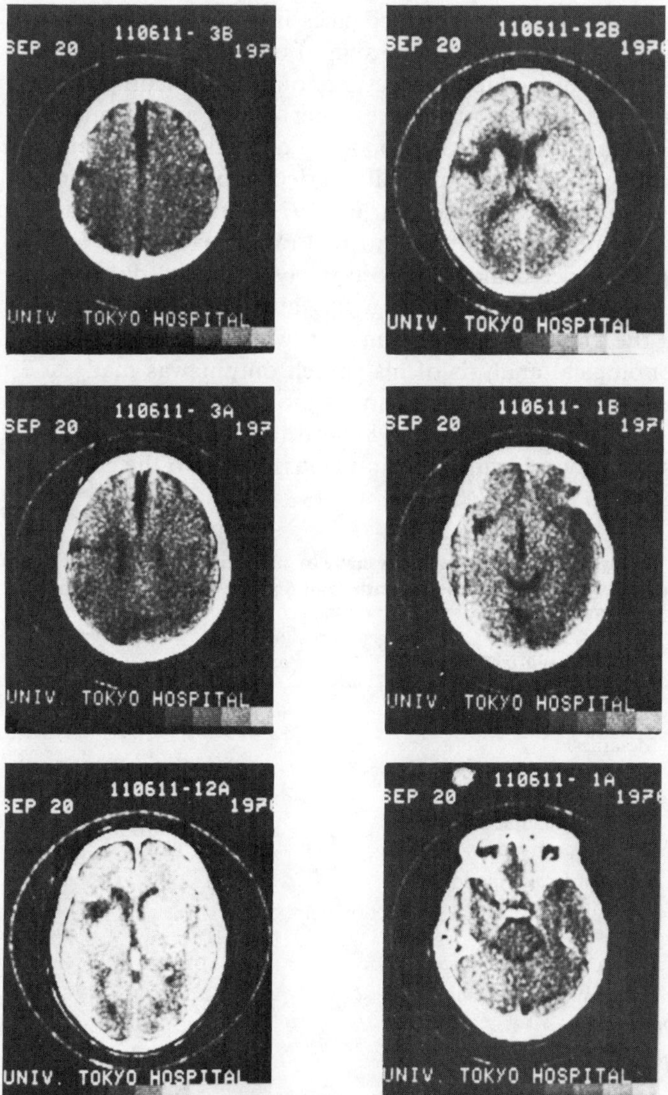

FIGURE 5-1
Computer tomograms of the apraxic patient, T.K.

An extensive speech and language examination was conducted 7 months after the onset of the illness when the patient was first referred to one of the authors. On a comprehensive aphasia test battery, he responded at a near-normal level in all modalities except in oral production where he exhibited marked impairment in articulation as well as in prosody, without any sign of disturbances in the muscular control of the speech mechanism. There was no sign of oral apraxia. His auditory comprehension was judged to be intact; he could follow complex oral instructions with accuracy and promptness, performed at a normal level on the Token Test and made no errors on a test of auditory perception of words and phrases which were minimally varied phonemically (similar to one described by Aten, Johns, & Darley, 1971). In reading and writing, his test scores were well within the normal range, except for a slight reduction in speed of performance. Subjectively, he believed that the reduction in speed of reading and writing was attributable to the difficulty in handling the kana-transcribed function words in the sentences.

A phonological analysis of his speech output was made at 7 months postonset and again at 6 years and 4 months postonset. On each occasion, T.K.'s oral reading of a 298-word text was tape-recorded, and his error responses were transcribed and classified into the categories shown in Table 5-1.

TABLE 5-1
Frequency and type of articulation errors made by the apraxic subject (T.K.) on the task of oral reading of a 298 word text at 7 months and 6 years, 4 months postonset

*Categories**	*7 Months Postonset*	*6 Years, 4 Months Postonset*
I. Substitution		
1. Metathesis		
(1). Within-word		
a. Adjacent	18	1
b. Nonadjacent	2	0
(2). Between-words	3	0
2. Backward Assimilation		
(1). Within-word	14	0
(2). Between-words	7	0
3. Forward Assimilation	4	1
4. Random Substitution	13	2
II. Addition	4	0
III. Omission	2	0
IV. Repetition	1	0
Totals	68	4

*Distortions and self-corrections were not tabulated, although a great many were observed.

It can be seen from Table 5-1 that, at 7 months postonset, the most predominant type of error was the "substitution" of a syllable or a phoneme (88.2% of the total of 68 instances of phonemic errors), while syllabic additions (5.9%), syllabic omissions (4.4%), and a syllabic repetition (1.5%) accounted for the rest of the errors. Among these substitutions, metatheses were the greatest in number (38.3% of the total substitutions), followed by backward (anticipatory) assimilations (35.0%), random substitutions (20.0%), and forward (perseverative) assimilations (6.7%). The metatheses (either adjacent or nonadjacent) took place not only with respect to syllables, phonemes, or distinctive features within the boundary of a word, but also across word boundaries. A few occasions of metatheses of words and short phrases were also observed. A similar characteristic was observed in the backward assimilations: two-thirds of them took place within a word and the rest across word boundaries, often across several word boundaries.

In other words, the predominant types of articulatory errors made by T.K. at 7 months after the onset of the illness were metatheses and backward assimilations, the majority of which (especially nonadjacent or between-word types) could be explained as errors in the selection or retrieval of target phonemes in the process of speech production (Fromkin, 1973; Garrett, 1975). Based on this observation, it was suggested that the impairment might not be confined to the motor aspsects of speech but might extend into the linguistic (but almost exclusively phonological spheres as well). The table also indicates that those errors which initially reflected a phonological (linguistic) impairment had diminished to almost zero by the time the second analysis was made at 6 years and 4 months postonset.

It should also be noted, however, that at 7 months postonset T.K. exhibited, on the level of phonetic analysis, a considerable number of "distortions" as well. Furthermore, his prosodic disturbances in the initial test were quite conspicuous, showing such symptoms as an overall reduction of the speaking rate, stuttering-like hesitations and blocks, and abnormal pitch contour, tending toward monotonous pitch and stress control. Most of these prosodic features were quite resistant to therapy, and they were still observable at 6 years and 4 months postonset.

The three experiments with T.K. reported in this chapter will be: fiberscopic observation of velar movements (Experiment 1), x-ray microbeam observation of the temporal organization of different articulators (Experiment II), and voice onset time analysis (Experiment III). These experiments were conducted over the 11-month period from 6 years and 4 months to 7 years and 3 months postonset of his illness.

EXPERIMENT I. FIBERSCOPIC (FIBEROPTIC) OBSERVATION OF VELAR MOVEMENTS

Movements of the velum in T.K. were examined by means of the fiberoptic technique and were compared with those of a normal control subject and two fluent aphasic patients. The normal control subject was a 51-year-old male who was free from any speech or hearing disorders. The fluent aphasic subjects were two male patients with Wernicke's aphasia, K.K. and N.S. Table 5-2 summarizes the age, cause of brain damage, site of lesion, and postonset time of K.K. and N.S. Diagnosis of both patients was made based on the overall pattern of their linguistic impairment as revealed by the Tokyo Metropolitan Institute of Gerontology Test for the Differential Diagnosis of Aphasia plus neurological findings which included CT scan data.

TABLE 5-2
The age, cause of brain damage, site of lesion, and postonset time of the two Wernicke's aphasic patients

Subject	*Age (ys)*	*Cause of Brain Damage*	*Site of Lesion**	*Postonset Time*
K.K.	51	Operational removal of ruptured aneurysm	Posterior region of the temporal lobe of the left hemisphere	2 years, 11 months
N.S.	67	Operational removal of hematoma	Superior temporal gyrus, optic radiation, angular gyrus and corona radiata of the left hemisphere	5 years, 3 months

*Identified by CT scan.

Procedure

Fiberscopic observation of the subjects' velar movements during speech was made according to the procedure developed by Sawashima and Ushijima (1971) and Sawashima, Ushijima, and Hirose (1976). The velar view was photographed with a 16-mm cinecamera at a rate of 50 frames per sec with simultaneous recording of the speech signal and synchronization time marks. Oscillographic traces of the speech signal with the time marks were made to obtain the correspondence between the film frames and the speech sounds. The photographed film frames were examined, frame by frame, by means of a motion picture analyzer.

Two kinds of speech materials were prepared: nonsense syllables and meaningful words. The nonsense syllables were /teNteNteNteN/, where /N/ was the syllable final nasal in Japanese. The meaningful words were combinations of the vowel /e/, the nasal sounds /n/ and/or /N/, or nonnasal consonants /d/, /s/, or /t/: /deenee/, /deedee/, /seeneN/, /teeneN/, /teedeN/, /see'eN/, and /see'ee/. These words were embedded in a carrier phrase of /. . . desu/("it is. . ."). The subjects were requested to read these speech materials at their conversational rate. They read the nonsense syllables three times and each of the meaningful words in the carrier phrase five times in random order.

Results and Discussion

The patterns of velar movements during speech obtained from the normal control and the Wernicke's aphasic subjects are in general agreement with those obtained from the normal subjects in Sawashima et al. (1976). T.K. exhibited various unique articulatory movement patterns of the velum.

Consistency in the pattern of velar movements. Figures 5-2 and 5-3 compare the superimposed patterns of the velar movements for three repetitions of /teNteNteNteN/ and for five repetitions of /deeneedesu/, respectively, in the normal subject (a), the apraxic subject T.K. (b), and Wernicke's aphasic subjects K.K. (c) and N.S. (d). The ordinate gives an arbitrary scale for the velar height and the abscissa the time course. The short vertical bars across the curve indicate the vowel onset or offset, which were obtained from the audio signal. The long vertical bars indicate the onset of /e/ after the initial nonnasal consonant, which served as the line-up point for a comparison among the several velar patterns of a given sequence of sounds.

The normal control shows regular oscillatory movements of the velum /teNteNteNteN/ (Figure 5-2a). It is also noted that there is a high degree of agreement in the patterns of velar movements for the three repetitions of the task for the normal subject. In contrast, the apraxic performance is characterized by less regular oscillatory velar movements with a marked variation in velum height and segmental duration (Figure 5-2b). In addition, the velar movement pattern varies considerably throughout the three repetitions of the task.

Similar results were obtained from repetitions of /deeneedesu/. While the normal subject exhibited a high degree of consistency through five repetitions of /deeneedesu/ (Figure 5-3a), T.K. showed a great variability in the pattern of velar movements, accompanied by a phonetic change from [n] to [d] (Figure 5-3b). In spite of this variability, however, note that the general successional pattern of the apraxic patient's velar

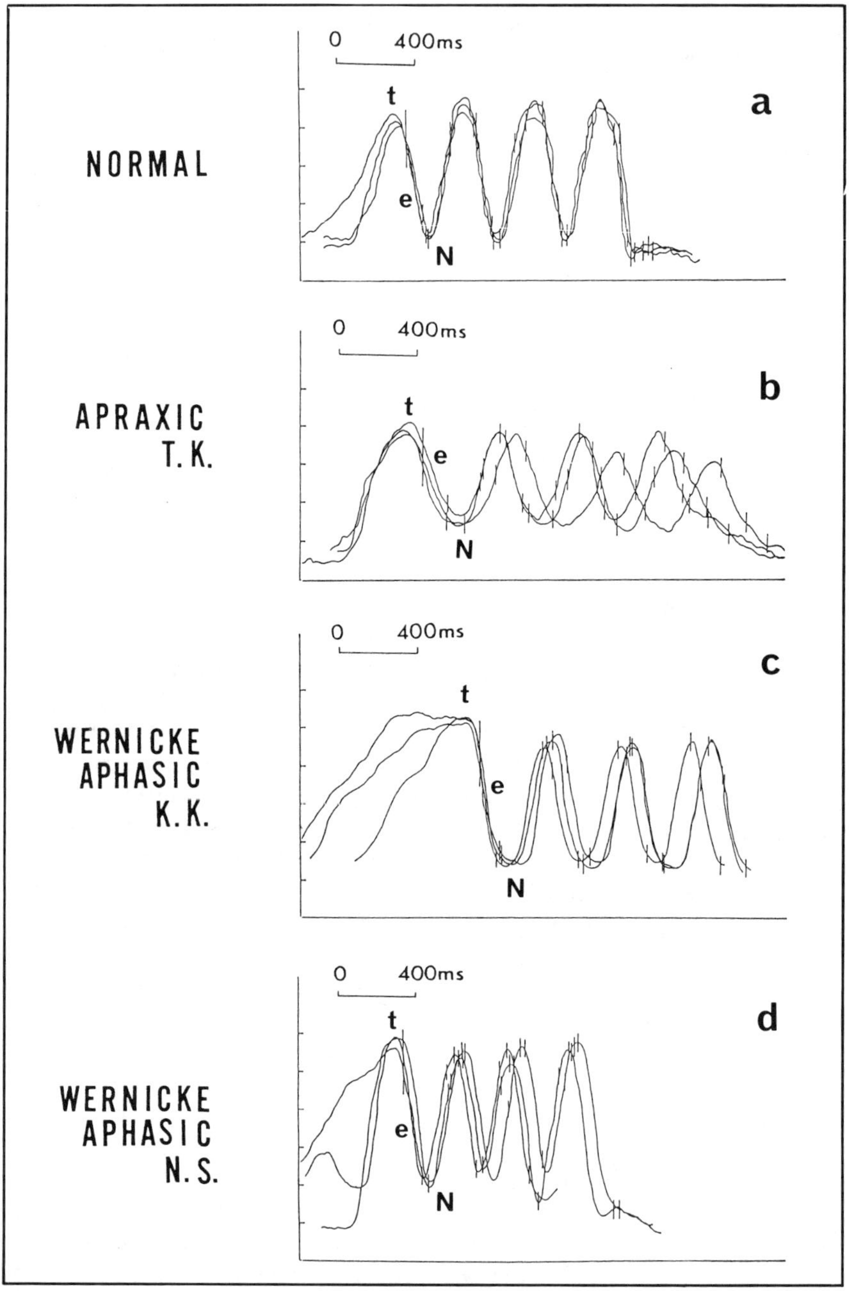

FIGURE 5-2
Superimposed patterns of the velar movements for three repetitions of /teNteNteNteN/.

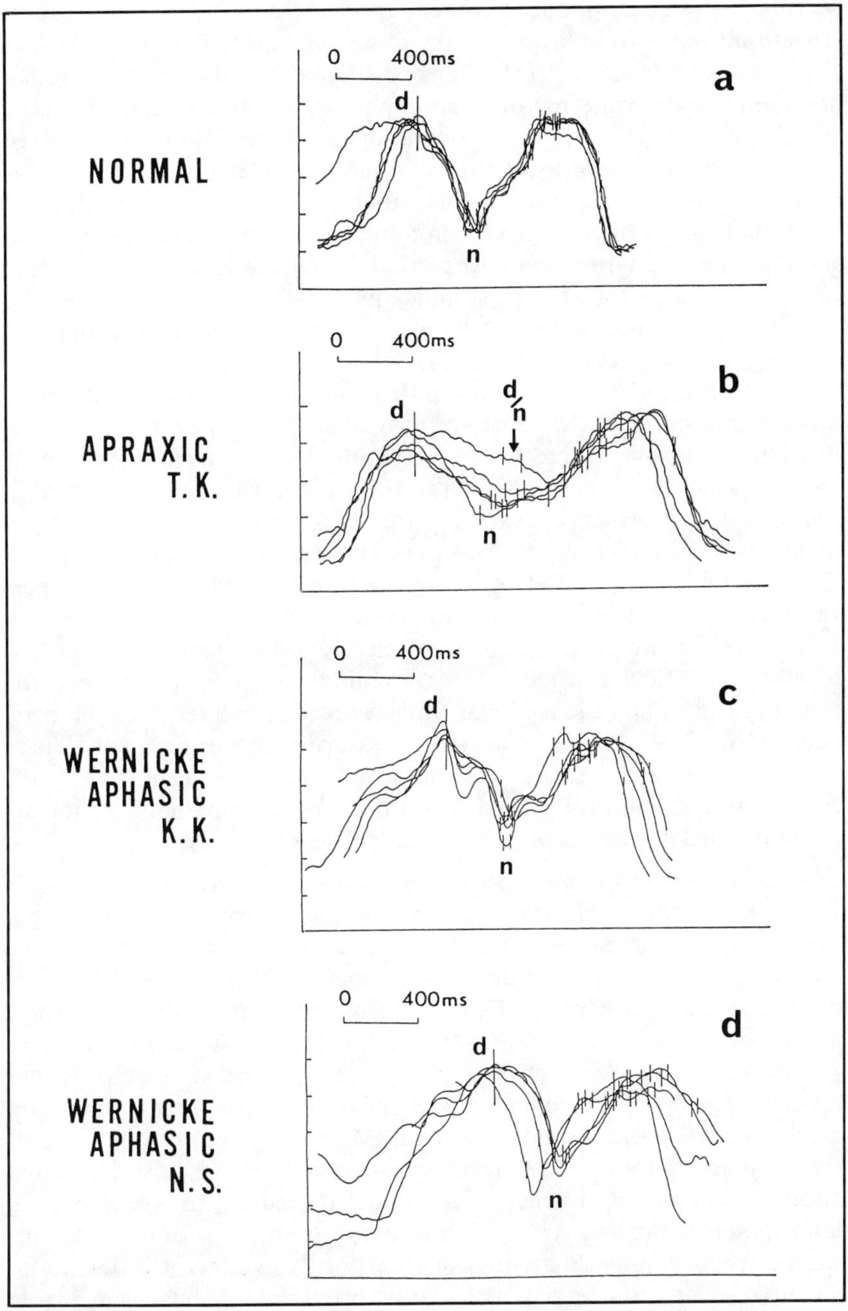

FIGURE 5-3
Superimposed patterns of the velar movements of five repetitions of /deeneedesu/.

gestures for a given phonetic context approximated the normal pattern. This result seems to indicate that the observed variation in the pattern of velar movements and the resultant phonetic change do *not* stem from a selection or retrieval error of a target phoneme in the process of speech production, namely, an error of phonological processing. If the observed phonetic change from [n] to [d] were due to a selection error, the successive pattern of velar movements should have been different; that is, the velum would have been kept in a high position because of the nonnasal phonetic environment /dee*d*eedesu/. We interpret, therefore, that this type of behavior in T.K. is indicative of a "motor" impairment in the process of programming "the positioning of speech musculature" (Darley, Aronson, & Brown, 1975).

Figures 5-2 and 5-3 also indicate that one of two patients with Wernicke's aphasia, K.K., exhibited a fairly high consistency in velar movement patterns over three or five repetitions of a given sequence of sounds, which is in sharp contrast to the marked variability observed in the apraxic performance. Although the performance of the other Wernicke's aphasic patient, N.S., was somewhat variable in comparison with the consistency of normal performance, the variability in N.S.'s performance was not large enough to result in any phonetic changes.[1] In fact, there was no single occasion of any phonetic changes that are indicative of difficulty in motor programming for speech in either of the two Wernicke's aphasic patients, while we often observed such phonetic changes in T.K., the apraxic patient, during the experiment. These results can be interpreted as indicating that the mechanism responsible for the organization (or reorganization) of neural commands to the articulators in Wernicke's patients is functioning properly.

Velar movement patterns during the process of speech sound error in Wernicke's aphasic patients. One of the two Wernicke's aphasic patients, N.S., made several speech sound errors and the other patient, K.K., made one such error during the experiment. N.S. was well aware of his errors and attempted to correct them immediately. Figures 5-4 and 5-5 depict two such instances. In Figure 5-4, N.S. produced /deedee/ for /dee*n*ee/ and then corrected it. The pattern of the anticipatory velar lowering for /n/ occurred immediately after /d/ on the first attempt, but on the second attempt the velum was kept in a high position because of the nonnasal phonemic environment /deedeedesu/. Figure 5-5 shows another example: in this case, N.S produced /teedeN/ for /tee*n*eN/ and immediately corrected it. Again the two patterns are quite different. Both of these results clearly indicate that this type of error is due not to an impairment at the level of articulatory programming but to an error in the selection or retrieval of a target phoneme.

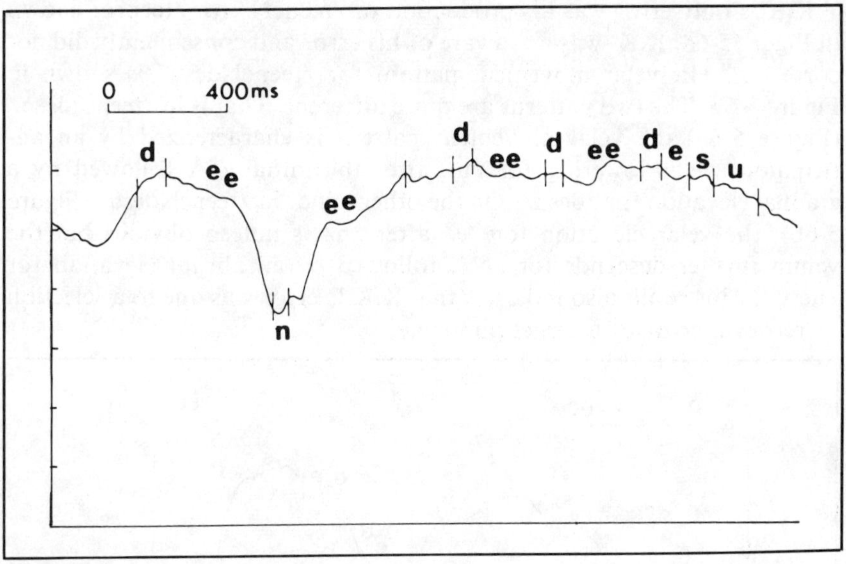

FIGURE 5-4
Movements of the velum during the speech sound error and self-correction process of the Wernicke aphasic patient, N.S., for /deedeedesu/.

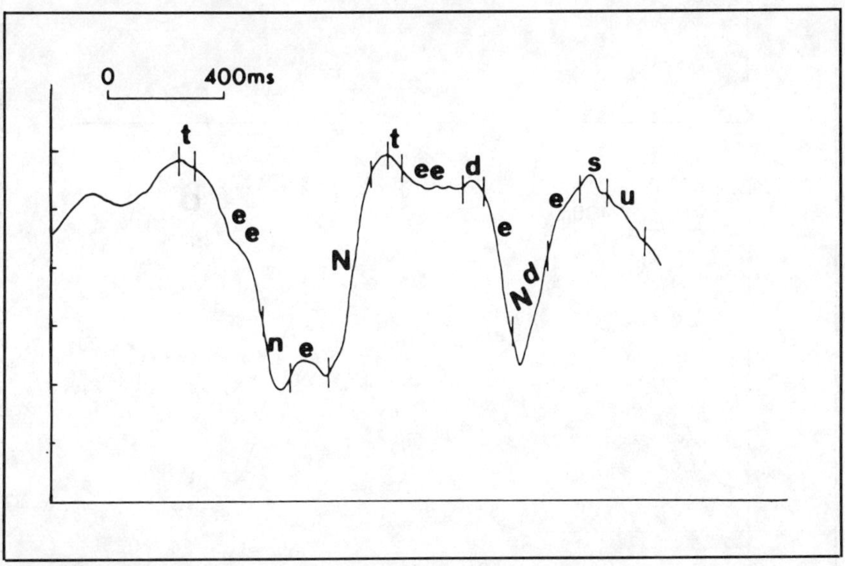

FIGURE 5-5
Movements of the velum during the speech sound error and self-correction process of the Wernicke aphasic patient, N.S., for /teedeNdesu/.

K.K.'s only error was his production of /teeneN/ for /teene*e*/ shown in Figure 5-6a. K.K. was not aware of his error and consequently did not correct it. His velar movement pattern for /teeneNdesu/ is shown in Figure 5-6b. The two patterns are quite different. That is in /teeneedesu/ (Figure 5-6a) the velar movement pattern is characterized by an anticipatory velar lowering for /n/ after the initial /t/, followed by a gradual elevation for /desu/. On the other hand, in /teeneNdesu/ (Figure 5-6b), the velar elevation for /e/ after /n/ is not so obvious but the velum further descends for /N/, followed by an abrupt elevation for /desu/. This result also indicates that K.K.'s error was due to a selection or retrieval error of a target phoneme.

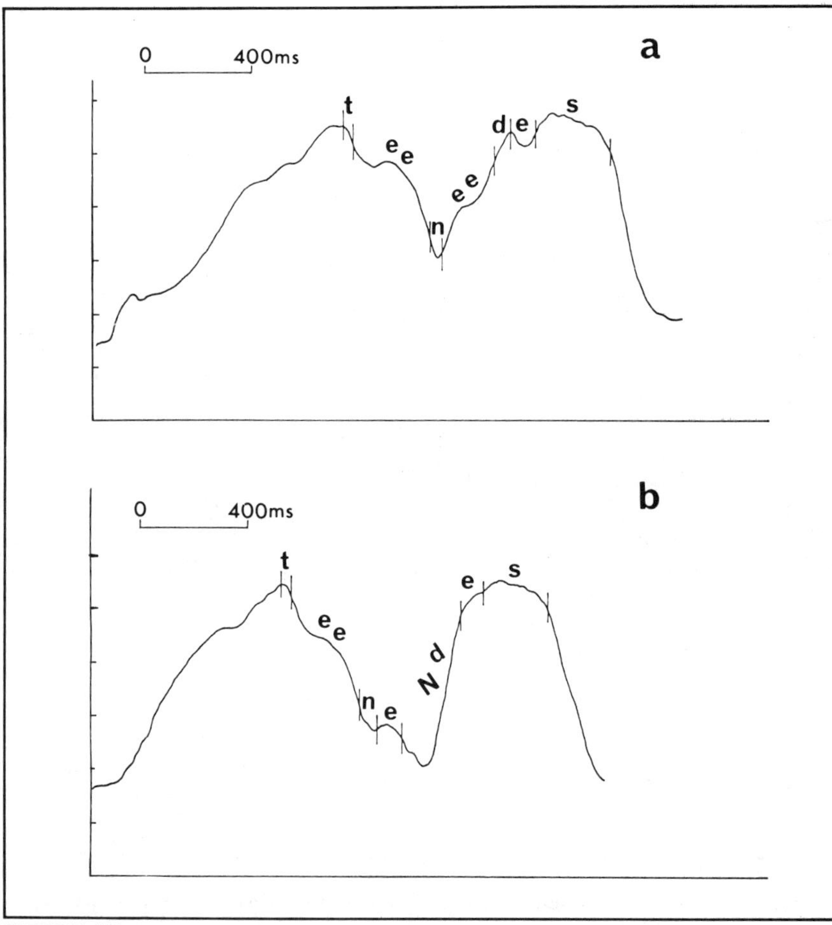

FIGURE 5-6
The velar movements in the Wernicke aphasic patient, K.K., for /teeneedesu/ (top) and for /teeneNdesu/ (bottom).

EXPERIMENT II. X-RAY MICROBEAM OBSERVATION OF THE TEMPORAL ORGANIZATION OF DIFFERENT ARTICULATORS

The temporal organization of articulatory movements in the apraxic patient T.K. was further explored by means of pellet tracking techniques using an x-ray microbeam system. The velocity of the articulators during speech was also estimated. In addition, the data obtained from the apraxic patient were compared with the data obtained from dysarthric patients so as to discover differences, if any, in articulatory movements between the two kinds of motor speech disorders. Control data were obtained from a 40-year-old normal male subject.

Procedure

A simultaneous observation of the movements of several articulators was made by means of an x-ray microbeam system, which was developed at the Research Institute of Logopedics and Phoniatrics, University of Tokyo. The detailed description of the system has been reported elsewhere (Kiritani, Itoh, & Fujimura, 1975). Essentially, the system employs a high-voltage, flying-spot-type x-ray microbeam generator with the rating of 150 kV-2mA controlled by a PDP-9 computer. Through the use of this system, the movement of the articulators can be observed by tracking lead pellets, about 3 mm in diameter, attached to the surface of the articulators. Up to 6 pellets can be tracked simultaneously at a rate of 120 to 170 frames per sec. During the tracking, movements of the pellets are displayed on an oscilloscope in real time. Coordinate values of the pellet positions at each frame as well as trajectories of the pellet movements can be reproduced on an oscilloscope for off-line analyses. The velocity of the articulators' displacement is obtained by differentiating the displacement.

For the present observation, pellets were attached to the lower lip, the lower incisor, the tongue tip, the tongue dorsum, and the nasal surface of the velum of the subjects. It was impossible to observe the tongue tip movement of T.K., however, because he had metal dentures which disturbed the tracking of the pellet on the tongue tip. Pellets were pasted to the surface of these articulators with a biomedical adhesive (Allonalpha).

The subjects were asked to utter a meaningful Japanese test word /deene/ embedded in a carrier phrase/ sono. . .desu/ (it is the. . .or)/ii. . . desu/ (it is good. . .) several times at a normal conversational rate indicated by the experimenter. In addition, the subjects were asked to repeat the nonsense syllables /pa/, /ta/, /ka/, and /teN/ at their fastest rate of speech.

Results and Discussion

Figure 5-7 compares the movement patterns of several articulators in the normal subject who uttered /deenee/ in a carrier phrase /sono... desu/ (it is the...) on two occasions, where the up and down displacements of several articulators are plotted as a function of time. The rate was controlled by timing signals given to the subject through a set of earphones. The vertical lines in the figure indicate the moment when the velum lowering for the /n/ of /deenee/ was at its maximum and can be used to compare the timing of the movements among the different articulators. It can be seen from the figure that there was an apparent temporal correspondence among the several articulators, that is, the velar lowering for /n/ corresponds well with the upward movement of the tongue tip for the apical closure.

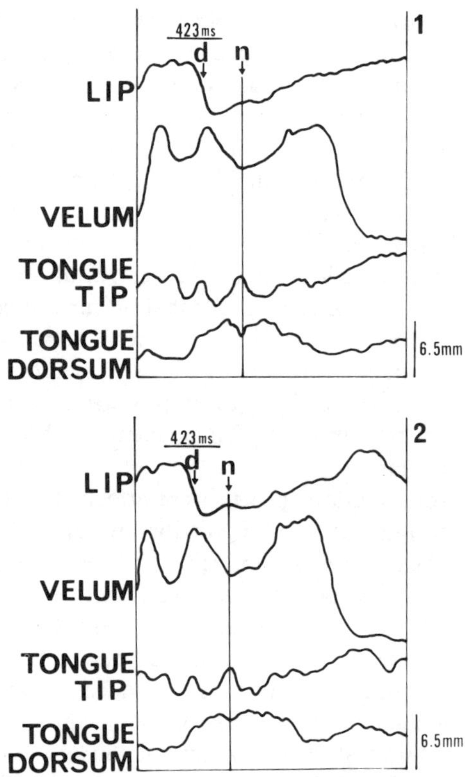

FIGURE 5-7

Up and down displacements of several articulators of the normal subject as a function of time during two productions of /deenee/ in the carrier phrase /sono...desu/ (it is the...). The vertical lines indicate the movement when the velum lowering was at its maximum.

Figure 5-8 illustrates that in T.K., the apraxic subject, there was an apparent disorganization of timing among the several articulators. Although T.K.'s tongue tip movement was not observed, the movement pattern of the tongue dorsum allows us to infer an upward movement of his tongue tip for the closure of /n/.[2] That is, the movement pattern of T.K.'s tongue dorsum for /n/ was characterized by a marked dip, and this makes it possible to examine the timing relationship between the velar lowering and the tongue tip movements for /n/ (i.e., by comparing the moment when the velum lowering for /n/ was at its maximum with the dip in the movement pattern of the tongue dorsum). Furthermore, an idiosyncratic pattern in the lower lip movement of T.K. (an upward movement for /n/, then a downward movement for the segments following /n/, resulting in a sort of peak) can be utilized for examining the timing relationship between the velum and lip movements.

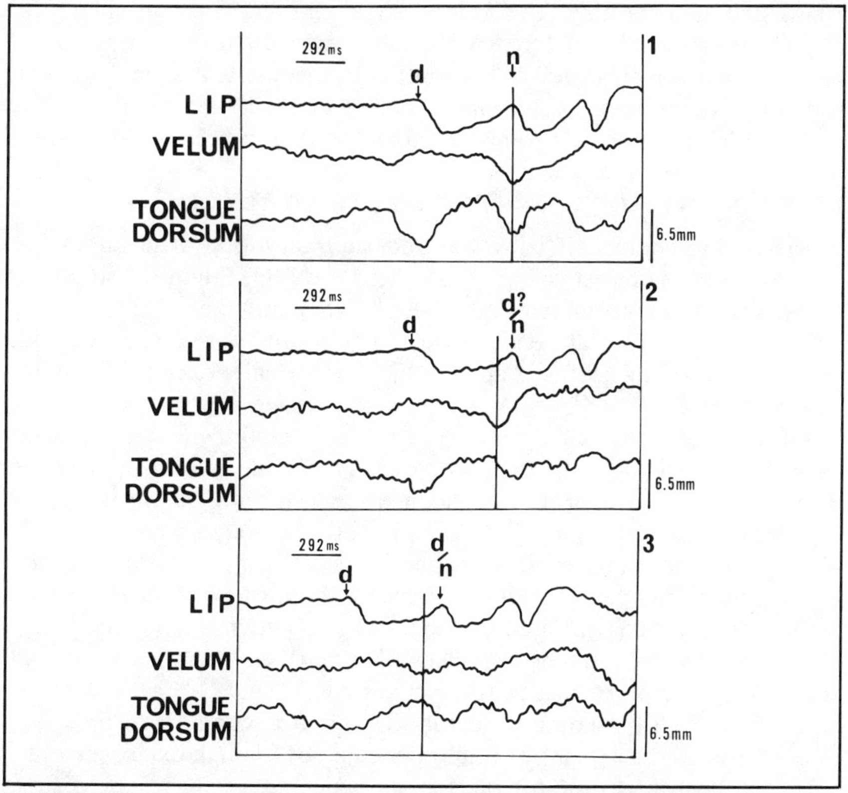

FIGURE 5-8

Up and down displacements of several articulators of the apraxic patient, T.K., as a function of time during three productions of /deenee/ in the carrier phrase /ii. . .desu/ (it is good. . .). The time scale of this figure is different from that shown in Figure 5-7.

It can be seen in Figure 5-8 that there was great variability in terms of the timing relationship between the velar lowering and lip and tongue movements for /n/ when the same word /deenee/ in the carrier phrase/ii... desu/ was repeated three times. In the first utterance (1), the dip of the velar lowering for /n/ corresponds well with the peak of the lip elevation and the dip of the tongue dorsum movement (presumably the peak of the tongue tip elevation). Such a timing relationship cannot be observed in the second utterance (2), where the dip of the velar lowering for /n/ preceded the peak of the lip elevation and the dip of the tongue dorsum movement. In this case /n/ was denasalized to some degree. In the third utterance (3), the velar lowering for /n/ preceded again the peak of the lip elevation and the dip of the tongue dorsum movement. It can also be noticed that the velum did not descend as much as in the first and second utterances and [n] changed to [d]. This finding seems to indicate that the motor programming for the temporal organization of different articulators becomes difficult in apraxia of speech under certain conditions resulting in inconsistent articulation errors. It remains to be determined, however, what the conditions are under which the time programming for articulation becomes difficult.

EXPERIMENT III. VOICE ONSET TIME ANALYSIS

The timing control of laryngeal and supralaryngeal articulatory adjustment was examined using voice onset time (VOT) data for stop consonants in the monosyllables /de/, /te/, /ge/, and /ke/ obtained from T.K. and three other apraxic subjects. The results were compared with those obtained from six fluent aphasic and five normal speakers. All the subjects were male.

All the apraxic patients, exhibited a marked impairment in articulation as well as in prosody. Two of these patients including T.K., demonstrated a relatively "pure" form of apraxia of speech without any symbolic disturbance due to aphasia, while the other two patients had mild aphasia in addition to apraxia of speech. According to the classification of aphasia by Schuell (Jenkins, Jiménez-Pabón, Shaw, & Sefer, 1975), the type of aphasia exhibited by the latter two patients can be classified as "aphasia with persisting dysfluency." The fluent aphasic patients included four Wernicke's aphasics, including K.K. and N.S. who were examined in the fiberscopic observation, and two conduction aphasics. Table 5-3 gives the age, type of aphasia, cause of brain damage, site of lesion, and postonset time for the four apraxic and six fluent aphasic patients. The normal subjects, aged 66 to 72 years, were volunteers from local senior citizen groups and had normal speech and hearing for their ages.

TABLE 5-3
The age, type of aphasia, cause of brain damage, site of lesion, and postonset time for the four apraxic patients and the six fluent aphasic patients

Subject	Age (ys)	Type of Aphasia	Cause of Brain Damage	Site of Lesion*	Postonset Time
Apraxic					
C1**	61	——	CVA	Near the anterior tip of the Sylvian fissure of the left hemisphere, both cortical and subcortical	6 years, 7 months
C2	66	——	CVA	Near the inferior frontal gyrus of the left hemisphere, both cortical and subcortical	4 years, 11 months
C3	45	Mild aphasia with persisting dysfluency	CVA	Near the anterior tip of the Sylvian fissure of the left hemisphere, both cortical and subcortical	6 months
C4	40	Mild aphasia with persisting dysfluency	Brain tumor	Parietal lobe of the left hemisphere	2 months
Fluent Aphasic					
B1	50	Wernicke's	CVA	Temporal lobe of the left hemisphere	3 months
B2	50	Wernicke's	CVA	Temporal lobe of the left hemisphere and the internal capsule of the right hemipshere	11 months
B3***	50	Wernicke's	Operational removal of ruptured aneurysm	Posterior region of the temporal lobe of the left hemisphere	1 year, 6 months
B4****	66	Wernicke's	Operational removal of hematoma	Superior temporal gyrus, optic radiation, angular gyrus and corona radiata of the left hemisphere	3 years, 9 months
B5	65	Conduction	CVA	Temporal and parietal lobes of the left hemisphere	2 years, 3 months
B6	49	Conduction	Operational removal of hematoma	Temporal and parietal lobes of the left hemisphere	4 years, 6 months

*Identified by CT scan. **This patient is T.K. ***This patient is K.K. ****This patient is N.S.

Procedure

Each subject read a randomized list of the Japanese monosyllables /de/, /te/, /ge/, and /ke/. The list contained 25 occurrences of each of these syllables for a total of 100 items in the test. Subjects were instructed to indicate when they misread any item. If any subject indicated such a misreading, he was asked to reread the item.

Wide-band spectrograms of the 25 productions of each syllable were made from the recordings. The VOT measurements were made according to the procedure used by Lisker and Abramson (1964). VOT measurements obtained from the spectrograms of each syllable were grouped into 10-msec intervals and frequency distributions were plotted for each subject.

Results and Discussion

Figures 5-9, 5-10, and 5-11 present individual data for each subject from the three subject groups in the form of the frequency distributions of the VOT values for /de/ and /te/ (left), and /ge/ and /ke/ (right). The abscissa represents the VOT values in milliseconds and the ordinate represents the total number of occurrences. The black columns indicate the VOT values for the voiced targets /de/ and /ge/, and the blank columns indicate those for the voiceless targets /te/ and /ke/.

As Figures 5-9 and 5-10 indicate, voiced and voiceless productions by the normal subjects as well as by the fluent aphasic subjects are distributed into relatively discrete areas of VOT, although there are sporadic occurrences of overlap between the VOT values for the two voicing categories. These results suggest that the timing relation between the articulatory release and the onset of the vocal fold vibration for the voiced and voiceless cognates is distinctively controlled in the normal and fluent aphasic subjects.

In contrast, the group of apraxic subjects exhibited a considerable overlap in VOT distribution between the voiced and voiceless cognates (Figure 5-11). It is also clear that there was a greater dispersion of productions along the continuum for both the voiceless and voiced stops among the apraxic subjects in comparison with the other subject groups. This result can be interpreted as indicating that the control over the timing of laryngeal and supralaryngeal articulatory events is disturbed in this subject group.

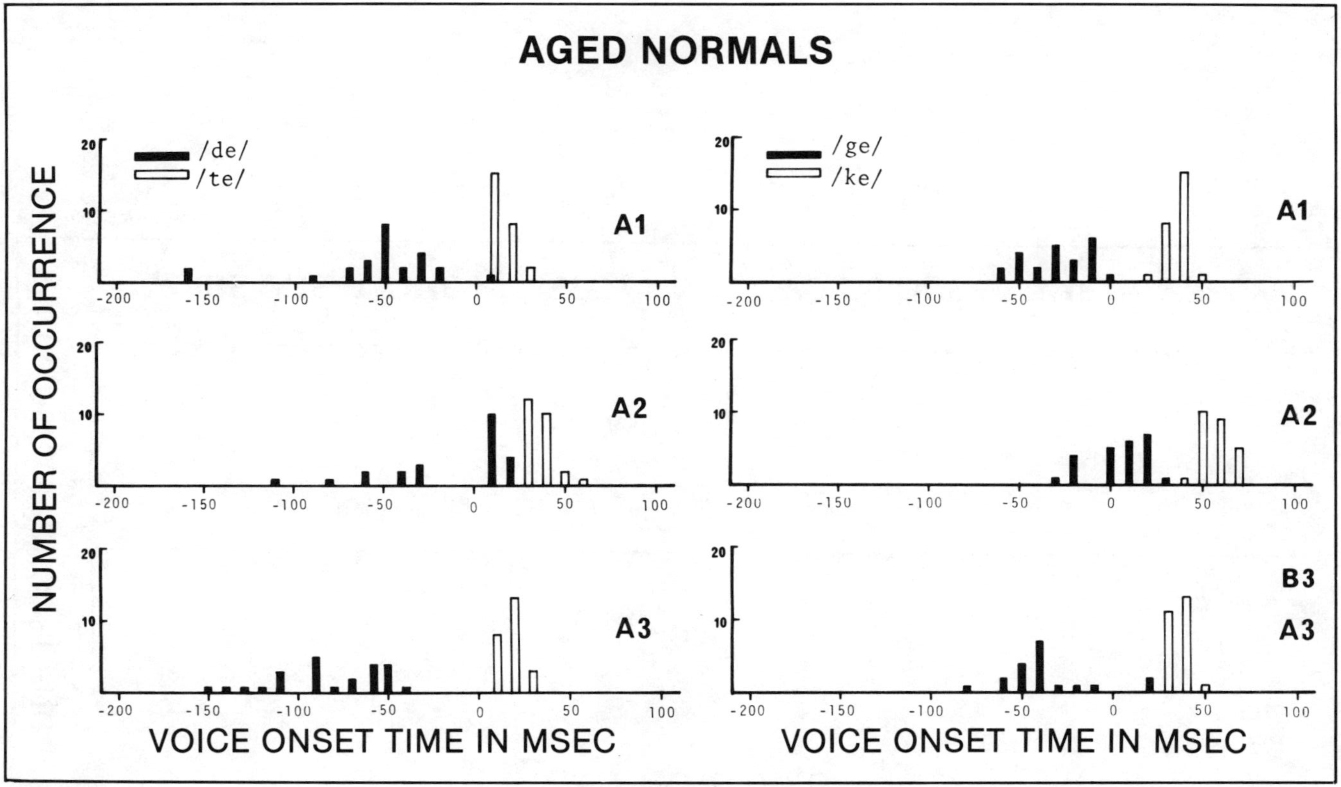

FIGURE 5-9
VOT distributions of the five normal subjects for /de/ and /te/ (left), and /ge/ and /ke/ (right).

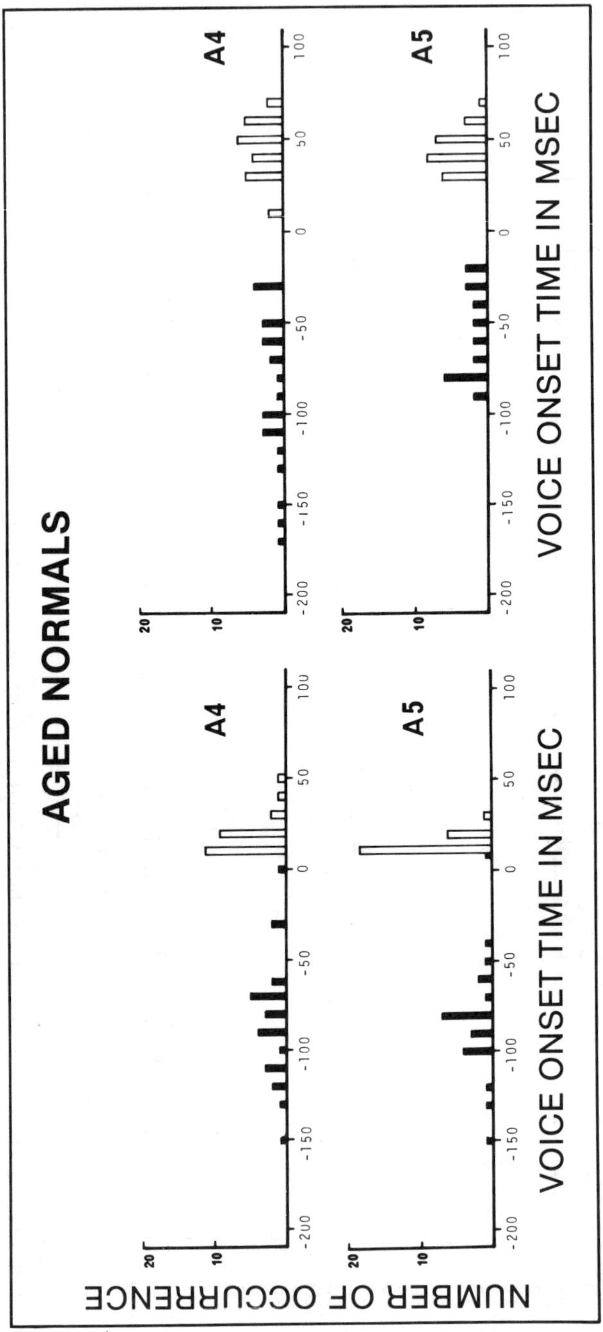

FIGURE 5-9 continued

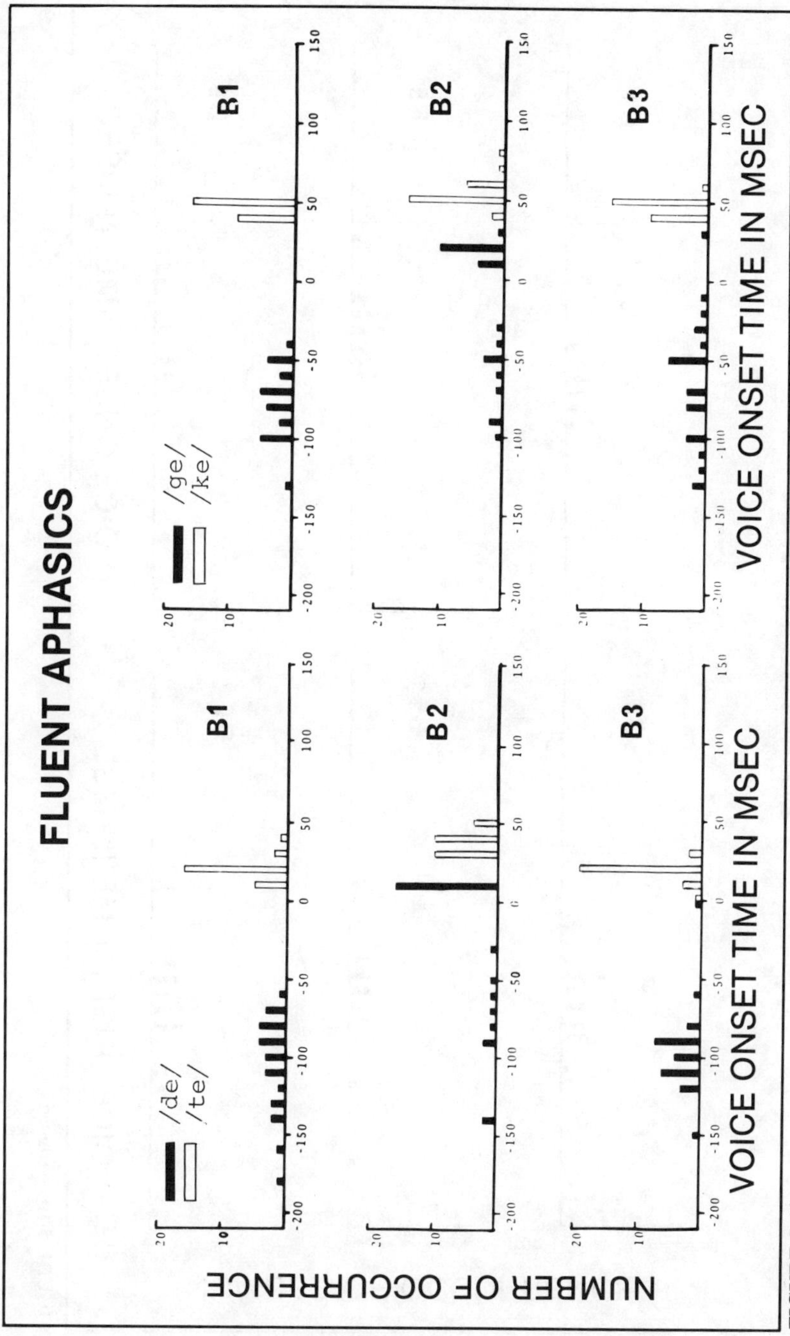

FIGURE 5-10
VOT distributions of the six fluent aphasic subjects for /de/ and /te/ (left), and /ge/ and /ke/ (right).

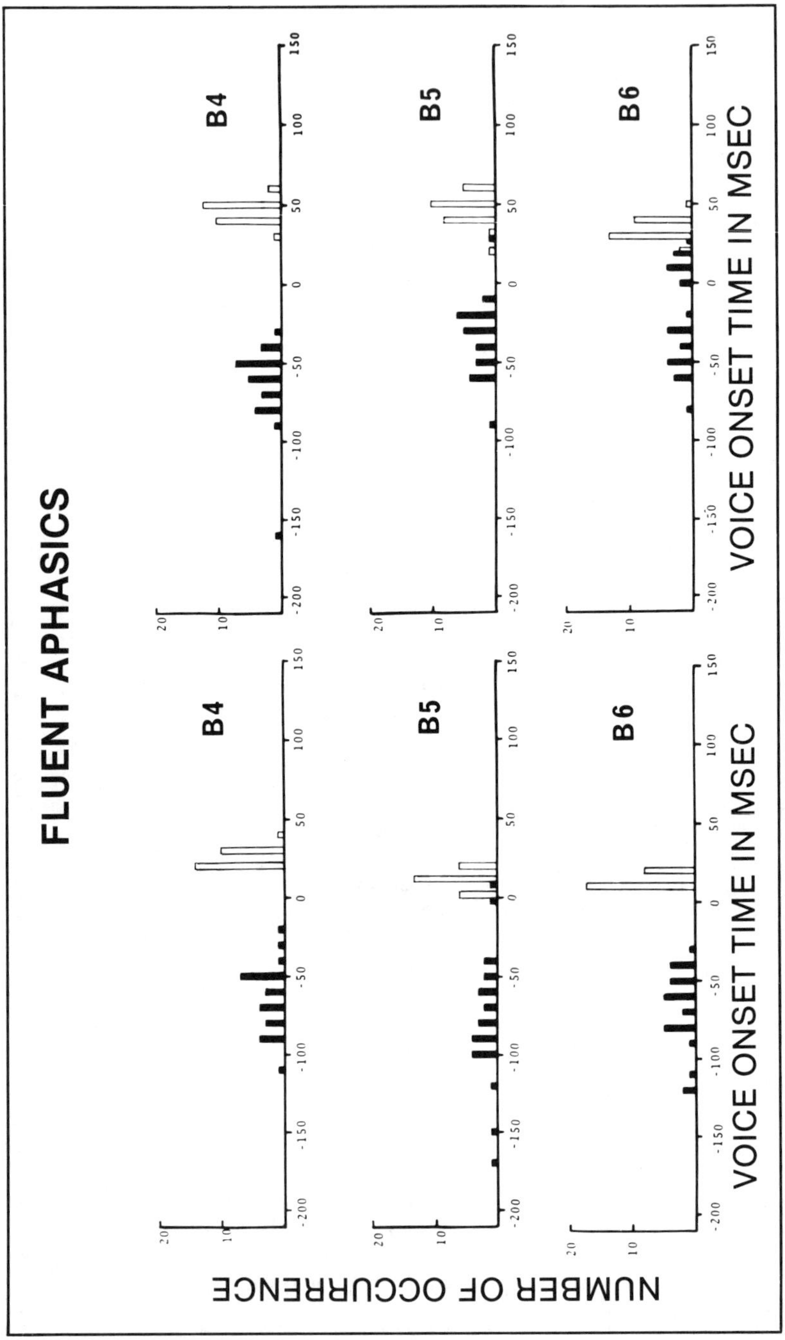

FIGURE 5-10 continued

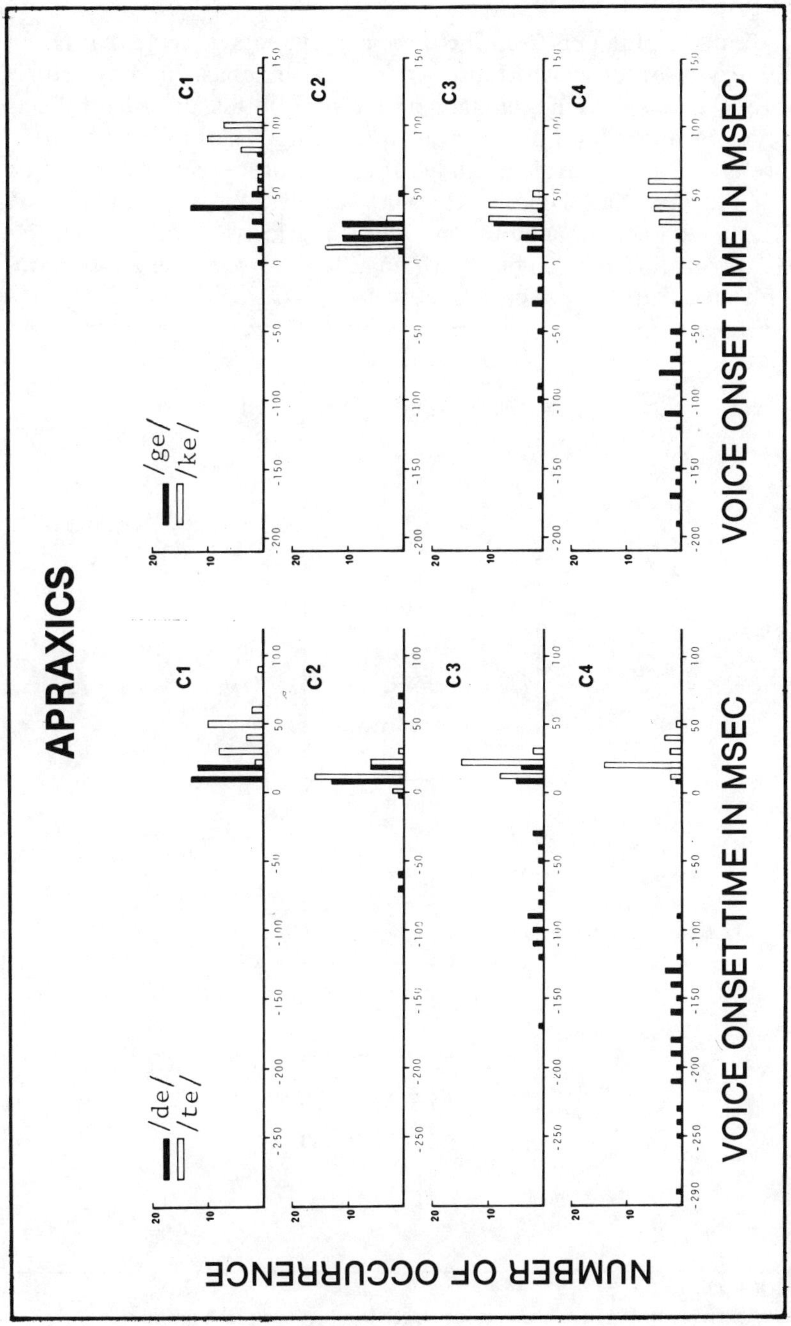

FIGURE 5-11
VOT distributions of the four apraxic subjects for /de/ and /te/ (left), and /ge/ and /ke/ (right).

GENERAL DISCUSSION

Our findings obtained from the three experiments indicate that (1) an articulatory disorder which is distinct from both aphasia and dysarthria can occur due to brain damage, and that (2) this disorder reflects malfunctions at the level of the motor programming of the articulators. With reference to a prevalent model of speech production suggested by various authors (e.g., Dubois, Hecaen, Angelergues, de Chatellier, & Marcie, 1973; Lecours & Rouillon, 1976), the locus of impairment indicated by our findings can be identified at Level 3, the level of programming for articulatory movement (Figure 5-12).[3]

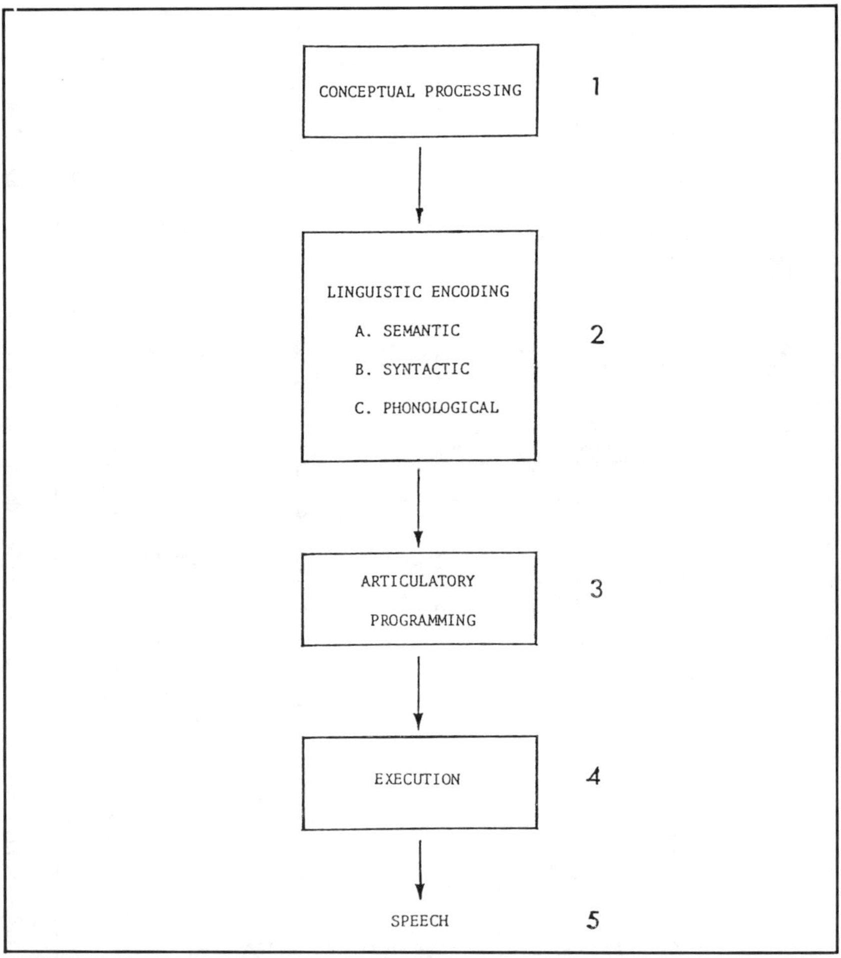

FIGURE 5-12
A schematic representation of the various stages involved in speech production.

There are some investigators, however, who claim that what we consider to be "apraxia of speech" is actually a language problem (Dunlop & Marquardt, 1977; Martin, 1974; Martin & Rigrodsky, 1974). According to these authors, the articulatory characteristics described by Johns and Darley (1970) represent a malfunction at the level of phonological (linguistic) processing (Level 2-c in Figure 5-12) because the sound errors exhibited by the patients are rule governed, showing target relatedness when analyzed in terms of distinctive features. Needless to say, this unsettled controversy over the nature of the disorder has crucial bearing not only on the model of speech production but also, and more directly, on the decisions that have to be made in the clinical management of the patients afflicted by the impairment.

What implications do the results of our studies with T.K. have in relation to this controversy and to the differential diagnosis of the disorder? They appear to point to the two fundamental issues that, in our view, consititute a major source of the controversy. One has to do with selection of experimental subjects for the study of apraxia of speech, and the other with the need for delimiting the core signs of apraxia of speech.

Subject Selection

Our patient, T.K., in the latter period of his clinical course can safely be considered to represent a rare example of a "pure" form of apraxia of speech. Thus, we are quite certain that the experimental data obtained from him constitute fairly representative samples of articulatory movement patterns in apraxia of speech. As most of the investigators will admit, however, it is the exception rather than the rule to find a "pure" form of apraxia of speech in a clinical setting. That is to say, it is highly probable that the majority of the patients who served as subjects in the previous studies on apraxia of speech were in fact those who at the same time showed various types and degrees of linguistic involvement, usually Broca's or nonfluent aphasia.[4] In other words, those articulatory characteristics of apraxia of speech set forward by Johns and Darley (1970) which have been confirmed by many investigators since then, in fact, might be reflecting an underlying impairment which is not confined to the level of motor programming (Level 3 in Figure 5-12), but extend into the level of linguistic (phonological) processing (Level 2-c in Figure 5-12) as well.

More rigorous criteria for subject selection in research will be mandatory if we are to extract only those articulatory characteristics which are the direct acoustic results of apraxic movements per se and nothing else. Note that our patient T.K. at 7 months postonset, after the comprehensive language examination, was judged to be "relatively" free from linguistic impairment, and yet his speech production (on the oral reading task) revealed a large proportion of adjacent and nonadjacent metatheses and backward assimilations, the majority of which could be interpreted to be linguistically (phonologically) based. This would mean that even those subjects who have been reported in the literature as exhibiting a "relatively pure" form of apraxia of speech might, in fact, be patients whose speech symptoms are not completely free from linguistically based errors.

In a clinical setting, therefore, it might appear that we clinicians require a sharpened awareness of the likelihood that the majority of the patients we judge as having the characteristics of apraxia of speech might exhibit, in addition, various types of phonologically based speech errors. An awareness of this kind might constitute a first step toward improved precision in diagnosis of apraxia of speech.

What is the Core Symptom of Apraxia of Speech?

There seems to be wide agreement among investigators that substitution errors (with and without assimilatory influences) constitute the most prevalent type of articulation error observed in apraxia of speech. It is true, however, that most of us clinicians have, at one time or another, experienced moments of uncertainty in trying to make a judgment as to whether a given instance of speech error in an apraxic patient should be classified as a case of "substitution" of the target phoneme or of "distortion."

Our findings with T.K. are clearly in support of the view that faulty programming of speech musculature constitutes the base of the symptom complex called "apraxia of speech" and that the most natural and reasonable end products of this underlying deficit are (phonetic) distortions. As was shown by T.K. in a phonetic change from [n] to [d] in Experiment I, it is distortion errors (taking place at Level 3, in Figure 5-12) rather than (phonemic) substitutions (taking place at Level 2-c), that constitute the inevitable consequences of faulty programming of speech musculature. This interpretation is also verified by VOT studies of our own Experiment III as well as by those of other authors (Blumstein, Cooper, Zurif, & Caramazza, 1977), indicating that the majority of errors that have been perceptually classified and labeled as "substitution" errors in the previous transcription studies with apraxic subjects might in fact be distortion errors. Nevertheless, even trained listeners tend to perceive these phonetic (distortion) errors as phonemic (substitution) errors, because the errors happen to cross the perceptual boundary of the target phoneme into another phonetic category, and because our ears have an unavoidable tendency toward categorical listening (Liberman & Studdert-Kennedy, 1978; MacNeilage, 1982).

On the other hand, our fiberscopic observation of articulatory velar movements with two Wernicke's aphasic patients (Experiment I) supports the view that speech errors exhibited by fluent aphasics are "true" substitution errors confined to Level 2-c, that is, the level of phoneme selection and sequencing.

Additional support for this interpretation will be found in a study by Monoi, Fukusako, Itoh, and Sasanuma (in press). These authors conducted phonemic and subphonemic analyses of speech sound errors exhibited by three conduction (fluent) and three Broca's (nonfluent) aphasic patients on naming and word repetition tasks. All of the patients were mild to moderate in terms of aphasic involvement. In addition, Broca's patients exhibited mild to moderate motor speech symptoms indicative of apraxia of speech. Three major findings were: (1) in the nonfluent patients, errors occurred selectively in consonants in both the naming and word repetition tasks, while in the fluent patients errors occurred equally often in consonants and vowels; (2) "substitution" errors constituted the majority of errors in the nonfluent patients, while in the fluent patients "transposition" errors (defined as the production of a phoneme that was a constituent elsewhere in the target word, e.g., /tamago/, /ta*g*ago/, /ta*gam*o/, /ta*go*/, etc.), occurred almost as often as substitution errors; (3) the nonfluent patients, as compared to the fluent patients, exhibited a markedly higher number of substitution errors occurring between phonemes separated by a single subphonemic feature on the naming task.

Of particular relevance to our discussion is their interpretation of "substitution" errors. In their view, the functional loci of the occurrence of substitution errors can be traced to at least two different levels of speech production: Level 2-c, which is the level of phoneme selection and sequencing, and Level 3, which is the level of the motor programming of articulatory gestures. That is, substitution errors exhibited by the fluent patients reflected an impairment which is more or less confined to Level 2-c whereas the substitution errors shown by the Broca's patients reflected an impairment which is not confined to Level 2-c but extends to Level 3 where programming for articulatory movement is carried out. The basis for this inference was their finding (3) above that, as compared to the fluent aphasic patients, nonfluent aphasic patients exhibited a greater number of single feature "substitution" errors in the naming task. According to Monoi et al., many of these one-feature errors in the nonfluent patients are, in fact, "deviation" (distortion) errors due to a malfunction at the level of articulatory programming. However, these deviation errors tend to be perceived and classified as single-feature substitution errors because the errors are allophones of neighboring phonemes and not allophones of the target phonemes. The so-called substitution errors exhibited by nonfluent patients, therefore, could in fact be of two (or even three) types with different origins: (1) those taking place at the level of phoneme selection, or "true" substitution errors; (2) those taking place at the level of articulatory programming, and thus, in fact, phonetic distortions which tend to be perceptually classified as one-feature substitutions; and perhaps (3) those taking place at both of these levels which tend to be classified as multiple-feature errors. The second of these three types of "substitution" errors — those which are, in fact, phonetic in nature arising from a malfunction in motor programming of articulators — appears to constitute an important factor contributing to the markedly high number of single-feature errors in the nonfluent patients. Of interest is that Martin (1974) and Martin and Rigrodsky (1974), on the basis of the target relatedness of error sounds exhibited by their aphasic patients, arrived at a very different conclusion, viz., that the existence of such a relation indicates a possible interaction of the characteristic errors of "apraxia of speech" with the linguistic component. It is important to note in addition, however, that 14 of their 15 subjects were classified as belonging to Schuell's Group I, while the remaining subject appeared to fit the description of her Group III patients. In other words, only one of their subjects possibly exhibited some features of apraxia of speech in addition to severe reduction of language.

How should we settle this controversy over the nature of apraxia of speech? We believe that there is a definite need for more research in the direction of specifying articulatory movements in apraxia of speech; in particular, direct observations of articulatory gestures in apraxic patients, and hopefully replications of our own experiments by other investigators. The information gained from such studies will provide a firmer basis with reference to which to delimit and specify the symptomatology of apraxia of speech with increased precision.

On the other hand, in a clinical setting we can probably start by sharpening our awareness of the core symptom of apraxia of speech, that is, articulatory distortions, and by sharpening our "ears" accordingly. Since most of the patients whom we may encounter in a clinical setting are likely to show a mixture of symptoms arising from multiple-level deficits in speech production processes, we have to tease apart this core symptom (i.e., articulatory distortions which are phonetic in nature) and accompanying symptoms such as phonemic substitutions of linguistic origin. The task of this phonetic/phonemic differentiation in a clinical setting is not always easy, because of our intrinsic tendency to perceive speech sounds categorically. However, there is some other information that can be of help in the differentiation. For instance, the presence of metatheses and backward assimilations of adjacent and, in particular, of a nonadjacent type in these patients, may indicate the presence of linguistic components as an underlying deficit. On the other hand, interpretation of similarity of the error sound to the target sound in terms of the subphonemic (or distinctive) feature framework may be tricky because it can indicate the motor origin of the impairment rather than the linguistic origin. Phonetic distortions can, of course, be indicative of a malfunction at the level of motor execution (Level 4 in Figure 5-12), or dysarthric involvement as well, especially when these errors are consistent.[5]

Finally, it is hoped that a continued effort be made to develop a method of application by means of which the high-precision techniques for the direct observation of articulatory gestures, now available only in the laboratory, can be brought into the clinical setting so as to aid in the diagnosis of apraxia of speech.

NOTES

[1]The reason for the variation in N.S.'s performance remains to be determined. One possible source of this variation, however, could be some changes in utterance speed on different trials since his performance is characterized mainly by a variation in segmental duration.

[2]As seen in Figure 5-7, in the normal subject the tongue dorsum usually moved downward when the tongue tip moved upward for the closure for /n/ of /deenee/ and then moved upward for the subsequent segments /ee/, resulting in a dip in the movement pattern.

[3]This level seems to correspond to what is called the level of "third articulation" (or phonetic level) by Lecours and Rouillon (1976) and the level of "second articulation" by Dubois et al. (1973).

[4]We will not get into the problem of dysarthric involvement here, although we are well-aware of the problem.

[5]Apraxic and dysarthric distortions have different origins and could be distinguished by the consistency of their errors. Dysarthric distortions are highly consistent, whereas apraxic distortions are highly variable (i.e., when T.K. repeated /deeneedesu/ five times in Experiment I, one of his utterances was completely free from any distortion, while the rest of his utterances were distorted to different degrees).

REFERENCES

Aten, J. L., Johns, D. F., & Darley, F. L. Auditory perception of sequenced words in apraxia of speech. *Journal of Speech and Hearing Research,* 1971, *14,* 131–143.

Blumstein, S. E., Cooper, W. E., Zurif, E. B., & Caramazza, A. The perception and production of voice onset time in aphasia. *Neuropsychologia,* 1977, *15,* 371–383.

Darley, F. L., Aronson, A. E., & Brown, J. R. *Motor speech disorders.* Philadelphia: Saunders, 1975.

Dubois, J., Hécaen, H., Angelergues, R., de Chatellier, A. M., & Marcie, P. Neurolinguistic study of conduction aphasia. In H. Goodglass & S. Blumstein (Eds.), *Psycholinguistics and aphasia.* Baltimore: Johns Hopkins University Press, 1973.

Dunlop, J. M., & Marquardt, T. P. Linguistic and articulatory aspects of single word production in apraxia of speech. *Cortex,* 1977, *13,* 17–29.

Fromkin, V. A. *Speech errors as linguistic evidence.* The Hague: Mouton, 1973. pp. 213–242

Garrett, M. F. The analysis of sentence production. In G. H. Bower (Ed.), *The psychology of learning and motivation: Advances in research and theory* Vol. 9. New York: Academic Press, 1975. pp. 133–177.

Itoh, M., Sasanuma, S., & Ushijima, T. Velar movements during speech in a patient with apraxia of speech. *Brain and Language,* 1979, *7,* 227–239.

Itoh, M., Sasanuma, S., Hirose, H., Yoshioka, H., & Ushijima, T. Abnormal articulatory dynamics in a patient with apraxia of speech: X-ray microbeam observation. *Brain and Language,* 1980, *11,* 66–75.

Itoh, M., Sasanuma, S., Tatsumi, I. F., Murakami, S., Fukusako, Y. & Suzuki, T. Voice onset time characteristics in apraxia of speech. *Brain and Language,* 1982, *17,* 193–210.

Itoh, M., Sasanuma, S., Hirose, H., Yoshioka, H., & Sawashima, M. Velar movements during speech in two Wernicke aphasic patients. *Brain and Language,* 1983, *19,* 283–292.

Jenkins, J. J., Jiménez-Pabón, E., Shaw, R. E., & Sefer, J. W. *Schuell's aphaşia in adults: Diagnosis, prognosis, and treatment.* New York: Harper & Row, 1975, 2nd ed.

Johns, D. F., & Darley, F. L. Phonemic variability in apraxia of speech. *Journal of Speech and Hearing Research,* 1970, *13,* 556–583.

Kiritani, S., Itoh, K., & Fujimura, O. Tongue-pellet tracking by a computer-controlled x-ray microbeam system. *Journal of Acoustical Society of America,* 1975, *57,* 1516–1520.

LaPointe, L. L., & Johns, D. F. Some phonemic characteristics in apraxia of speech. *Journal of Communication Disorders,* 1975, *8,* 259–269

Lecours, A. R., & Rouillon, F. Neurolinguistic analysis of jargonaphasia and jargonagraphia. In H. Whitaker, & H. A.Whitaker (Eds.), *Studies in neurolinguistics* (Vol. 2). New York: Academic Press, 1976.

Liberman, A. M., & Studdert-Kennedy, M. Phonetic perception. In R. Held, H. Leibowitz, & H. L. Teuber (Eds.), *Handbook of sensory physiology Vol. VIII: Perception.* Heidelberg: Springer-Verlag, 1978, pp.143–178.

Lisker, L., & Abramson, A. S. A cross-language study of voicing in initial stops: Acoustical measurements. *Word,* 1964, 20, 384–422.

MacNeilage, P. F. Speech production mechanisms in aphasia. In S. Grillner, B. Lindblom, J. Lubker, & A. Perrson (Eds.), *Speech motor control* (Wenner-Gren Center International Symposium Series, Vol. 36). New York: Pergamon Press, 1982.

Martin, A. D. Some objections to the term apraxia of speech. *Journal of Speech and Hearing Disorders,* 1974, *39,* 53–64.

Martin, A. D., & Rigrodsky, S. An investigation of phonological impairment in aphasia, part 2: Distinctive feature analysis of phonemic commutation errors in aphasia. *Cortex,* 1974, *10,* 329–346.

Monoi, H., Fukusako, Y., Itoh, M., & Sasanuma, S. Speech sound errors in conduction and Broca's aphasics. *Brain and Language,* (in press).

Rosenbek, J. C., Wertz, R. T., & Darley, F. L. Oral sensation and perception in apraxia of speech and aphasia. *Journal of Speech and Hearing Research,* 1973, *16,* 22–36.

Sawashima, M., & Ushijima, T. Use of the fiberscope in speech research. *Annual Bulletin, Research Institute of Logopedics and Phoniatrics, University of Tokyo,* 1971, *5,* 25–34.

Sawashima, M., Ushijima, T., & Hirose, H. Movements of the velum in speech articulation. *Transactions of the Committee on the Speech Research, Acoustical Society of Japan,* 1976, *S75–56,* (In Japanese).

Shankweiler, D., Harris, K. S., & Taylor, M. L. Electromyographic studies of articulation in aphasia. *Archives of Physical Medicine and Rehabilitation,* 1968, *49,* 1–8.

Trost, J. E., & Canter, G. J. Apraxia of speech in patients with Broca's aphasia: A study of phoneme production accuracy and error patterns. *Brain and Language,* 1974, *1,* 63–69.

6

Apraxic Speakers' Vowel Duration In Consonant-Vowel-Consonant Syllables

Joseph R. Duffy
Carol A. Gawle

Historically, there has been considerable debate about the underlying nature of the communication disorder frequently called apraxia of speech. A persistent and major focal point of this debate has been whether apraxic speech reflects improper selection or ordering of the abstract phonemes of the language, or inadequate selection, timing, or sequencing of the movements required for their physical realization. Detailed reviews of these competing intepretations can be found in Rosenbek, Kent, and LaPointe's essay in this volume (Chap. 1) and in several other sources (Aten, Darley, Deal & Johns, 1975; Blumstein, 1981; Buckingham, 1981a, 1981b, 1979; Darley, 1982; Johns & LaPointe, 1976; Martin, 1974; Martin, Wasserman, Gilden, Gerstman, & West, 1975).

Most of our current knowledge about the phonological and phonetic characteristics of apraxic speech, and much of the modern-day debate about the nature of the disorder, are based on broad phonetic transcriptions and distinctive feature analyses. These descriptive methods have the advantages of relative simplicity and direct and easy applicability to clinical diagnosis and management. However, they are subject to unreliability and tend to "force" the perception of articulatory events into phonological categories. Such approaches are also insensitive to potentially valuable information lying below the observer's perceptual threshold. Finally, broad transcription methods cast data in a manner several steps removed from the specific acoustic properties and movement dynamics of speech, a potentially incomplete or misleading representation on which to base theoretical interpretations, particularly for a problem often interpreted as "motor" in nature.

In recent years, several investigators have turned from descriptive data bases to relatively objective acoustic and physiological methods of analysis. Of special import is the notion that acoustic and physiological analyses do not require abstract categorization of the data, but, under the right circumstances, do permit inferences about the integrity of both the linguistic and movement control systems. For example, voice onset time (VOT) associated with the production of syllable-initial prevocalic stops is an acoustically measurable property of speech whose temporal characteristics are well-described for non-brain-injured adults. VOT normally varies as a function of the linguistic voicing feature of syllable-ititial prevocalic stops, and there are distinct and perceptually important boundaries between phonemes perceived as voiced and voiceless. Although temporal-acoustic analyses of speech must be interpreted cautiously with respect to inferences about the presence and nature of linguistic and motor control problems, studies of VOT in aphasic, apraxic, and/or aphasic-apraxic speakers have contributed to descriptions of the temporal characteristics of apraxic speech and theories about its underlying nature (Blumstein, Cooper, Zurif, & Caramazza, 1977; Blumstein, Cooper, Goodglass, Statlander, & Gottlieb, 1980; Freeman, Sands, & Harris, 1978; Jaffe, 1977).

The present investigation focuses on another acoustically measurable property of speech known to vary as a function of phonological differences. Specifically, we focused on the duration of vowels preceding syllable-final stops. In English, vowel duration varies consistently as a function of the voicing feature of the final consonant, with vowels preceding voiced final consonants ranging from 20 to 90 percent longer — and averaging 40 to 50% longer — than vowels preceding voiceless final consonants (Chen, 1970; House, 1961; House & Fairbanks, 1953; Klatt, 1973, 1976; Malecot, 1958; Peterson & Lehiste, 1960; Raphael, 1972; Umeda, 1975). This average durational difference is consistently produced by normal adult speakers and has been shown to be a major

(House, 1961) and sometimes necessary (Raphael, 1972) cue to the voicing feature of the following consonant; it is also employed by esophageal speakers (Gandour & Weinberg, 1980), by children as young as 3 years (Krause, 1982), and by some children who omit word-final stops (Weismer, Dinnsen, & Elbert, 1981). Of considerable importance is the fact that vowel duration variation as a function of the voicing feature of the following consonant is not simply a physiological byproduct, but rather is primarily phonologically conditioned, that is, a reflection of a phonological "rule" regarding the voicing distinction (Klatt, 1976; House, 1961; Chen, 1970; Lehiste, 1970). Consequently, analysis of vowel duration preceding syllable-final stops can be used as an index of both phonological adequacy and proper motor control. That is, normal maintenance of vowel duration differences preceding voiced and voiceless final stops permits an inference that phonological "selection" of the final consonant voicing feature is adequate. At the same time, correct "patterns" of vowel duration — in terms of average duration and variability — presumably reflect adequate motor control. Therefore, failure to maintain durational differences, under some circumstances, can be viewed as a reflection of a phonological breakdown, while inability to maintain normal absolute durational average and variability can be viewed as reflecting impaired motor control.

The above rationale was central to the purpose and methods used in this study. Specifically, we asked (1) if aphasic patients with apraxia of speech differ from non-brain-injured adults and aphasic patients without apraxia of speech in their vowel duration preceding voiced and voiceless final stops and (2) if aphasic patients with apraxia of speech differentiate vowel duration preceding voiceless final stops from those preceding voiced final stops and, if so, if they do so in the same manner as non-brain-injured adults and aphasic patients without apraxia of speech. The resultant data were examined relative to their consistency with linguistic and motor control explanations of apraxia of speech.

METHOD

Subjects

A group of adults without brain injury (Normals), a group of adults with aphasia and apraxia of speech, and a group of adults with aphasia without apraxia of speech were studied. All subjects passed perception and production pretests which are described below. Subjects in the brain-injured groups had medical evidence of a single, unilateral left-hemisphere lesion with a cerebral vascular etiology. For the sake of brevity, subjects with aphasia and apraxia of speech will be referred to as "apraxic subjects," while subjects with aphasia but without apraxia will be called "aphasic subjects."

Criteria for establishing the presence of apraxia of speech were similar to those frequently described in the literature (Darley, 1982; Darley, Aronson, & Brown, 1975; Rosenbek, 1978; Wertz, 1978; Rosenbek, Kent, & LaPointe, this volume, Chap. 1). They included: effortful groping for articulatory postures; inconsistent and variable articulatory errors; apparent substitutions, additions, repetitions, and prolongations, usually in excess of omissions and distortions; better articulatory performance on automatic versus volitional speech; increased errors with increasing length of utterance; presence of errors on spontaneous and imitative tasks, with imitative sometimes poorer than spontaneous (a diagnosis of apraxia in this study, however, required apraxic features in both spontaneous and imitative speech).

Diagnosis of apraxia was based on a sample of spontaneous speech and imitation of sounds, syllables, multisyllabic words, words series, sentences, alternating motion rates (AMRs) for "puh," "tuh," and "kuh," and sequential motion rates (SMRs) for "puh-tuh-kuh." All diagnoses were made independent of performance on the experimental task.

TABLE 6-1
Summary of aphasic (APH) and apraxic (APX) subjects' characteristics and test results

Subjects	*OA PICA Percentile*	*PICA Verbal Percentile*	*BDAE Fluency Rating*	*BDAE Severity*
APH1	60	55	Pred. NonFl.	2
APH2	73	56	Fluent	4
APH3	57	51	Fluent	3–4
APH4	58	46	Pred. NonFl.	1–2
APX1	Not avail.	Not avail.	Pred. NonFl.	2
APX2	42	27	Nonfluent	1
APX3	86	80	Pred. Fl.	4
APX4	50	50	Nonfluent	1–2
APX5	40	42	Nonfluent	1

Note. Porch Index of Communicative Ability (PICA) overall percentile; PICA verbal percentile; Boston Diagnostic Aphasia Examination (BDAE) fluency rating from the Rating Scale Profile of Speech Characteristics; and the BDAE severity rating scale where 0 = no usable speech or auditory comprehension, and 5 = minimal discernable handicaps. Pred. NonFl. = predominantly nonfluent.

Table 6-1 summarizes the performance of each group of brain-injured subjects on the Porch Index of Communicative Ability (PICA) (Porch, 1967), the severity rating scale of the Boston Diagnostic Aphasia Examination (BDAE) (Goodglass & Kaplan, 1972), and the Rating Scale Profile of Speech Characteristics of the BDAE. Fluency ratings of "predominantly fluent" or "predominantly nonfluent" indicate that a subject's speech was consistent with a fluent or nonfluent profile, respectively, as described in the BDAE manual, on at least four but not all six of the characteristics rated on the BDAE scale. Additional characteristics of subjects in each group are described below.

Normals. Two males and three females without neurological damage: Their mean age was 62 with a range of 58 to 66 years.

Aphasic. Four males with a diagnosis of aphasia without apraxia of speech: Their mean age was 62 with a range of 60 to 65 years. Mean time postonset was 35 months with a range of 26 to 45 months.

In addition to characteristics summarized in Table 6-1, some additional features of some of the aphasic subjects are relevant. The fluency rating of aphasic Subject 1 (APH1) as predominantly nonfluent, instead of nonfluent, was due to his always intelligible speech and largely unimpaired "articulatory agility," with the exception of mild breathiness and consistent, mild consonant imprecision (importantly, the voicing feature of some of his consonants were occasionally ambiguous) — he may have had a mild unilateral upper motor neuron dysarthria.

APH3 had a clearly nonapraxic, fluent pattern of conversational speech, but did have difficulty sequencing SMRs and exhibited substitutions, additions, omissions, and some postural groping during repetition of some multisyllablic words and word groups; he was aware of these errors. Although these errors were apraxic-like, their absence in spontaneous speech was not felt to warrant a diagnosis of apraxia. This mismatch between imitative and spontaneous speech was not inconsistent with that reported for patients with so-called "conduction aphasia" (Goodglass, 1981; Goodglass & Kaplan, 1972).

APH4, like APH1, was rated predominantly nonfluent, instead of nonfluent, because of largely unimpaired articulation. However, he did exhibit a prosodic pattern characterized by excess and equal stress, a rate which was somewhat slow, and gave the impression of articulating "carefully." Also, some articulatory substitutions, omissions, and subtle groping were noted on multisyllabic word and word series imitation. Our impression was that he may have been a "recovered" or well-compensated apraxic, but his overall behavior in both conversation and imitation did not consistently match the characteristics typically associated with apraxia of speech.

Apraxic. Two males and three females with diagnoses of aphasia and apraxia of speech: Their mean age was 56 with a range from 45 to 63 years. Time postonset averaged 75 months and ranged from 12 to 275 months.

All subjects in this group were clearly apraxic. In addition to the characteristics summarized in Table 6-1, the following are of relevance. APX1 had a marked apraxic impairment which rendered a number of conversational utterances unintelligible. Her rating of predominantly nonfluent, instead of nonfluent, was due to her fairly frequent use of phrases of five or more words and occasional complex grammatical constructions, in spite of significant articulatory impairment and prosodic restrictions. She exhibited nearly all of the characteristics of apraxia of speech noted above as criteria for diagnosis.

APX2 had severe apraxia which resulted in largely unintelligible speech, handicapping her well beyond the verbal limitations imposed by her moderately severe aphasia. Her ratings on the BDAE fluency scale were clearly nonfluent for articulation, prosody, and phrase length; nonfluent ratings for grammatical variety, paraphasia, and word finding required considerable inference because of her unintelligibility. Her articulatory errors were quite consistent and unvarying, at least partially because of her restricted repertoire of consonants. Consonants in conversational and imitative responses were almost exclusively stops and nasals, with an occasional glide or /l/. As a result, many errors were articulatory simplifications. In addition, her speech did not improve on automatic tasks. Although these characteristics do not correspond to the criteria described above for diagnosis of apraxia, her speech was consistent with those of patients with severe apraxia of speech, as described by Rosenbek (1978). Rather than exclude her because she did not correspond to criteria established by studies which generally excluded severe impairments for purposes of experimental "purity," she was included for the opportunity to compare her performance on the experimental task to patients meeting more traditional criteria for identifying apraxia.

APX3 was mildly aphasic and apraxic. His predominantly fluent rating was a product of his mild language impairment, although his articulation and prosody were rated in the nonfluent range. While he had more distortions than is typically described for apraxia of speech, he exhibited most of the other criterion characteristics of apraxia.

APX4 had a marked apraxic impairment, only slightly less severe than that of APX1; her language, however, was slightly more impaired. Her fluency rating was consistent with a rating of nonfluent.

APX5 had a marked apraxia, similar in severity to that of APX1. His fluency profile was unambiguously nonfluent. With the exception of very few articulatory additions or complications during conversation, he exhibited all of the criterion characteristics for apraxia of speech.

Pretests

Two perception and one production pretest were administered. Perception Pretest 1 assessed subjects' ability to discriminate between voiced and voiceless final consonants in consonant-vowel-consonant (CVC) syllables. In this test each of the six experimental stimulus words (beet, bead, pick, pig, cop, cob) was paired with itself or its minimally contrasting counterpart (e.g., beet-beed). The test consisted of 12 items, with one "same" judgement for each of the six words, and two "different" judgements for each of the three minimally different pairs. Test items were recorded and presented to each subject at 5-sec intervals. Subjects indicated their same-different judgement verbally or by nodding.

In Perception Pretest 2, the ability to recognize the meaning of the six stimulus words was assessed. Stimulus words were recorded and presented along with a picture of the word and its minimally different counterpart. Subjects pointed to the picture of the word they felt they heard. Each word was presented twice; items were randomly ordered.

The production pretest was devised to eliminate individuals whose speech would preclude valid analysis of experimental test responses. Each of the six experimental stimuli were recorded twice, randomized, and presented at 5-sec intervals. Subjects repeated the stimulus. If the subject responded with a CVC in which the vowel was perceived as phonologically accurate, and the initial and final consonants were stops, the response was considered correct.

To be included in the study a minimal score of nine (75%) on each of the three pretests was required. This minimal score was exceeded (perfect scores were most typical) by all subjects on all pretests with the exception of APH1 and APX4 who received scores of nine on Perception Pretest 1.

Experimental Test

Six real word CVC syllables (beet, bead, pick, pig, cop, cob), three with voiced final consonants and three with voiceless final consonants, served as stimuli. Each word was recorded by an adult female with no pronounced regional speech differences. Vowel durations were measured oscilloscopically to assure that they conformed to typical adult values reported for the preconsonantal position (Peterson & Lehiste, 1960; Raphael, 1972; Umeda, 1975; Klatt, 1976). The master tape containing these stimuli was then used to create a test tape which contained 10 randomly ordered presentations of each of the six stimulus words interspersed at 10-word intervals with one of six nontest real CVC words. Five-second intervals separated each word. The 66-item tape was played twice to each subject, generating 20 responses to each of the six stimulus words.

Administration

The stimulus tape was presented at a comfortable listening level in the sound field. Responses were recorded on a second high-quality recorder with the microphone placed approximately 6 in. from the mouth. Stimuli were repeated once if requested, and the stimulus tape was halted if additional time was required to respond; this rarely was necessary.

Analysis

Vowel duration was measured to the nearest 5 msec with a storage oscilloscope (Tektronix, 5103N). Vowel duration was defined as the time from the onset of periodic oscillation following the release of the initial stop to cessation of periodic oscillation preceding the final stop, in the voiceless environment; offset of the vowel in the voiced environment was at the point where signal amplitude was significantly lessened preceding the final consonant.

At least five responses per subject were measured from wide-band spectrograms (Voice Identification 7000) in order to verify oscilloscopic readings. Spectrograms were also made when oscilloscopic readings were difficult to interpret. A response was considered unanalyzable when it did not contain an initial stop, did not contain a final stop, or was not unambiguously measurable oscilloscopically or spectrographically. APH1 had 9 (8%) unanalyzable responses; APH4 had 6 (5%); APX1 had 16 (13%); APX2 had 2 (2%); and APX4 had 14 (12%). All other subjects had no unanalyzable responses.

Reliability of Measurements

To assess interjudge reliability, the two authors made independent vowel duration measurements of 25 randomly selected responses from each of six subjects. The six subjects included two randomly chosen subjects from each of the three subject groups. Measurements by the two authors within 10 msec of each other were considered to be in agreement.

Agreement of vowel duration measures for the six subjects ranged from 84 to 100% and averaged 94%.

RESULTS

Results will be discussed first with respect to average vowel duration and variability in the voiced and voiceless consonant environments. This will permit references about motor control adequacy in the aphasic and apraxic subjects irrespective of the linguistic effects of such control (or lack thereof). Vowel durations preceding voiced final consonants will then be compared to those preceding voiceless final consonants to determine if aphasic and apraxic subjects maintain phonologically important durational differences.

Vowel Duration Preceding Voiced Final Stops

Table 6-2 contains the means, standard deviations, and coefficients of variation for vowel duration preceding voiced final stops (voiced environments) for all normal (N), aphasic, and apraxic subjects. Mean duration can be viewed as an average "target" value accomplished by subjects, while standard deviation (*SD*) can be viewed as a gauge of precision of motor control relative to the "target". The coefficient of variation (CV) (standard deviation divided by the mean) also is a measure of motor control precision and is particularly useful when mean duration varies substantially among subjects; in effect, it makes variability about means of different magnitudes more directly com-

TABLE 6-2
Mean, standard deviation *(SD)*, and coefficient of variation *(CV)* of vowels preceding voiced final consonants for normal, aphasic, and apraxic subjects

	BEAD			*COB*			*PIG*		
	$\overline{X}$	*SD*	*CV*	$\overline{X}$	*SD*	*CV*	$\overline{X}$	*SD*	*CV*
N1	401	38	.10	372	22	.06	203	22	.11
N2	262	31	.12	297	17	.06	163	17	.11
N3	273	21	.08	249	18	.07	154	23	.15
N4	294	19	.06	295	16	.05	158	15	.10
N5	284	23	.08	267	19	.07	139	21	.15
N Group	303	26	.09	296	18	.06	163	20	.12
APH1	224*	45	.20*	194*	33*	.17*	155	22	.14
APH2	316	46	.15	313	71*	.23*	199	38	.19
APH3	225*	31	.14	251	14	.06	145	13	.09
APH4	258	30	.11	213*	13	.06	176	52*	.29*
APX1	159*	40	.25*	240	42*	.17*	104*	23	.22
APX2	224*	35	.15	251	45*	.18*	120	28	.24*
APX3	263	20	.07	259	14	.05	209	9	.04*
APX4	229*	60*	.26*	181*	57*	.32*	87*	22	.25*
APX5	164*	22	.14	152*	27	.18*	98*	17	.17

Note. Starred means are equal to or less than the mean minus 1 *SD* of the normal subject with the shortest mean for that word. Starred *SD* and *CV* are 50% or more greater (or less) than that of the normal subject with the largest (or smallest) *SD* or *CV* for that word.

parable by expressing precision as a percentage of variability around the mean. Because the "precision of durational control may vary with mean duration even in normal talkers" (Kent, Netsell, & Abbs, 1979, p. 638), the CV may, in fact, be a more valid measure of relative precision than the *SD*.

Durations for "bead", "cob", and "pig" among the normal subjects were quite homogeneous except for N1 who had considerably longer durations than the other normal subjects. Their average duration of about 300 msec for the inherently long vowels /i/ and /a/, and 163 msec for the inherently short vowel /ɪ/, are consistent with values reported in the literature for long and short vowels (House, 1961; Klatt, 1976; Peterson & Lehiste, 1960; Port and Rotuno, 1979). *SDs* and *CVs* among these subjects were relatively homogeneous and they presumably reflect the normal range of precision of durational control; the *SDs* of the normal subjects also are consistent with those reported in the literature for vowels in similar environments (Peterson & Lehiste, 1960; Raphael, 1972, Umeda, 1975).

Testing for group differences was considered inappropriate because of the small number of subjects and the large individual differences among brain-injured subjects. Therefore, analysis of individual data was undertaken to determine if any aphasic or apraxic subject differed appreciably from normal subjects. Because N1 had mean vowel durations which were considerably higher than other normal subjects, the group mean was not considered a good measure of central tendency on which to base judgements of deviancy in the brain-injured subjects. That is, because brain-injured subjects tended to have shorter than normal durations, use of an upwardly biased normal group mean for comparisons would inflate the number of deviances found. Therefore, aphasic and apraxic subjects were considered to have deviant mean durations if their mean was equal to or less than the mean duration minus 1 *SD* of the normal subject with the shortest mean duration for the vowel in question (or equal to or greater than the mean duration plus 1 *SD* of the normal subject with the longest mean duration for the vowel in question). For example, for "bead," N2 had the shortest normal duration (262) and a *SD* of 31, so any brain-injured subject with a mean vowel duration equal to or less than 231 msec was considered deviant for that word. It should be noted that these criterion values for determining deviancy were, for all six words, more stringent than if the normal group mean minus 2 *SD* had been used.

The *SDs* and *CVs* of aphasic and apraxic subjects were considered deviant when they: exceeded by 50% or more the largest *SD* or *CV* obtained by normal subjects for the stimulus word in question; or, fell short by

50% or more the shortest *SD* or *CV* obtained by normal subjects for the stimulus word in question. These criteria for establishing differences in variability are considered conservative, and they probably agree with or underestimate the number of differences which would be considered "clinically significant."

Aphasic subjects did not fall consistently within the means and variability values for normal subjects. APH1's average durations of 224 and 194 msec in "bead" and "cob," respectively, were notably shorter than those of the normal subject with the shortest duration for those vowels (262 msec for N2 in "bead"; 249 msec for N3 in "cob"). In addition, his *CV* for "bead" (.20) and his *SD* (33) and *CV* (.17) for "cob" were more than 50% greater than the normal subject with the greatest variability for each of those vowels. His average vowel duration and variability for "pig" were within normal values. APH3 and APH4 had within normal average durations for two of the three vowels but shorter than normal duration for one vowel (APH3 in "bead" and APH4 in "cob"). APH3 had normal variability values for all three vowels, while APH4 had a very deviant *SD* and *CV* for "pig." APH2 had normal means and variability for all vowels, except for greater than normal *SD* and *CV* for "cob."

Apraxic subjects also did not fall consistently within normal means and variability values and, for many measures, were also more deviant than all the aphasic subjects. One exception was APX3, the most mildly impaired aphasic and apraxic subject in the study, who had normal durational averages and variability for all voiced environment vowels with the exception of his *CV* for "pig," which was more than 50% less than the smallest *CV* for normal subjects. APX1 had shorter than normal durations for "bead" and "pig," and APX2 had shorter than normal duration for "bead." For APX1 the duration for both of those words, and for APX2 the duration for "pig," were also shorter than that of any aphasic subject. For APX1, the *SD* and/or *CV* were greater than normal in "bead" and "cob"; for APX2 *SD* and/or *CV* were greater than normal in "pig" and "cob." APX4 and APX5 had shorter than normal durations for all three vowels, with two of the three vowels for APX4 and all three vowels for APX5 being shorter than those of any aphasic subject. APX4 also had greater than normal *SD* and *CV* for all vowels with the exception of her *SD* for "pig." APX5, in contrast, had normal variability values with the exception of a large *CV* for "cob."

The differences among the three groups of subjects are best summarized by plotting the average duration against the *CV* for each subject. This has been done in Figure 6-1 for "bead"; similar group and subject differences would be apparent in plots for "cob" and "pig." Figure 6-1 shows that the control group is more homogeneous than the aphasic and especially the apraxic group (the area on the figure covered by the control subjects is smaller). Only APH4 and APX3 fall within or near the distribution of normal subjects for both mean and *CV*. The remaining three aphasic subjects are more variable than the controls and two have shorter durations. The remaining four apraxic subjects have shorter than normal durations and greater than normal variability, with APX1 having a shorter duration and APX1 and APX4 having greater variability than any aphasic subject.

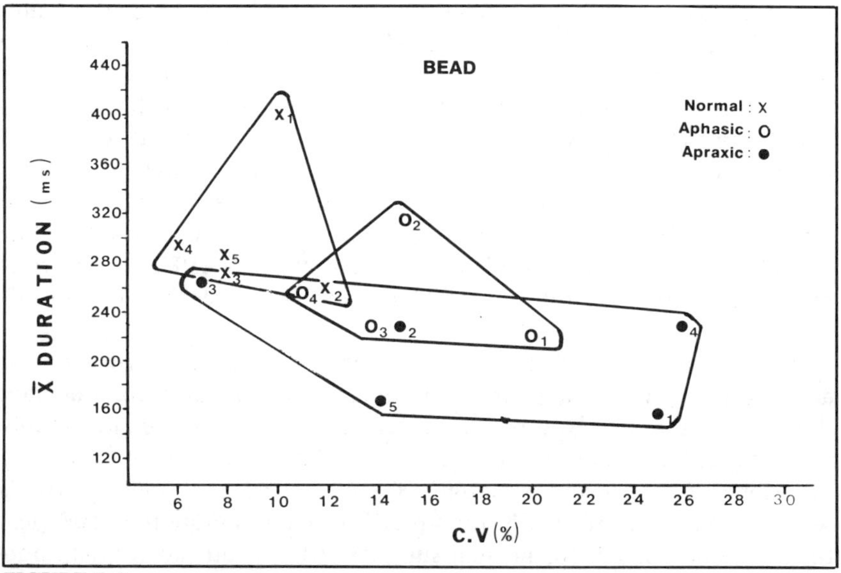

FIGURE 6-1
Mean vowel duration plotted against coefficient of variation (CV) for "bead" for normal, aphasic, and apraxic subjects.

Vowel Duration Preceding Voiceless Final Stops

Table 6-3 contains the mean, *SD*, and *CV* for all subjects' durations preceding voiceless final stops (voiceless environments). As found for the voiced environments, normal subjects were quite homogeneous in their mean durations, with the exception of N1 who had the longest mean duration for each vowel. *SDs* and *CVs* also were homogeneous and relatively small, presumably reflecting normal motor control precision. The average duration of 178 msec for the inherently long vowels /i/ and /a/, and of 102 msec for the inherently short vowel /I/, as well as their associated *SDs*, are consistent with those reported in the literature for

TABLE 6–3
Mean, standard deviation *(SD)*, and coefficient of variation *(CV)* of vowels preceding voiceless final consonants for normal, aphasic, and apraxic subjects

	BEAT			*COP*			*PICK*		
	$\overline{X}$	*SD*	*CV*	$\overline{X}$	*SD*	*CV*	$\overline{X}$	*SD*	*CV*
N1	209	13	.06	237	16	.07	112	8	.07
N2	153	13	.09	213	17	.08	109	11	.10
N3	167	17	.10	164	15	.09	99	10	.10
N4	163	13	.08	182	16	.09	97	10	.10
N5	146	13	.09	146	13	.09	92	11	.12
N Group	168	14	.08	188	15	.08	102	10	.08
APH1	180	30*	.17*	156	31*	.20*	133*	18*	.13
APH2	186	23	.12	197	27*	.14*	129*	14	.11
APH3	139	11	.08	180	15	.08	96	10	.11
APH4	156	27*	.17*	170	21	.12	103	23*	.22*
APX1	105*	28*	.27*	146	21	.14*	82*	22*	.26*
APX2	137	39*	.29*	146	30*	.20*	75*	15	.21*
APX3	128*	15	.12	155	12	.08	122*	17*	.14
APX4	106*	23	.22*	108*	41*	.38*	60*	15	.26*
APX5	108*	17	.16*	106*	15	.14*	62*	15	.24*

Note. Starred means are equal to or less (or more) than the mean minus (or plus) 1 *SD* of the normal subject with the shortest (or longest) mean for that word. Starred *SD* and *CV* are 50% or more greater (or less) than that of the normal subject with the largest (or smallest) *SD* or *CV* for that word.

vowels in similar environments (House, 1961; Klatt, 1976; Peterson and Lehiste, 1960; Port and Rotunno, 1979; Raphael, 1972; Umeda, 1975).

For the aphasic subjects, vowel duration in voiceless environments was typically normal, except for APH1 and APH2 whose average durations in "pick" of 133 and 129 msec, respectively, were more than 1 *SD* greater than that of the control subject with the longest mean for that vowel (112 msec for N1). APH3 had normal *SD* and *CV* for all vowels, while APH1 had greater than normal *SD* and/or *CV* for all three vowels. APH2 had a deviant *SD* and *CV* in "cop," and APH4 had a deviant *SD* and *CV* in "beet" and "pick."

The apraxic subjects exhibited deviances from normal which were similar to the patterns found for the voiced environments. APX1 had a deviantly short duration in "beet," with "beet" and "pick" being shorter than that of any aphasic subject; his *SD* and/or *CV* were greater than normal for all three vowels. APX2 had shorter than normal duration in "pick" and this was shorter than for any aphasic subject. APX3, while performing quite normally in voiced environments, had shorter than normal duration in "beet" and longer than normal duration in "pick." His variability, however, was usually within normal limits, with the exception of a deviantly large *SD* for "pick." APX4 and APX5 had shorter than normal duration and greater than normal *SD* and/or *CV* for all three vowels, and their durations were shorter than for any aphasic subject.

Figure 6-2 plots average duration against *CV* for "beet" (once again, similar and no less apparent differences would be evident in plots for "cop" and "pick"). As was evident in Figure 6-1 for "bead," the control group is more homogeneous than the aphasic and especially the apraxic group. Aphasic subjects fall within normal mean durations but three of four are more variable than normal. The apraxic group is distinguished completely from both the control and aphasic groups, with all apraxic subjects having shorter durations than all normal and aphasic subjects, and three of five apraxic subjects being more variable than all aphasic subjects.

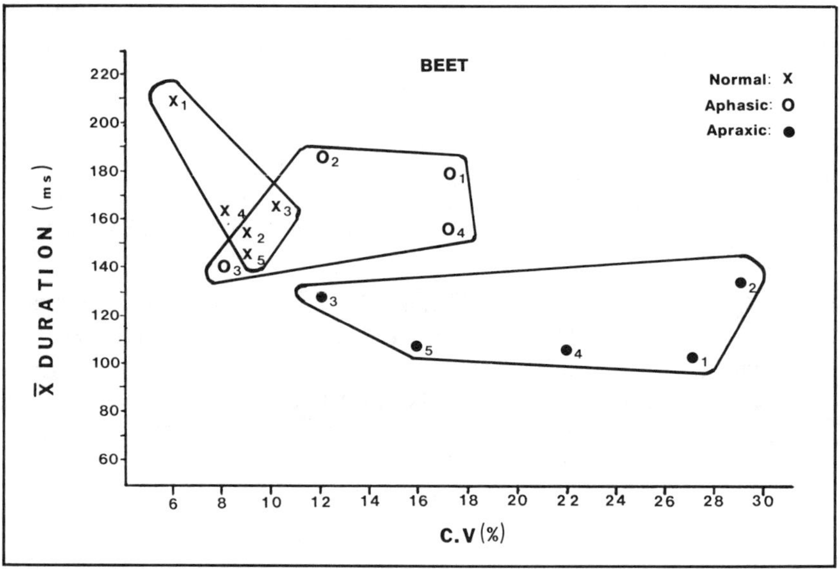

FIGURE 6–2
Mean vowel duration plotted against coefficient of variation (CV) for "beet" for normal, aphasic, and apraxic subjects.

Summary of Performance in Voiced and Voiceless Environments

The above findings establish that neither the aphasic nor the apraxic subjects, as groups, were normal in their vowel duration or in their precision of vowel duration control. Patients with apraxia of speech generally were more frequently and dramatically deviant from normal than were aphasic patients without apraxia. Unexpectedly, the durational deviation for apraxic subjects was almost always in the direction of shorter than normal duration, with all but APX3 having shorter than normal durations on at least two of the six words. In addition, three of the five apraxic subjects (1, 2, and 4) had less absolute precision (as measured by *SD*) than normal subjects for three of the six stimulus words, and all but APX3 had less relative precision as measured by *CV* on four or more of the six words.

It should be noted that greater than normal variability of the apraxic (and some aphasic) subjects cannot be interpreted as an artifact of their shorter than normal average durations. First, there are data that suggest that variability normally is less, not greater, with shorter duration (Kent & Forner, 1980), including those from control subjects in this study, whose *SDs* in voiced environments were larger than their voiceless counterparts, in which vowel duration is relatively short. In fact, this also was generally true for our aphasic and apraxic subjects. In contrast, all subjects had relatively comparable *CVs* when voiced and voiceless environment durations were compared. This suggests that all subjects tended to have greater absolute vowel variability in voiced environments than voiceless environments but comparable relative variability in the two environments. Second, when comparable average durations for normal and apraxic subjects are compared — irrespective of the specific vowel or environment — the apraxic subjects are still more variable than normal. For example, while durations for APX1 and APX2 for "cop" were not significantly different from normal, their *SD* and/or *CV* were significantly greater than normal; similarly, while average duration for APX4 in "cob" (181 msec) was nearly identical to the average duration for N4 in "cop" (182 msec), both the *SD* and *CV* for APX4 were more than three times greater than normal (*SD* of 57 versus 16; *CV* of .32 versus .09).

All of these findings suggest the presence of some type of motor control deficit in a number of the aphasic and apraxic subjects, with such deficits clearly more frequent and prominent in the apraxic subjects. However, the linguistic significance of these durational findings must be assessed before it can be concluded that phonological (linguistic) deficits can be ruled out as a major explanation for the durational deviances.

Differences between Vowels in Voiced and Voiceless Environments

The general "knowledge" of subjects regarding the voicing feature of the final stop can be assessed by comparing their vowel duration preceding voiced final stops to those preceding voiceless final stops. As indicated in the introduction, vowels preceding voiced final consonants are typically 40% or more longer than vowels preceding voiceless final consonants.

Table 6-4 gives vowel duration ratios for each pair of word stimuli. Ratios achieved by normal subjects equalled or exceeded 1.4 for all word pairs, indicating that averaged voiced environment vowels were at least 40% greater than averaged voiceless environment vowels. For aphasic subjects, ratios equalled or exceeded 1.2 for all vowels, and only APH1 had ratios consistently below 1.4 (it should be noted that ratios as low as 1.2 and 1.3 have occasionally been reported for normal subjects (e.g., Krause, 1982)). If the ratios of APH1 are interpreted as a "blurring" of the linguistic distinction between voiced and voiceless final consonants, however, it does not necessarily establish a phonological basis for his problem. APH1, as noted previously, probably had a mild dysarthria and, in fact, showed a tendency to neutralize vowel duration. That is, the difference between his shortest average duration (133 msec in "pick") and his longest average duration (224 msec in "bead") of 91 msec was

TABLE 6–4
Vowel duration ratios (voiced environment duration divided by voiceless environment duration) for each syllable pair for normal, aphasic, and apraxic subjects

	Bead/Beet	*Cob/Cop*	*Pig/Pick*	*Average Ratio*
N1	1.9	1.6	1.8	1.8
N2	1.7	1.4	1.5	1.5
N3	1.6	1.5	1.6	1.6
N4	1.8	1.6	1.6	1.7
N5	1.9	1.8	1.5	1.7
APH1	1.3	1.2	1.2	1.2
APH2	1.7	1.6	1.5	1.6
APH3	1.6	1.4	1.5	1.5
APH4	1.7	1.3	1.7	1.6
APX1	1.5	1.6	1.3	1.5
APX2	1.6	1.7	1.6	1.6
APX3	2.1	1.7	1.7	1.8
APX4	2.2	1.7	1.5	1.8
APX5	1.5	1.4	1.6	1.5

the smallest durational range found for any subject, and only about half that typically exhibited by control subjects. It is possible, therefore, that his low ratios resulted from some physiological restriction of his ability to vary vowel duration. Listener transcriptions of his responses (see next section) also suggest that his relatively low ratios were not the result of phonological errors.

Apraxic subjects had ratios which equalled or exceeded 1.4 in all cases, except for APX1 who had a ratio of 1.3 for the "pig-pick" distinction. The implications of this finding will be discussed later.

In general, these ratios indicate that the aphasic and, most notably, the apraxic subjects varied vowel duration as a function of the postvocalic consonant's voicing feature, and they did so to a degree comparable to normal. Importantly, a number of our apraxic (and aphasic) subjects accomplished this linguistic goal in the presence of durational deviances and poor precision of motor control.

Differences in vowel duration preceding voiced and voiceless final consonants can be appreciated further by examining Figure 6-3 which plots the mean and *SD* for each subject's vowel in "bead" and "beet." Once

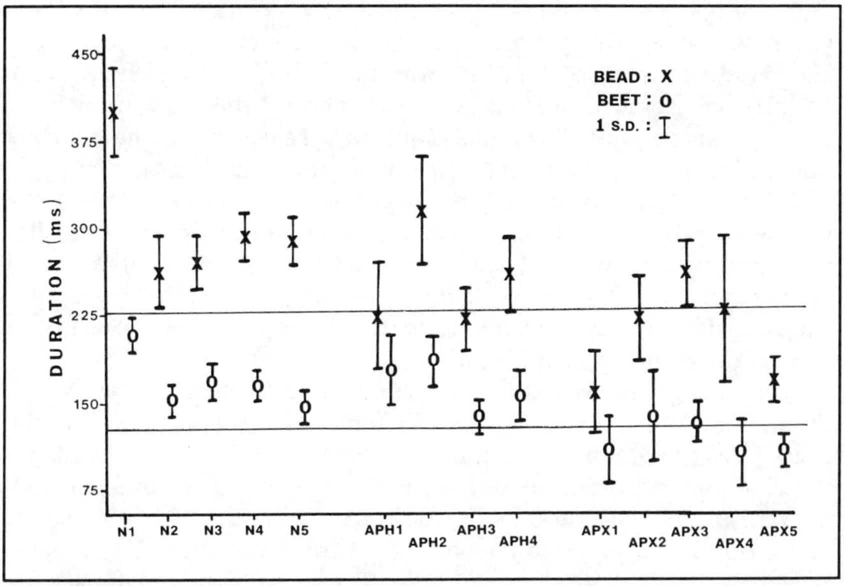

FIGURE 6-3

Mean vowel duration and 1 standard deviation range for "bead" and "beet" for each normal (N), aphasic (APH), and apraxic (APX) subject. Upper horizontal line separates lower border of normal subjects' voiced environment vowels from upper border of voiceless environment vowels. Lower horizontal line is at lower border of normal subjects' voiceless environment vowels.

again, a similar general pattern of results would be derived for similar analyses of the other word pairs. It is clear in Figure 6-3 that normal subjects' mean values and distributions (the vertical lines in the figure encompass plus or minus 1 *SD* from the mean) for the vowels in the voiced environment are always longer than for the voiceless environment, and that there is no overlap in the distributions for any subject in the group. In the aphasic group, APH2 and APH4 have fairly normal patterns. APH3 has vowel durations in "bead" which fall noticeably within control subjects' distributions for "beet," although his distributions for the two words are clearly separable (his ratio was 1.6). APH1 has a distribution for "bead" which also falls noticeably within the control distribution for "beet" and, in fact, clearly overlaps his own distribution for "beet" (his ratio was only 1.3). This overlap also is apparent for the other word pairs, except that for the short vowel /ɪ/ in "pig" and "pick" the overlap takes place within the normal subjects' range for the voiced environment (i.e., he appears to have shortened his long vowels and lengthened his short ones, in line with his apparent neutralization of duration described previously).

The apraxic group differs from both the control and aphasic group. Only APX3 has distributions which clearly separate his voiced and voiceless environment productions from one another without overlap of his voiced environment durations with control subject durations for the voiceless environment (his voiceless environment duration, however, is shorter than normal). The remaining four apraxic subjects have shorter than normal durations and all four have voiced environment durations which fall within normal subjects' ranges for voiceless environment productions. In fact, for APX1 and APX5, the voiced environment distribution (represented by the 1-*SD* range) falls entirely within the normal range for the voiceless environment. However, APX1 is the only apraxic subject with any appreciable overlap between his own voiced and voiceless environment durations.

When integrated with the vowel duration ratio data, this analysis of durational distributions leads to one conclusion and a testable prediction. The generally normal ratios and the lack of significant overlap in the distributions of voiced and voiceless environment durations for the apraxic and aphasic subjects demonstrate "knowledge" of the voicing distinction between voiced and voiceless final consonants. This suggests that the "phonological conditioning" of durational differences is reasonably intact, even in the presence of marked-to-severe apraxia in some cases. However, the occurrence among apraxic subjects of vowel durations for voiced environments which fall noticeably or largely within normal distributions for vowels in voiceless environments leads to a prediction that, for these subjects, a significant number of voiceless for voiced substitutions should be perceived by listeners. Thus, the conclusion and the prediction are paradoxical. On one hand, the data indicate phonological intactness, while on the other they lead to a prediction that voicing "substitutions" will be perceived.

Additional Analyses: Relation of Perceptual Judgments to Durational Data

To test the prediction from durational data that voiceless for voiced errors should be perceived in the apraxic subjects, the authors, independently of one another and without access to durational data, transcribed the 120 responses of each subject with respect to the final consonant voicing feature. Decisions about the voicing feature were based on the authors' judgment of the feature likely to be perceived by listeners if asked to respond to each response independently of all others. Final stop voicing was scored as correct, incorrect, or ambiguous. For reliability purposes, responses rated as ambiguous by one judge and incorrect by the other were considered to be in agreement and were considered "errors." Agreement between the two judges ranged from 98–100% and averaged 99% for the control subjects; for aphasic subjects ranged from 90–100% and averaged 95%; for apraxic subjects ranged from 83–95% and averaged 89%.

Table 6-5 summarizes the perceptual data for the aphasic and apraxic subjects; no errors were perceived for any control subjects. A response

TABLE 6–5

Number of responses from aphasic and apraxic subjects rated by two judges as incorrect or ambiguous with regard to the voicing feature of the final consonant (20 responses per subject per word)

	Beet	*Bead*	*Pick*	*Pig*	*Cop*	*Cob*	*% VL/V*	*% V/VL*
APH1	2	—	—	—	4	—	0	10
APH2	—	—	—	—	—	—	0	0
APH3	—	5	—	—	—	—	8	0
APH4	—	—	—	—	—	—	0	0
APX1	—	8	—	19	—	16	72	0
APX2	—	11	—	4	1	2	28	2
APX3	—	13	—	1	—	3	28	0
APX4	—	1	—	4	—	1	10	0
APX5	—	5	—	2	—	5	20	0

Note. Also shown are the percentages of all voiced final stops rated as voiceless or ambiguous (%VL/V) and the percentage of all voiceless final stops rated as voiced or ambiguous (%V/VL).

was considered an "error" only if both judges rated it as ambiguous or incorrect with regard to the final consonant voicing feature (approximately 70% of errors were rated as ambiguous by the judges).

Few errors were perceived for aphasic subjects. For APH1 it is of interest that his 10% error rate consisted solely of voiced for voiceless errors, and that they occured for "beet" and "cop," whose durations were normal. Also, in spite of the fact that his "bead" and "cob" durations fell within normal ranges for voiceless environments, no voiceless for voiced substitutions were perceived. He clearly had to have provided cues other than vowel duration to explain correct perception of voiced final stops and incorrect perception of a small number of voiceless stops. It is of interest that the tendency for errors to be perceived as voiced for voiceless is consistent with findings for some individuals with dysarthria (Farmer, 1977). In contrast, the 8% voiceless for voiced error rate of APH3 was consistent with his distributional overlap between "beet" and "bead," the pair generating the only perceived errors for him. Although errors for APH3 were few, because their pattern was consistent with that for apraxic subjects, it is noteworthy that he exhibited apraxic-like behaviors on imitative speech tasks during diagnostic testing, although his conversational speech was free of such errors.

The perceptual data for the apraxic subjects were overwhelmingly consistent with the durational prediction. Ninety-nine percent of the voicing errors perceived for the group were voiceless for voiced, with the percentage of errors perceived for voiced environments ranging from 10% for APX4 to 72% for APX1. The large percentage of errors for APX1 is consistent with her degree of durational overlap between voiced and voiceless environments within the normal voiceless environment range.

Of special interest is the fairly large percentage of errors perceived for APX3, the least impaired apraxic subject clinically and the one with the most normal durational values. He apparently exhibited deviant characteristics other than vowel duration which explain perception of voicing errors (we believe his frequent unvoiced and aspirated release of voiced final stops explain the perceived errors).

While durational data predict quite well the general direction of perceived errors, it also is of value to examine if they predict individual errors, and if durations associated with perceived errors have a distributional location suggestive of phonological selection errors or durational (motor) control errors. Figures 6-4 through 6-7 represent distributions for "bead" and "beet" for N3, APX1, APX2, and APX3. N3 has clearly separated and generally normally distributed durations which are representative of all normal subjects. APX3 also has clearly separated durations. His 13 voiceless for voiced errors clearly cannot be

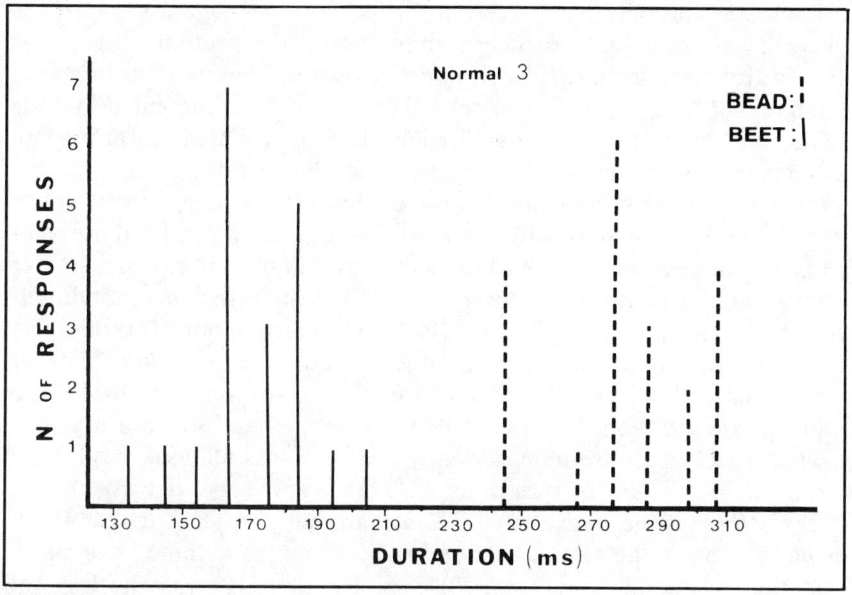

FIGURE 6–4
Distribution of vowel durations in "bead" and "beet" for normal Subject 3.

attributed to vowel duration, and the normal and separate distributions for the two environments indicate adequate phonological selection of the voicing feature, further suggesting the presence of another behavior leading to perceived ambiguities or errors in voicing.

APX1 has overlapping but somewhat separate distributions which are both almost entirely within the range of normal voiceless values. Durations for which errors were perceived are spread over the distribution for the voiced environment and suggest that perceived errors are due to durational control problems. That is, if all errors were due to phonological substitution of a voiceless for voiced stop, the associated vowel durations should be distributed similarly to that of vowels for correctly produced voiceless final stops; also, the distribution for voiced environment productions should be bimodal, with one mode associated with correctly produced voiced stops and the other with incorrectly selected but correctly produced voiceless stops. However, his errors are clearly distributed within or beyond the upper end of the voiceless environment distribution and do not appear bimodally distributed (it could be argued that the error perceived between 100 and 110 msec does represent a phonological substitution).

APX2 has a pattern similar to that of APX1. Perceived errors are distributed within or beyond the upper end of the voiceless environment distribution and only one perceived error (between 140 and 150 msec) is likely to have resulted from a clear phonological substitution.

It is also clear from the distributions shown in Figure 6-5 through 6-7 (and for all other apraxic subjects) that voiced environment durations falling within the normal range for voiceless environment durations are often perceived as correct. This suggests that these subjects often are able to signal correctly the voicing feature of the final stop, in spite of vowel duration more consistent with the voiceless cognate (for most of our subjects we suspect that these cues lie within final stop closure and/or release). This possibility has been shown to exist for normal individuals (Malecot, 1958; Wardrip-Fruin, 1982). Indirect support for this also comes from transcription of our subjects' responses by a naive listener who was asked to identify the final stops of our subjects. She listened to all responses, without knowledge of the stimulus, and was not asked to evaluate each response independently (i.e., she was allowed to "learn" from subjects' previous responses). Her errors, in contrast to the authors' ratings, never exceeded 11% for any subject, although they consistently were in the same direction predicted by the authors' judgments and the durational data (i.e., 80% of her errors were voiceless for voiced). This implies that our subjects were, with some regularity, differentiating voiced from voiceless final stops not only by vowel duration,

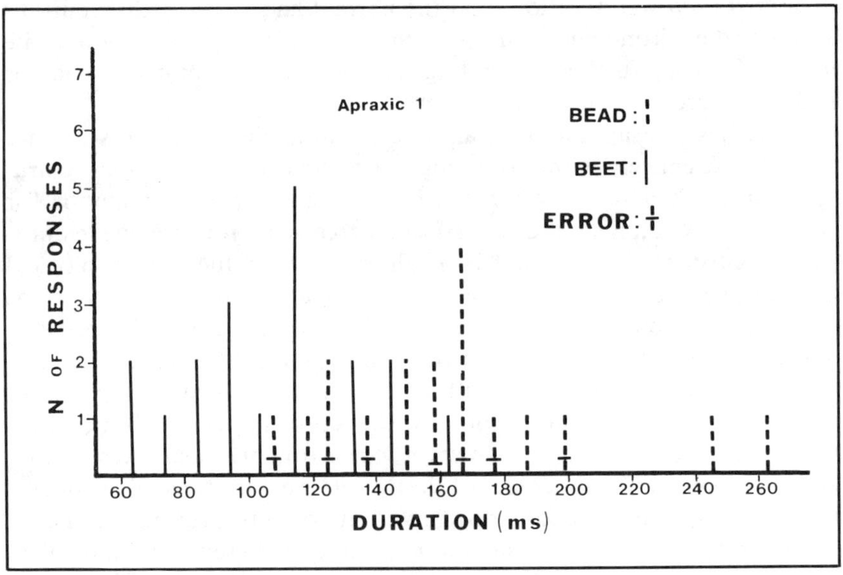

FIGURE 6–5

Distribution of vowel durations in "bead" and "beet" and identification of durations associated with perceived voicing errors for apraxic Subject 1.

but also by other cues to final stop voicing. Finally, these data also indicate that acoustic analysis may identify abnormal temporal (phonetic) characteristics when broad transcription implies accuracy and normalcy of production.

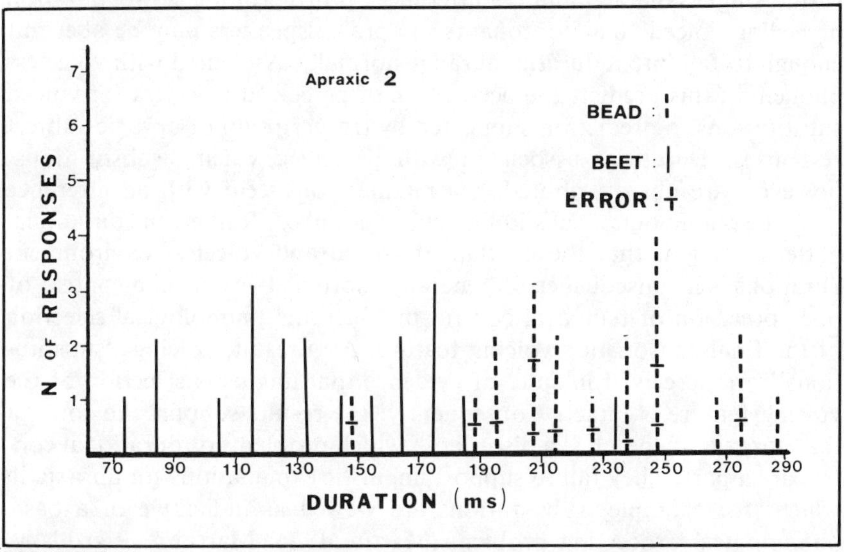

FIGURE 6–6
Distribution of vowel durations in "bead" and "beet" and identification of durations associated with perceived voicing errors for apraxic Subject 2.

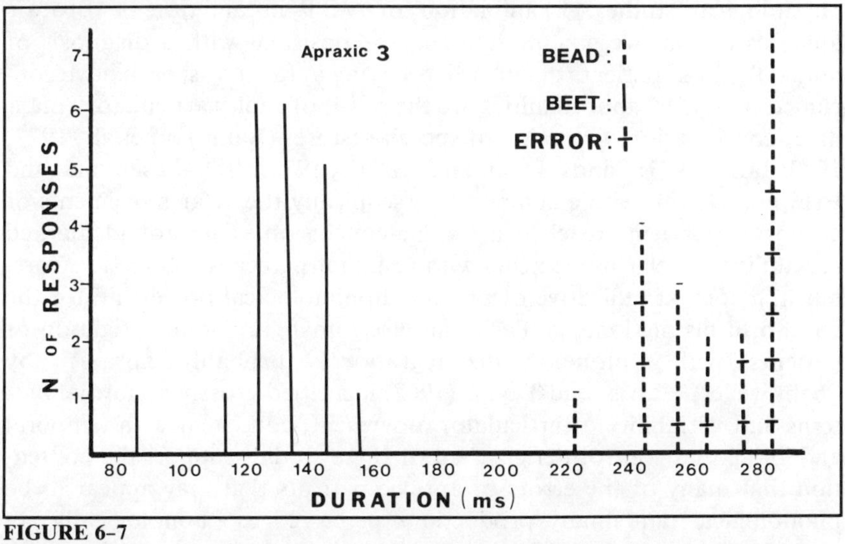

FIGURE 6–7
Distribution of vowel durations in "bead" and "beet" and identification of durations associated with perceived voicing errors for apraxic Subject 3.

DISCUSSION

The results of this study indicate that apraxia of speech can be associated with abnormally short and highly variable vowel durations within single-syllable imitative utterances. Furthermore, vowel duration preceding voiced final consonants in apraxic speakers may be aberrant enough to fall into a durational range normally associated with voiceless phonemes; this predicts the occurrence of perceived voiceless for voiced substitutions, a prediction supported by transcription of apraxic subject responses. Durations associated with perceived voicing substitutions, however, are not distributed in a manner consistent with an inference that true phonological substitutions have occurred. Rather, the durational patterns suggest that the overlap of voiced and voiceless environment durations is a consequence of generally shortened vowels in a context of poor precision of temporal control but accurate phonological selection of the final consonant's voicing feature. As a result, voicing "substitutions" are perceived in spite of evidence that linguistic selection of the voicing feature is intact. Consequently, the results support the concept that apraxia of speech is a disorder in which problems of durational control are a part. They fail to support linguistic explanations for apraxia in which, for example, substitutions are viewed as indicative of a basic phonological processing problem (Martin, 1974; Martin & Rigrodsky, 1974a & 1974b; Martin et al., 1975).

The above conclusions are consistent with several acoustic and physiological studies. Examination of VOT in anterior or Broca's aphasics (whom we assume had speech consistent with a diagnosis of apraxia) and in patients diagnosed as having apraxia of speech have concluded that VOT abnormalities are the result of faulty articulatory planning, coordination, or timing of speech gestures (Blumstein et al., 1977, 1980; Jaffe, 1977; Sands, Freeman & Harris, 1978). Itoh, Sasanuma, and Ushijima (1979), who examined fiberscopically the velar movements of an apraxic patient, reached a similar conclusion. They found marked variability of velar movements with resultant perceived phonetic errors, but in a context indicative of preserved phonological processing for the nasal-oral distinction. Similarly, an electromyographic investigation of patients with "phonetic disintegration" (probably apraxic) by Shankweiler, Harris, and Taylor (1968) identified grossly abnormal patterns and variability of articulator movement, consistent with temporal and/or spatial control deficits. All of these studies support the contention that many of the errors of apraxic patients that may appear to be phonological (and many productions perceived as phonologically accurate) are more accurately described as phonetic in nature. They also suggest that many clinical descriptions of apraxia of speech as being relatively free of "distortions" (particularly in contrast to the dysarthrias) (Darley, Aronson, & Brown, 1975; Johns & Darley, 1970) may need clarification or modification in light of emerging acoustic and physiological evidence to the contrary. Resolution of this discrepancy also will have to address the extent to which "distortions" in apraxia of speech are different from those existing in the dysarthrias. This obviously requires a great deal of additional research.

It is important to repeat that none of the apraxic subjects in this study had "pure" apraxia; all had some degree of aphasia. This obviously raises questions about the role of aphasia in their vowel duration abnormalities. However, there was considerable overlap between the apraxic and aphasic subjects both in severity of aphasia and fluency classifications (the tendency toward lower PICA and BDAE severity ratings in the apraxic group is probably explained by the additional handicap imposed by their apraxia and not their language impairment). In spite of this overlap the apraxic subjects emerged as generally more deviant in both duration and variability than aphasic subjects. This separation of apraxic from aphasic subjects is noteworthy in light of the fact that APH3 and APH4 presented somewhat difficult diagnostic challenges during original subject classification; both exhibited some apraxic-like symptoms during diagnosis, with APH3 resembling patterns described for "conduction aphasia," and APH4 perhaps being a well-recovered apraxic. In spite of this, we did not feel a diagnosis of apraxia of speech was justified for them. The vowel duration results tended to support this decision. While both APH3 and APH4 exhibited some deviances, they were less pervasive and severe than for our apraxic subjects, with the exception of APX3 who was mildly impaired. In effect, the durational analysis helped validate our diagnostic decisions; this cross-validation represents a significant potential contribution of acoustic studies to clinical diagnosis. It also suggests that apraxia can be studied in patients with aphasia, under some circumstances, without severely confounding the results. If this interpretation is valid, it would permit the study of severe apraxia of speech, which rarely occurs in the absence of some degree of aphasic impairment. Of relevance in this regard are the findings for APX2, who had a moderately severe aphasia and severe apraxia, but did not correspond to traditional criteria for identifying apraxia. Her vowel duration behavior was consistent with those of the other apraxic subjects, lending support to her diagnosis as apraxic. However, she was not the most deviant apraxic subject in her vowel duration, suggesting that vowel duration may not be a precise index of judged clinical severity.

Although the aphasic and apraxic subjects were generally distinguished by vowel duration measures, the finding of some abnormalities in all aphasic subjects cannot be ignored. This is particularly significant for APH2, for whom there were no clinical signs or history of apraxia or dysarthria, but who had abnormally large variability for some test words and — in contrast to all apraxic subjects but mildly impaired APX3 — longer than normal duration on one word. Such findings suggest that all aphasic patients may exhibit some deviations in temporal control (cf. Blumstein et al., 1980), in spite of the fact that only some have enough of an impairment to warrant a diagnosis of apraxia of speech. Whether the "subtle" vowel duration abnormalities in nonapraxic subjects reflect a clinically nonsignificant apraxia of speech or some other problem cannot be answered by these data.

The finding of shorter than normal vowel duration among apraxic subjects is surprising in light of findings by Collins, Rosenbek, and Wertz (1978) and Ryalls (1981) of longer than normal vowel and word durations in apraxia as well as typical clinical descriptions of apraxic speech as slow, effortful, and pause filled (Darley, Aronson, & Brown, 1975; Darley, 1982). In fact, the apraxic subjects in this study clearly exhibited these typical clinical characteristics. Several comments are relevant in this context. First, we examined vowel duration — not syllable duration — and the results do not establish that word duration is typically shorter than normal. Second, we examined duration in a single-syllable imitation task and do not know if similar results would emerge from examination of longer utterances and/or spontaneous speech tasks. Third, there are some data in agreement with the present findings. Bauman (1978), after accounting for differences in overall speech rate among subject groups, concluded that her Broca's aphasia group had "shorter than normal relative vowel duration yet longer than normal consonant duration" (p. 181). DiSimoni and Darley (1977), in a study of one apraxic patient's phoneme duration in utterances of varying length, found evidence for an increase of intrasyllabic articulatory rate.

Regardless of some precedent for a finding of reduced vowel duration, it remains unclear as to why such a reduction occurs. Because it is extremely difficult to separate the direct effects of the motor impairment on durational control from compensations in response to that impairment (Kent, Netsell, & Abbs, 1979), it is not even possible to establish if reduced vowel duration is a direct product of the apraxic impairment, an indirect result of a primary deficit more directly associated with consonant gestures, or the product of efforts to compensate in some way for impaired motor control. It is clear that continued study of both vowel, consonant, and syllable duration is necessary both to validate the present findings and develop explanatory models for the results.

Although the finding of shortened vowel duration was unexpected, the resultant prediction and confirmation of predominant voiceless for voiced substitutions is consistent with several clinical studies. Trost and Canter (1974) reported that 67.5% of voicing errors were voiceless for voiced substitutions and that their occurrence was more prominent in the final position of monosyllabic words. Similar patterns of voicing errors have been reported by Fry (1959), Johns and Darley (1970), and Shankweiler and Harris (1966), although the latter two studies did not distinguish errors in the initial and final positions. LaPointe & Johns, 1975, found no differences between voiced and voiceless errors but did not separate errors in the initial and final positions. To the extent that vowel duration is a major cue to the final consonant's voicing feature, the clinical literature tends to have predicted the findings of this study, although the preponderance of voiceless for voiced errors in our apraxic subjects was far greater than reported in previous work.

Our findings also raise the issue of whether vowel duration should receive attention in the clinical management of apraxia. Of particular interest is whether it already receives attention within some currently employed treatment strategies. For example, if reduced vowel duration is an integral part of the apraxic disorder — and not a compensatory response to it — to what extent is it "treated" by melodic intonation therapy (MIT, Sparks, 1981; Sparks & Holland, 1976) and contrastive stress drills (Darley, Aronson, & Brown, 1975; Rosenbek, 1978). Both of these methods are frequently employed with apraxic speakers and involve marked prosodic alterations (e.g., increased vowel duration, particularly in MIT). If such methods, in addition to promoting articulatory accuracy, also help "normalize" vowel duration, or exaggerate it, to what extent does that normalization contribute to articulatory improvements of surrounding consonants? This issue could be addressed by documenting the degree and sequence of change in vowel duration and articulatory accuracy in response to various treatment approaches.

Finally, while vowel abnormalities in apraxia of speech seldom cross phonological boundaries and are far less frequently perceived to be "in error" than consonants (Darley, Aronson & Brown, 1975; Johns & Darley, 1970; LaPointe & Johns, 1975), the findings of this study indicate that temporal abnormalities in vowels may be a common occurrence in apraxia of speech. It appears that more attention to durational (and other) characteristics of vowels than has occurred to date is warranted for its potential to contribute to our understanding of the nature of apraxia of speech and its clinical diagnosis and management.

REFERENCES

Aten, J. L., Darley, F. L., Deal, J. L., & Johns, D. F. Comment on A. D. Martin's "Some objections to the term apraxia of speech." *Journal of Speech and Hearing Disorders,* 1975, *40*, 416–420.

Bauman, J. A. *Sound duration: A comparison between performances of subjects with central nervous system disorders and normal speakers.* Ph.D. dissertation, University of Colorado, 1978.

Blumstein, S. Phonological aspects of aphasia. In M. T. Sarno (Ed.), *Acquired aphasia.* New York: Academic Press, 1981.

Blumstein, S., Cooper, W. E., Goodglass, H., Statlender, S., & Gottlieb, J. Production deficits in aphasia: A voice-onset-time analysis. *Brain and Language*, 1980, *9*, 153–170.

Blumstein, S., Cooper, W. E., Zurif, E., & Caramazza, A. The perception and production of voice-onset time in aphasia. *Neuropsychologia*, 1977, *15*, 371–383.

Buckingham, H. W. Explanation in apraxia with consequences for the concept of apraxia of speech. *Brain and Language*, 1979, *8*, 202–226.

Buckingham, H. W. Explanations for the concept of apraxia of speech. In M. T. Sarno (Ed.), *Acquired aphasia.* New York: Academic Press, 1981. (a)

Buckingham, H. W. Phonological aspects of aphasia. *Topics in language disorders,* 1981, *4*, 29–40. (b)

Chen, M. Vowel length variation as a function of the voicing of consonant environment. *Phonetica*, 1970, *22*, 129–159.

Collins, M., Rosenbek, J. C., & Wertz, R. T. *Spectrographic analysis of vowel and word duration in apraxia of speech.* Paper presented at the American Speech-Hearing-Language Association Convention, San Francisco, 1978.

Darley, F. L. *Aphasia.* Philadelphia: Saunders, 1982.

Darley, F. L., Aronson, A. E., & Brown, J. R. *Motor speech disorders.* Philadelphia: Saunders, 1975.

DiSimoni, F. G., & Darley, F. L. Effect of phoneme duration control on three utterance-length conditions in an apractic patient. *Journal of Speech and Hearing Disorders*, 1977, *42*, 257–264.

Farmer, A. Stop cognate production patterns in adult athetotic cerebral-palsied speakers. *Folia Phoniatrica*, 1977, *29*, 154–162.

Freeman, F. J., Sands, E. S., & Harris, K.S. Temporal coordination of phonation and articulation in a case of verbal apraxia: A voice onset time study. *Brain and Language,* 1978, *6*, 106–111.

Fry, D. B. Phonemic substitutions in an aphasic patient. *Language & Speech,* 1959, *2*, 52–61.

Gandour, J., & Weinberg, B. Influence of postvocalic consonants on vowel duration in esophageal speech. *Language and Speech*, 1980, *23*, 149–158.

Goodglass, H. The syndromes of aphasia: Similarities and differences in neurolinguistic features. *Topics in Language Disorders*, 1981, *1*, 1–14.

Goodglass, H., & Kaplan, E. *Boston Diagnostic Aphasia Examination.* Philadelphia: Lea and Febiger, 1972.

House, A. S. On vowel duration in English. *Journal of the Acoustical Society of America.* 1961, *33*, 1174–1178.

House, A. S., & Fairbanks, G. The influence of consonant environment upon the secondary acoustical characteristics of vowels. *Journal of the Acoustical Society of America,* 1953, *25*, 105-113.

Itoh, M., Sasanuma, S., & Ushijima, T. Velar movements during speech in a patient with apraxia of speech. *Brain and Language*, 1979, *7*, 227-239.

Jaffe, D. W. *Acoustic analysis of voice onset time characteristics of apraxic, aphasic, and non-brain-injured adults.* Master's thesis, University of Massachusetts, 1977.

Johns, D. F., & Darley, F. L. Phonemic variability in apraxia of speech. *Journal of Speech & Hearing Research*, 1970, *13*, 556-583.

Johns, D. F. & LaPointe, L. L. Neurogenic disorders of output processing: Apraxia of speech. In H. Whitaker & H. A. Whitaker (Eds.), *Studies in neurolinguistics* (Vol. 1). New York: Academic Press, 1976.

Kent, R. D., & Forner, L. L. Speech segment durations in sentence recitations by children and adults. *Journal of Phonetics*, 1980, *8*, 157-168.

Kent, R. D., Netsell, R., & Abbs, J. H. Acoustic characteristics of dysarthria associated with cerebellar disease. *Journal of Speech & Hearing Research,* 1979, *22*, 613-626.

Klatt, D. H. Interaction between two factors that influence vowel duration. *Journal of the Acoustical Society of America*, 1973, *54*, 1102-1104.

Klatt, D. H. Linguistic uses of segmental duration in English: Acoustical and perceptual evidence. *Journal of the Acoustical Society of America*, 1976, *59*, 1208-1221.

Krause, S.E. Developmental use of vowel duration as a cue to postvocalic stop consonant voicing. *Journal of Speech and Hearing Research*, 1982, *25*, 388-393.

LaPointe, L. L. & Johns, D. F. Some phonemic characteristics in apraxia of speech. *Journal of Communication Disorders*, 1975, *8*, 259-269.

Lehiste, I. *Suprasegmentals.* Cambridge: MIT Press, 1970.

Malecot, A. The role of releases in the identification of released final stops. *Language*, 1958, *34*, 370-380.

Martin, A. D. Some objections to the term apraxia of speech. *Journal of Speech & Hearing Disorders*, 1974, *39*, 53-64.

Martin, A. D. & Rigrodsky, S. An investigation of phonological impairment in aphasia, part I. *Cortex*, 1974, *49*, 317-328. (a)

Martin, A. D. & Rigrodsky, S. An investigation of phonological impairment in aphasia, part 2: Distinctive feature analysis of phonemic commutation errors in aphasia. *Cortex*, 1974, *49*, 329-346. (b)

Martin, A. D., Wasserman, N. H., Gilden, L., Gerstman, L., & West, J. A. A process model of repetition in aphasia: An investigation of phonological and morphological interactions in aphasic error performance. *Brain and Language*, 1975, *2*, 434-450.

Peterson, G. E., & Lehiste, I. Duration of syllable nuclei in English. *Journal of the Acoustical Society of America*, 1960, *32*, 673-703.

Porch, B. *The Porch Index of Communicative Ability.* Palo Alto, CA: Consulting Psychologists Press, 1967.

Port, R. F., & Rotunno, R. Relation between voice-onset time and vowel duration. *Journal of the Acoustical Society of America*, 1979, *66*, 654-662.

Raphael, L. J. Preceding vowel duration as a cue to the perception of voicing of American English consonants in word final position. *Journal of the Acoustical Society of America*, 1972, *51*, 1296–1303.

Rosenbek, J. Treating apraxia of speech. In D. F. Johns (Ed.), *Clinical management of neurogenic communicative disorders*. Boston: Little, Brown, 1978.

Ryalls, J. H. Motor aphasia: Acoustic correlates of phonetic disintegration in vowels. *Neuropsychologia*, 1981, *19*, 365–374.

Sands, E. S., Freeman, F. J., & Harris, K. S. Progressive changes in articulatory patterns in verbal apraxia: A longitudinal case study. *Brain and Language*, 1978, *6*, 97–105.

Shankweiler, D., & Harris, K. S. An experimental approach to the problem of articulation in aphasia. *Cortex*, 1966, *49*, 277–292.

Shankweiler, D., Harris, K. S. & Taylor, M. L. Electromyographic studies of articulation in aphasia, *Archives of Physical Medicine and Rehabilitation*, 1968, *49*, 1–8.

Sparks, R. W. Melodic intonation therapy. In R. Chapey (Ed.), *Language intervention strategies in adult aphasia*. Baltimore: Williams & Wilkins, 1981.

Sparks, R. W., & Holland, A. Method: Melodic intonation therapy. *Journal of Speech & Hearing Disorders*, 1976, *41*, 287–297.

Trost, J., & Canter, G. Apraxia of speech in patients with Broca's aphasia: A study of phoneme production accuracy and error patterns. *Brain and Language*, 1974, *1*, 63–79.

Umeda, N. Vowel duration in American English. *Journal of the Acoustical Society of America*, 1975, *58*, 434–445.

Wardrip-Fruin, C. On the status of temporal cues to phonetic categories: Preceding vowel duration as a cue to voicing in final stop consonants. *Journal of the Acoustical Society of America*, 1982, *71*, 187–195.

Weismer, G., Diennsen, D., & Elbert, M. A Study of the voicing distinction association with omitted, word final stops. *Journal of Speech & Hearing Disorders*, 1981, *46*, 320–328.

Wertz, R. T. Neuropathologies of speech and language: An introduction to patient management. In D. F. Johns (Ed.), *Clinical management of neurogenic communicative disorders*. Boston: Little, Brown, 1978.

ACKNOWLEDGMENT

The authors would like to express their gratitude to Mrs. Ezmat Ezzat, Director of the Department of Speech Pathology and Audiology at Holyoke Hospital, Holyoke, Mass. for her help in identifying and facilitating the testing of the patients who served as subjects in this study.

7

An Analysis of Voice Onset Time (VOT) in Aphasic and Normal Subjects

Cynthia M. Shewan
Herbert A. Leeper, Jr.
John C. Booth

Problems in the phonological-articulatory[1] systems, which can manifest themselves to a large extent as articulation errors, have both been referred to by a myriad of terms and studied in a variety of brain-damaged patient populations. When patients with anterior left-hemisphere lesions, those occurring in and surrounding Broca's area, have been studied these articulation errors frequently have been subsumed under the terms apraxia of speech or verbal dyspraxia. Although occurring in isolation, these problems are most frequently accompanied by aphasia and are often considered as part of the syndrome of Broca's aphasia (Blumstein, Cooper, Goodglass, Statlender, & Gottlieb, 1980; Trost & Canter, 1974). The phonological-articulatory production problems of posterior lesion patients, which also manifest themselves as articulation errors, are typically referred to as literal or phonemic paraphasias. They occur primarily in conduction aphasic patients and, to a lesser degree, in Wernicke's aphasic patients (Burns & Canter, 1977; Goodglass & Kaplan, 1972).

Traditionally, in these aphasic groups the phonological-articulatory problems have been described as clinically different and have been suggested to stem from different neurological bases. In Broca's type, the problems have been described as the result of programming problems in the sequencing of neuromotor commands which drive the articulatory musculature. In this case, the linguistic message to be produced is intact but the programming of it is defective and misarticulations are heard in the spoken message. The types of errors observed have been described at length elsewhere (Shankweiler & Harris, 1966; Johns & Darley, 1970; Trost, 1970; Trost & Canter, 1974; LaPointe & Johns, 1975; Shewan, 1980; and this volume). Briefly, they include inconsistent phonemic substitutions, groping for correct articulatory posturing, particular problems with place of articulation, and increasing difficulty across vowels, singleton consonants, consonant clusters, and longer stimuli. The view that these problems are due solely to motor speech sequencing problems has recently been challenged since linguistic variables have been found to influence performance (Martin & Rigrodsky, 1974; Tonkovich & Marquardt, 1977) and since independent studies of voice onset time (VOT) have been interpreted as showing that Broca's aphasic speakers make both phonemic and phonetic errors (Blumstein, Cooper, Zurif, & Caramazza, 1977; Blumstein et al., 1980). Phonetic errors were characterized by VOTs which spanned the time zone between the two distinct VOT regions corresponding to normal voiced and voiceless categories. These errors were consistent with an interpretation of a motor speech programming impairment. The phonemic errors, while less common, were found in some Broca's aphasic patients and were clearly phonemic substitutions, interpreted as indicating impairment in phonological selection or an incorrect underlying phonological representation. A more recent report (Blumstein et al., 1980) corroborated these data and extended them by describing additional types of aphasic patients.

As part of their overall symptom complex, posterior lesion patients also demonstrate phonological-articulatory production problems which are thought to be the result of impairment in the phonological component of the linguistic system. The resulting articulation errors, phonemic substitutions, are thought to be due to phonemic selection problems, whereby the wrong phoneme is selected but programmed and produced accurately. Blumstein et al.'s (1980) recent study analyzing VOT showed that both conduction and Wernicke's aphasic groups made not only these phonemic errors but also phonetic errors. Therefore, the articulation errors in Broca's, conduction, and Wernicke's aphasic individuals appeared to be similar, that is, all groups demonstrated *both* phonetic and phonemic problems.

The present investigation extends beyond consideration of apraxia of speech as traditionally defined. It was designed to determine whether Broca's and conduction aphasic subjects showed similar or different phonological-articulatory problems, using an analysis of VOT. The aphasic groups were compared to age-matched normal controls to ensure that any differences were the result of brain damage and not of the aging process. The study further investigated whether older normal controls' productions were similar to or different from younger controls previously reported in the literature (Lisker & Abramson, 1964, 1967; Sweeting & Baken, 1978).

SUBJECTS

The 15 aphasic subjects were selected from a larger clinical population seen at several outpatient facilities. The diagnosis of aphasia was made by qualified, experienced speech-language pathologists, based on the results of clinical speech and language evaluations which included the Boston Diagnostic Aphasia Examination (BDAE; Goodglass & Kaplan, 1972) or the Western Aphasia Battery (WAB; Kertesz & Poole, 1974) and in one case the Minnesota Test for Differential Diagnosis of Aphasia (MTDDA; Schuell, 1965). Type of aphasia, either Broca's or conduction, was assigned by the speech-language pathologist using the profile of oral speech and language characteristics demonstrated by each aphasic subject. Severity of aphasia was similarly assigned using a clinical rating scale from mild to severe; the mild and moderate categories predominated (Table 7-1).

The Broca's group was composed of 9 subjects and the conduction group contained 6. All subjects, 10 males and 5 females, were English speakers. Etiology of aphasia was cerebrovascular accident (CVA) in all cases, with the exception of one head trauma. All aphasic subjects were stable at the time of testing, with a mean of 20 months postonset. All subjects passed an audiometric screening test using age appropriate norms. Age ranged from 34 to 72 years, with a mean of 59.13 years. The normal control group, containing 9 subjects, 6 females and 3 males, was comparable in age with the aphasic group. No subject had a history of any neurological disorder; all passed an audiometric screening test; and all were first-language users of English.

TABLE 7-1
Background data for aphasic and normal subjects

	Age	Sex	Months Postonset	Severity
Broca's Aphasics				
	47	M	16	Severe
	49	M	9	Severe
	49	F	9	Moderate
	52	M	3	Mod.-Sev.
	61	M	2	Mild
	62	F	11	Moderate
	64	M	51	Mild
	67	F	27	Moderate
	72	F	1	Moderate
Conduction Aphasics				
	34	M[a]	5	Mild
	54	F	86	Moderate
	65	M	34	Mild
	68	M	36	Mild
	71	M	1	Mild
	72	M	12	Mild
Normal Controls				
	48	F		
	54	F		
	59	F		
	61	F		
	61	M		
	62	F		
	67	M		
	68	F		
	77	M		

[a] = Traumatic etiology.

METHODOLOGY

Speech Materials

The speech samples consisted of 70 monosyllabic consonant-vowel-consonant (CVC) words containing, with approximately equal frequencies, the stop consonants /p,t,k,b,d,g/ in initial position, followed by a representative set of tense/lax vowels, and terminated by another consonant. The list, taken from Stevenson (1975), was identical to that used for an auditory discrimination task reported elsewhere (Booth, Leeper, &

Shewan, in preparation). Frequency of occurrence was not strictly controlled but the means for voiced and voiceless cognate words were comparable.

Administration

After passing screening tests, each subject was tested individually by the same examiner. The word list was randomized for every subject to avoid either facilitation or interference of word order. The subject produced the word after the examiner's prompt "Say____" while being shown the printed word. No response after three prompts eliminated any word. If a subject had initiation, repetition, or word retrieval difficulties after the third prompt, the item was repeated at the end of the list; a failure eliminated it from analysis.

All speech samples were tape recorded using a TEAC (model A-7300) reel-to-reel recorder and Electro Voice (model 664) microphone placed 30 cm from the speaker's mouth. All recordings were made in a sound-treated test suite at a tape transport speed of 19 cm/sec.

VOT Measurement

The voice onset time (VOT) measurements, taken from the initial stop consonant and vowel portion of each intelligible word, were derived from wide-band spectrograms made on a Kay Elemetrics (model 7071A) spectrograph. Measurement of VOT, using Lisker and Abramson's (1964) method, is the relative time period between the onset of energy (noise burst) which is acoustically representative of air release through the occlusal port for the stop and the first vertical striation (glottal pulse). The interval between the burst and the initiation of voicing was measured manually using calipers calibrated in millimeters and the obtained values then converted to milliseconds (to the nearest 5 msec). Voicing lead was defined as the time interval in which the glottal pulses occurred before the stop release and was assigned a negative (−) sign (negative VOT values are enclosed in angled parentheses throughout the text and tables). Voicing lag was defined as the time interval in which the onset of glottal pulsing occurred after the plosive burst and was assigned a positive (+) sign. Glottal pulses occurring at the same instant as the burst release were assigned a zero (0) value.

RESULTS

Normal and Aphasic Group VOT Measurements

The VOT values (milliseconds) for each of the six stop phonemes were examined for the three groups of subjects. For the normals, Table 7-2

TABLE 7-2
VOT measures for normal and aphasic groups

Group	*Number of Productions*	*Mean*	*Median*	*VOT Values (msec) Range*	*Standard Deviation*
Normal Controls					
p	114	72.51	62.65	0 - 168.00	37.77
t	117	90.42	84.11	23.10 - 190.20	35.33
k	133	101.31	92.48	37.80 - 319.20	42.05
b	121	<47.89>[a]	<0.28>	<252.00>- 67.20	72.62
d	113	<34.81>	7.42	<239.40>- 42.00	79.12
g	90	<24.72>	16.59	<226.80>- 151.20	80.90
All	688	29.60	41.88	<252.00>- 319.20	87.36
Broca's Aphasics					
p	111	50.93	41.99	<50.40>- 241.50	44.72
t	115	55.89	50.09	<197.40>- 352.80	47.52
k	126	70.35	63.20	<42.00>- 226.80	38.23
b	125	<34.10>	0.16	<407.40>- 75.60	84.88
d	109	<20.60>	16.19	<428.40>- 92.40	98.74
g	88	26.05	27.48	<159.60>- 247.80	45.12
All	674	24.82	31.50	<428.40>- 352.80	76.03
Conduction Aphasics					
p	75	49.73	49.88	<75.60>- 142.80	36.77
t	77	58.80	59.37	14.70 - 147.00	28.03
k	88	77.84	79.10	0 - 273.00	42.50
b	84	<39.50>	<9.45>	<210.00>- 33.60	56.32
d	77	<32.38>	<0.26>	<176.40>- 50.40	58.89
g	58	<2.57>	17.25	<134.40>- 46.20	45.69
All	459	19.85	25.17	<210.00>- 273.00	65.79

[a]< > = Negative portion of VOT continuum.

shows that the mean VOT values for the voiceless phonemes /p,t,k/ were all positive, (72.51, 90.42, 101.31 msec) with an increasing VOT lag as place of articulation proceeded from labial to velar. The corresponding values for /b,d,g/ were all negative, with means of ⟨ 47.89 ⟩, ⟨ 34.81 ⟩, and ⟨ 24.72 ⟩ msec, and accompanied by a decreasing VOT lead time from labial to velar. Therefore, shifts to the right along the VOT scale paralleled backing in place of articulation. The median VOT values were similar to the mean values for /p,t,k/, with less than 10 msec differences observed. The wider difference spread for /b,d,g/ indicated these VOT distributions were positively skewed.

The normal group's range in VOT values for each of the six phonemes was quite large, from 167.10 msec to 378.00 msec, with the larger ranges associated with the voiced phonemes. Their VOT values spanned the lead, the simultaneous, and lag portions of the VOT scale. The standard deviations, paralleling the trends found in their range data, varied from 35.33 to 80.90, with smaller deviations for /p,t,k/ than for /b,d,g/.

For the Broca's aphasic group (Table 7-2) the mean VOT values for /p,t,k/ were 50.93, 55.89, and 70.35 msec and for /b,d,g/ were ⟨ 34.10 ⟩, ⟨ 20.60 ⟩, and 26.05 msec. Parallel shifts to the right along the VOT continuum were observed as place of articulation proceeded from labial to velar. The median VOT values were close to the mean values for /p,t,k/ but were further displaced for /b,d,g/, showing positively skewed VOT distributions.

Ranges for phoneme production were large, 268.80 to 781.20 msec, with the smaller ranges characteristic of the voiceless phoneme triad. For the voiced phonemes, productions spanned both the lead and lag portions of the VOT scale. Standard deviations from 38.23 to 98.74 msec followed the range data, with smaller deviations for /p,t,k/ than for /b,d,g/.

VOT measures for the conduction aphasic group revealed mean values for /p,t,k/ of 49.73, 58.80, and 77.84 msec, respectively, all demonstrating a VOT lag (Table 7-2). The means for /b,d,g/ were ⟨ 39.50 ⟩, ⟨ 32.38 ⟩, and ⟨ 2.57 ⟩ msec, all showing a VOT lead. Place of articulation changes from labial to velar were associated with VOT shifts to the right along the VOT continuum. Median VOT values for /p,t,k/ were similar to the mean values. The greater differences for /b,d,g/ were in the direction of skewing the distributions positively.

The ranges for VOT values, 132.30 to 273.00 msec, were similar for /p,t,k/ and /b,d,g/, with both the smallest and largest ranges falling in the /p,t,k/ group. Standard deviations were smaller for /p,t,k/ than for /b,d,g/, with values spanning from 28.03 to 58.89 msec, indicating greater variability within the voiced triad.

Normal Group Comparisons with Previous Literature

To eliminate VOT values which were not representative of our normal group [Shewan–Leeper–Booth (SLB)], "standard" lower and upper bounds were established by eliminating those VOT values which constitute the bottom and top 5% of the frequency distribution for each stop phoneme.[2] These values, termed "standard" values, were then compared with VOT measurements from four young subjects reported by Lisker and Abramson (1964; LA; Table 7-3). For VOT ranges, SLB subjects extended the lower bounds for four of six phonemes, with three being the

TABLE 7-3
VOT values for initial stop consonants

Phoneme	*"Standard"[a] Current Data*		*Lisker and Abramson (1964)*		*Sweeting and Baken (1978)*		*Jaffe (1977)*	
	Range	*Mean*	*Range*	*Mean*	*Range[c]*	*Mean*	*Range[d]*	*Mean*
p	25.2 - 138.6	72.5	20.0 - 120.0	58.0	41.0 - 112.0	77.76		
b	<184.8>- 14.7	<104.4>	<130.0>- 5.0	<101.0>	4.0 - 31.0	12.95		
		5.5		1.0				
p-b gap[b]	10.5		15.0		10.0			
t	42.0 - 159.6	90.4	30.0 - 105.0	70.0			35.0 - 170.0	85.93
d	<222.6>- 25.2	<104.6>	<155.0>- 25.0	<102.0>			<185.0>- 42.0	94.47
		11.3		5.0				11.03
t-d gap	16.8		5.0				7.0[e]	
k	50.4 - 163.8	101.3	50.0 - 135.0	80.0				
g	<168.0>- 42.0	<114.5>	<150.0>- 35.0	<88.0>				
		23.3		21.0				
k-g gap	8.4		15.0					

[a]"Standard" refers to the upper and lower VOT values which include 90% of the frequency distribution for each phoneme for the normal subject group.
[b]Gap refers to the width in milliseconds on the VOT scalé corresponding to the separation of the two cognate phonetic categories.
[c]Ranges are approximate since they were calculated from the figures in the paper.
[d]Ranges are approximate since they were taken from histograms included in the thesis.
[e]This represents an overlap of 7.0 msec between the phonetic categories.

voiced /b,d,g/ triad, and extended the upper bounds for five phonemes. Although the extensions were small (≅10 msec) in half the cases, they appeared as large as 122.6 msec in others. The LA data reported a 15 msec VOT gap between the cognate phonetic categories for /p-b/ and /k-g/ (Table 7-3), with a 5 msec gap for /t-d/. SLB gaps were smaller for /p-b/ and /k-g/, with respective values of 10.5 and 8.4 msec, but larger for /t-d/, with a value of 16.8. Reasons for these differences will be discussed later.

SLB VOT means for the voiced phonemes are reported using both a negative (−) and a positive (+) mean value to coincide with the LA reporting method. For the voiceless triad, SLB mean VOTs were consistently larger than those of LA, with the mean increases varying from 14 to 21 msec. For the voiced phonemes, SLB negative means were very similar, except for /g/, which showed a longer lead time; the positive means were also similar differences ≅6 msec). In general, SLB VOT ranges were extended and means were higher, indicating a wider spread along the VOT continuum than characteristic of LA's data. The unavailability of the LA raw data precluded any statistical comparisons.

The VOT literature reported for older normals is limited but some consistency emerged when SLB data were compared with Sweeting and Baken (1978) and Jaffe (1977). All studies (Table 7-3) showed a consistent VOT lag and similar mean VOT values for /p,t/. Less consistency was found for /b,d/; some productions showed a VOT lead and some a short lag. Mean VOT values were also more variable.

The lower and upper cutoff values for the VOT continuum of ⟨ 150 ⟩ to +150 msec. have been frequently used in the literature (Blumstein et al., 1980). We examined whether productions from the SLB older normals consistently fell within this range. Overall, 9.46% of SLB productions were outside this range and it included all productions of only two of the nine subjects. For five subjects, up to 10% of their productions were outside this range and for the remaining two, greater than 25% were outside the range. There appeared to be no clear-cut tendency for any phoneme to be particularly vulnerable to deviations from this range, with percentages varying from 5.26 to 14.05.

SLB values were then compared with the more restricted VOT ranges of the younger subjects reported by Lisker and Abramson (1964) (Table 7-4). Overall, 22.71% of SLB productions fell outside the range for its respective phoneme. Of the six phonemes, the smallest percentage of outliers occurred for /g/ (2.33%) and the largest for /b/ (6.26%).

TABLE 7-4
Percent VOT productions outside specified VOT ranges

	Percent Outside Range	
Phoneme	*Blumstein, Cooper, Goodglass, Statlendar and Gottlieb (1980)* *<150> to + 150 msec*	*Lisker and Abramson (1964)*
p	5.26	2.77
t	7.76	4.80
k	8.27	3.49
b	14.05	6.26
d	12.39	3.06
g	8.89	2.33
Total	9.46	22.71

Comparison of Normal and Aphasic Groups

The VOT values for our normals were then compared with the values for the Broca's and conduction aphasic groups. Whether these three groups exhibited similar VOT values for the six phonemes studied was examined using an analysis of variance (ANOVA) for repeated measures. As seen in Figures 7-1, 7-2, and 7-3, the mean VOT values for the aphasic groups showed shorter VOT lag times than for the normals for /p,t,k,/ and shorter VOT lead times for /b,d,g/. A test of simple main effects indicated that the group factor was not significant, ($F\,(2,21) = .20$, $p = .82$); that is, these differences were not large enough to reach statistical significance. This finding did not imply that normals and aphasics were similar in all respects in phoneme production. Clearly, the aphasics made errors and their distribution of productions along the VOT continuum differed from the normals. Figures 7-1, 7-2, and 7-3 show that the VOT ranges[3] were frequently larger for the aphasic groups and that the voiced–voiceless phonetic categories overlapped.

As was expected, mean values for the six phonemes differed. This was statistically confirmed by the significant main effect of phoneme ($F\,(5,105) = 59.44$, $p = .0001$). All phonemes were significantly different from one another, except p-t, b-d, and t-k, using the post hoc analysis of Newman–Keuls' shortest significant range test. The significant Group × Phoneme interaction ($F\,(10,105) = 2.37$, $p = .01$) could be explained by the differences between phoneme means for the voiced-voiceless triads; as examination of Figures 7-1, 7-2, and 7-3 shows the patterns across the three subject groups were similar.

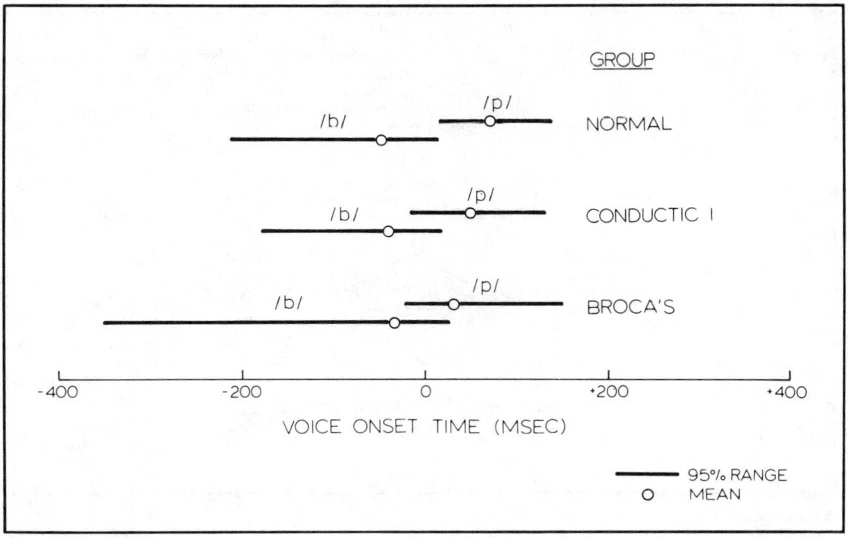

FIGURE 7–1
Ninety-five percent range and mean VOT values of /p,b/ for normal controls and Broca's and conduction aphasic groups

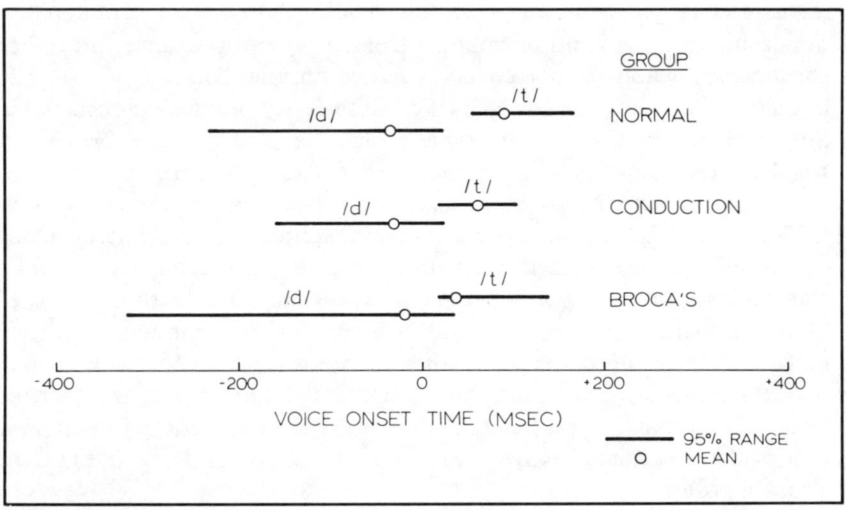

FIGURE 7-2
Ninety-five percent range and mean VOT values of /t,d/ for normal controls and Broca's and conduction aphasic groups

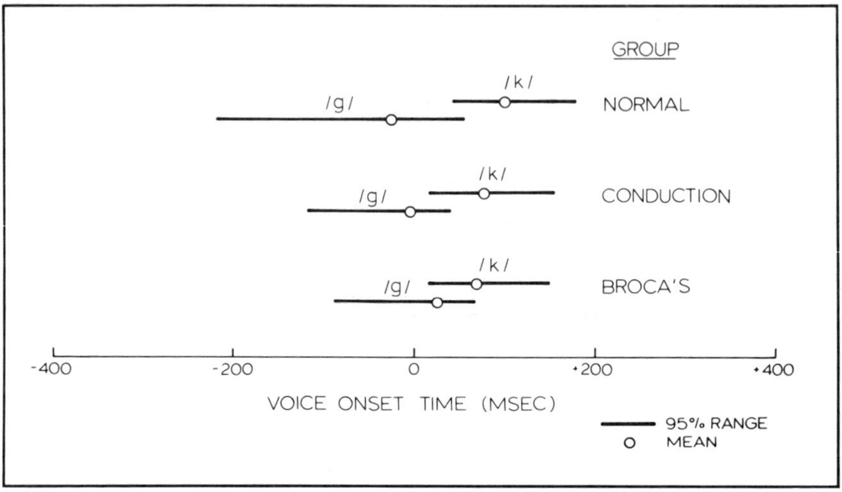

FIGURE 7-3
Ninety-five percent range and mean VOT values of /k,g/ for normal controls and Broca's and conduction aphasic groups

Blumstein et al. (1980) noted differences in the distributions of VOT for correct target productions among Broca's, Wernicke's, and conduction aphasic groups and normal controls. They noticed fewer prevoiced consonants, lead for voiced consonants, in the Broca's group than in the controls, but did not know how frequently prevoicing occurred in a normal group. Using a similar analysis, the percentage of prevoicing for the three subject groups in the present study was determined (Table 7-5). Prevoicing was defined as a VOT between the boundaries of ⟨ 500.0 ⟩ to ⟨ 2.0 ⟩ msec. For the normal subjects, prevoicing occurred on 38.89% of the voiced phonemes. The Broca's group consistently showed less prevoicing ($p < .01$) than the normal controls for each voiced phoneme while the opposite was evident for the conduction group ($p < .05$). Site of lesion in the conduction aphasic group could be verified by CT scan in only two cases, which prevented determining whether the prevoicing behavior was related to lesion site. The conduction aphasic group also exhibited significantly ($p < .01$) more prevoicing than the Broca's group.

Errors in Aphasic Groups

The subsequent analyses examined types and frequencies of errors in the aphasic groups. Any production errors for which a normal subject produced a voiced phoneme for its cognate and vice versa had been eliminated from their productions by using the 90% "standard" con-

TABLE 7–5
Percentage prevoicing for voiced consonants in aphasic and normal control groups

Group	*Percentage Prevoicing* *Phoneme* *b*	*d*	*g*	*Total*
Normal	48.76	33.63	32.22	38.89
Broca's	37.60	22.73	10.22	25.08
Conduction	52.38	48.05	31.03	45.21

cept. This had the effect of eliminating any extreme VOT values from both voiced and voiceless productions. These standard values from the normals were then used for comparison with the Broca's and conduction subjects' productions. For a voiceless target, if the aphasic subject produced a VOT value which was below the upper boundary for its voiced cognate, this was termed a phonemic B error. That is, the VOT value fell within the boundaries of a voiced phoneme and would be perceived as such by a listener depending on what other cues were present in the signal. If, for a voiced target, the aphasic subject produced a VOT value above the lower boundary for its voiceless cognate, this was termed a phonemic A error. If productions occurred in the area of separation between the voiced-voiceless cognates, where normals did not make productions, these were termed phonetic gap errors. Table 7-6 shows the percentage occurrence of these error types in the aphasic groups.

TABLE 7–6
Number and percentage phonetic gap and phonemic errors in Broca's and conduction aphasic groups

Cognate Pair	*Phonetic Gap* *No.*	*%*	*Phonemic A* *No.*	*%*	*B* *No.*	*%*	*Total* *No.*	*%*
Broca's Aphasics								
p-b	26	3.9	4	0.6	13	1.9	43	6.4
t-d	32	4.7	10	1.5	16	2.4	58	8.6
k-g	7	1.0	14	2.1	20	3.0	41	6.1
Total	65	9.6	28	4.2	49	7.3	142	21.1
Conduction Aphasics								
p-b	13	2.8	2	0.4	9	2.0	24	5.2
t-d	10	2.2	1	0.2	11	2.4	22	4.8
k-g	1	0.2	0	0.0	23	5.0	24	5.2
Total	24	5.2	3	0.6	43	9.4	70	15.2

The Broca's group made a total of 21.1% errors, with 9.6% phonetic gap errors, the type often ascribed to articulatory programming difficulties. Phonemic A errors accounted for 4.2% and Phonemic B errors 7.3%, indicating there were more phonemic than phonetic errors and, of the latter, more substitution errors of the voiced for voiceless phonemes. Similar error patterns were reflected for /p-b/ and /t-d/ cognate pairs, with more phonetic gap than phonemic errors, and among the phonemic, more B than A errors. The /k-g/ pair showed more phonemic than phonetic gap errors, although the pattern of more B than A errors held.

For the conduction aphasics, the total error percent was 15.2, with 5.2% phonetic gap errors, 0.6% phonemic A errors, and 9.4% phonemic B errors. The percent errors for phonemic versus phonetic gap was higher for the /t-d/ and /k-g/ cognate pairs, while there was a slightly larger percentage phonetic gap errors for /p-b/.

The effect of the type of aphasia on error production was examined using an analysis of variance. Because the data were not normally distributed, the percentages were transformed using the arc sine transformation. Since the outcome results were virtually identical for the transformed and the untransformed data, the results will be reported in their untransformed form for the sake of reader familiarity. The first analysis, grouping phonemic A and B errors into a single phonemic category, revealed no significant effects. That the main effect of the group did not emerge as significant ($F(1,13) = .44$, $p = .52$) indicated that the Broca's and the conduction aphasics did not differ in their overall mean percentage of errors. Type of error did not emerge as a significant effect ($F(1,13) = 2.94$, $p = .11$), suggesting that one type of error was not more prevalent than the other. Of particular interest was the interaction between group and error type. Also not significant ($F(1,13) = .97$, $p = .34$), this indicated that the two aphasic groups were performing similarly for the phonetic and phonemic error types.

Although there were no differences between the two major error types, further examination of the data substantiated the hypothesis of potential differences when phonemic A and B errors were treated separately. Error type (phonetic gap, phonemic A, phonemic B) emerged as a significant effect ($F(2,26) = 5.05$, $p = .01$). Post hoc analysis, using Newman-Keuls' shortest significant range test, indicated that there were significantly more phonetic gap and phonemic B errors than phonemic A errors ($p < .01$).

The contribution of place of articulation was examined by comparing the error percentages for labial (/p-b/), alveolar (/t-d/), and velar (/k-g/) positions. Results of the analysis of variance, although revealing no significant main effect for place of articulation, did reveal a significant interaction between error type and place (F (4,52) = 4.76, p = .002). Therefore, certain error types were more frequent for certain places of articulation. Post hoc analysis, using the Newman-Keuls' test, revealed that there were significantly more phonetic gap errors for /t-d/ and phonemic B errors for /k-g/ ($p < .05$) than phonemic A errors for /p-b/ and phonetic gap errors for /k-g/. All other groups were not significantly different from one another.

Whether voicing had an effect on error production was also measured. The analysis of variance revealed that voicing was a significant effect at the .07 level, indicating borderline significance (F (1,13) = 3.95). There were more errors for the voiceless triad /p,t,k/ than for their voiced cognates /b,d,g/.

DISCUSSION

When studying clinical problems in an older brain-damaged population, it is necessary to confirm that any manifest symptoms are due to the brain damage and not to the general aging process. This was particularly necessary in studying VOT because, like other speech production characteristics, such as vocal fundamental frequency, it may change with age (Hollien & Shipp, 1972; Kent & Burkard, 1981; Meyerson, 1976; Ryan, 1972; Schow, Christenson, Hutchinson, & Nerbonne, 1978).

Normal Control Group

Little VOT information is available for normal older subjects (Jaffe, 1977; Sweeting & Baken, 1978; Itoh, Sasanuma, Tatsumi, & Kobayashi, 1979) and previous studies comparing aphasic and normal subjects (Blumstein et al., 1977; Blumstein et al., 1980) have used the data from young adults as normal controls. The small number of normal subjects (largest group N = 5) and/or the restricted number of phonemes studied (Sweeting & Baken, 1978) further restrict the usefulness of the data. Employing a larger older normal control group enabled us to compare our data with those reported previously to examine whether age was a significant variable affecting VOT. Our observed differences and explanations offered can not be conclusive at this time since our data base too is limited. However, they do raise questions which further research should be designed to address.

Comparison of our SLB results with those of LA (four young normals) suggested some differences; however, insufficient LA data precluded statistical comparisons. The extended VOT production boundaries, the higher means for voiceless phonemes, and the large percentage SLB productions outside the LA ranges for their respective phonemes might be explained by a loss of precision in the operation of the physiological speech mechanism; that is, slowness in starting laryngeal vibration (glottal pulsing) or differences in respiratory and supraglottal physiological reactions to voiced and voiceless sound production (Hixon, 1982). This explanation is consistent with the longer VOT lag times for the voiceless stops but inconsistent with the long VOT lead times for the voiced stops. A better explanation, consistent with our data, is a difficulty in the ability of the vocal mechanism to shift rapidly from stop to vowel to the following stop consonant. Another possibility, that the four LA subjects did not produce VOTs representative of young adults, cannot be confirmed since data from additional speakers (Lisker & Abramson, 1967) corroborated these findings, while Sweeting and Baken's (1978) /p-b/ data contradicted it. Amidst this confusion what is certain, however, is that a larger data base is needed to establish reliable norms.

Further reports of the effects of aging on VOT will need to consider the structure and function of the respiratory, phonatory, articulatory systems, and their interactions since these systems are involved in VOT production and are affected by aging. Structural changes, such as atrophy (Corso, 1975; Fink, 1974; Kahane, 1981) and loss of tissue elasticity (Kahane, 1981) alter speech production related to voicing contrasts. Physiological changes, such as reduced efficiency and reduced control (Hixon, Mead, & Goldman, 1976; Kahane, 1981; Netsell, 1969; Turner, Mead & Wohl, 1968), may also affect VOT production. The relative importance of each system and whether effects occur both upstream and downstream also need consideration. The effects may also extend beyond the peripheral speech production mechanism to neuromotor control of the distinctive speech gestures necessary to produce distinctive VOT values.

The voicing lead used by all our normal subjects contrasted with previous reports. That voicing lead is more characteristic of citation speech than of sentence production (Lisker & Abramson, 1967) may explain our differences with Sweeting and Baken (1978) who used a carrier phrase with their samples. The age difference in the speakers may explain the general absence of voicing lead for Lisker and Abramson (1964).

Comparing SLB and LA data, the SLB gaps between cognate phonetic categories (Table 7-3) were smaller for phonemes whose places of articulation were at the peripheries of the vocal tract (/p-b, k-g/), with a reverse trend for the /t-d/ pair. Differences in measurement techniques and/or in instrumental error might be responsible. These considerations, however, would apply to all the published research in VOT.

Since 9.46% of our normals' productions fell outside the VOT bounds of ⟨ 150 ⟩ to +150 msec (Blumstein et al., 1980), caution should be exercised in using these cutoffs. The extended boundaries could also have resulted from the operation of a less precise mechanism or stimulus differences. Blumstein et al. included stop consonants plus the vowel /a/, whereas our data used a variety of vowels within the CVC format. Although Lisker and Abramson (1967) found no significant relationship between vocalic context and VOT, Weismer (1979) has noted that VOT may be a function of the additive effects of the vowel that follows — tense/ lax, and the characteristic of the following consonant — voiced/ voiceless; that is, with VOT being longer when the vowel is tense and the following consonant voiced. Since our CVC data were pooled and included both tense and lax vowels and voiced and voiceless final consonants, it is possible that a slight overall lengthening of VOT has resulted from these additive effects.

The VOT values for labial, alveolar, and velar stops showed parallel shifts for voiced and voiceless cognates. As place of articulation proceeded from labial to velar, VOT lag time increased for the voiceless stops and VOT lead time decreased for the voiced stops. This was consistent with both Lisker and Abramson (1964, 1967) and Blumstein et al. (1980), who based their values on the former study. Therefore, VOT appears to be sensitive to the place of closure in the vocal tract. As has been noted by Weismer (1980), this place effect may be related, not as an active control system, but rather as a passive control system related to aerodynamic function of the pressure drop across the glottis from sequentially smaller volumes of air from front to back place of articulation.

Aphasic Subject Groups

The aphasic and normal group mean VOT values showed no statistically significant differences, probably due to the large variability within each group. These results were consistent with Jaffe's finding for /t-d/ (1977). On the average, the aphasic subjects produced shorter VOT lead and lag times for members of all cognate pairs. They also produced utterances whose VOTs fell within the gap between phonetic categories, which had the result of converging mean VOT values toward the 0 point of the continuum.

Our measures for the aphasic groups suggested that, similar to Blumstein et al. (1980), VOT was sensitive to both place of articulation and voicing. Parallel shifts of shorter VOT lead and longer VOT lag for voiced and voiceless stops were seen as place proceeded from labial to velar.

The similarities between the two aphasic groups in the present study were striking. Their VOT values were similar and showed similar patterns to the normal controls. Both groups showed both types of errors with more phonemic B and phonetic gap errors than phonemic A errors. This pattern, contrary to most of the previous literature, was in agreement with the Blumstein et al. VOT study (1980) and her previous comparison (Blumstein, 1973) of phonological behavior in free speech.

Problems with Motor Sequencing and Phonemic Selection as Exclusive Explanations of Aphasic Group Data

The data for the Broca's and conduction aphasics in this study might be explained in several ways, which, in turn, depend on how the behavior is viewed. The error data were divided into phonemic and phonetic categories on the basis of standards from age-matched normal controls. That these represent different types of errors is perhaps more controversial for the Broca's aphasics than for the conductions. If one accepts that there are both phonetic and phonemic errors, the task becomes how to explain these errors in both groups of aphasic subjects. Whether the phonological-articulatory behaviors are viewed as the same or different and whether these can be explained by the same or different underlying causes presents four alternative hypotheses. The traditional view that Broca's aphasic groups demonstrate phonetic errors and conduction aphasic groups demonstrate phonemic errors was not supported by our data. Both groups made phonetic and phonemic errors, with the latter type predominant. This suggested that an explanatory hypothesis of different surface behaviors being explained by different underlying causes, that is, the unitary explanations of motor sequencing problems explaining Broca's aphasics' performance and phonemic selection problems explaining conduction aphasics', were not adequate.

A second alternative hypothesis that the same behavior, for example, phonemic errors, can be explained by the same underlying cause in both aphasic groups also encounters difficulties. A motor sequencing hypothesis can be invoked to explain the phonetic errors of the Broca's aphasics and it could be used for their phonemic errors by including these as severely disturbed neuromotor programs. A similar explanation for the conduction aphasics seemed improbable since phonetic errors were less predominant; no conduction subject had a predominance of phonetic errors. Further, the predominance of phonemic errors would indicate more abnormal motor programming in this group than in the Broca's aphasics. Such an explanation seems suspect in view of their fluent speech.

Similarly, a phoneme selection hypothesis encounters difficulty with the phonetic gap errors. English has no phonemic categories which correspond to these productions, therefore precluding selection of such a category. The phonetic gap errors of the conduction aphasic subjects are thereby difficult to reconcile. The timing problems seen in coordinating production systems in a patient with apraxia of speech (Itoh, Sasanuma, & Ushijima, 1979) argue against a simple phonemic selection view for Broca's aphasic subjects.

A third possibility that the different behaviors of the two aphasic groups are simply different surface manifestations of a single underlying cause also runs into difficulty. While phonetic and phonemic errors could be explained by different degrees of motor programming difficulties in the Broca's aphasic group, this association is circumspect for the conduction aphasic subjects.

The fourth possibility that the same behavior is explained by different underlying causes in the two groups also proves unsatisfactory. For example, phonetic gap errors can not be reconciled to motor programming problems in Broca's aphasics and to phoneme selection problems in conduction aphasics. What emerges from this discussion is that the phonological-articulatory problems in both groups can not be explained by a single underlying cause, that is, either motor programming or phoneme selection.

What seems apparent from this discussion is that the situation is more complex than assigning a particular behavior to a particular underlying cause for all subjects. Problems with such an assignment arise at all levels:

(1) *Behavioral.* Are phonemic and phonetic errors a reality? To determine this question conclusively, we need correlated data from various levels of analysis, perceptual, acoustic, and physiologic. Our data are limited to acoustic analysis with the single feature of the VOT. Additional data from other features are necessary to corroborate both types of problems that emerge.

(2) *Explanations.* Exclusive notions of motor sequencing or phoneme selection represent two possibilities, the ones which have been traditionally invoked as explanations. Readers are exposed to several additional ones outlined by Rosenbek, Kent, and LaPointe in this volume (Chap. 1). Our data were not designed to, and can not resolve all these issues.

(3) *Subjects.* Our data included two types of aphasic patients. When interpreting phonological-articulatory behaviors, this adds another dimension to be dealt with. Many other data bases have included only one type of patient, that is, apraxia of speech. Additional research extending beyond this group will be necessary to determine if subject groups are homogeneous or heterogeneous with regard to their phonological-articulatory production.

Conduction aphasic group. The conduction aphasics examined in the present study, if they made production errors, always demonstrated more phonemic than phonetic errors. Two subjects showed a 2:1 ratio for phonemic to phonetic errors while two others made no errors of either type. The generalizability of these patterns to all conduction aphasics is not possible since our sample size was small and included primarily mildly impaired conduction aphasics.

Our findings contrasted with the Blumstein et al. (1980) report of two conduction subgroups: one with more phonetic than phonemic errors; a second with more phonemic errors. Blumstein et al. suggested that the differing VOT patterns were correlated with different speech output which, in turn, was reflective of different lesion sites. CT scan corroboration revealed one "phonetic" conduction aphasic with a suprasylvian lesion and one "phonemic" with a subsylvian lesion. In our conduction group the one subject with a confirmed frontoparietal lesion did not show the predicted predominance of phonetic errors; the other with a parietotemporal lesion did show a predominance of phonemic errors. With only two CT scans available in both studies, it is hazardous to draw any conclusions and not possible to determine whether the groups were comparable with respect to lesion site and, correspondingly, error patterns.

Broca's aphasic group. When our Broca's aphasics' data were compared with the Blumstein et al. (1980) findings, both consistencies and inconsistencies were found. They did show less prevoicing for voiced consonants than the controls. However, we found shorter rather than longer VOT lag times for voiceless consonants and a greater percentage of phonemic than phonetic errors. Differences in number of subjects (Blumstein tested five Broca's) and/or severity of patients might contribute to these findings. That the pattern of Broca's errors could be explained by speech initiation difficulties seemed unlikely. We did not find longer VOT lag times for the voiceless phonemes and although VOT lead times for the voiced phonemes were smaller than for normals, the differences were not remarkable. Also, one might have expected more errors on the voiced phonemes: the opposite was observed.

Influence of Place of Articulation and Voicing

Percentage of errors was not affected by place of articulation in the aphasic groups. Place did interact with error type but no particular pattern emerged. Since the gap between the /k-g/ phonetic categories was very small (8.4 msec), fewer phonetic and more phonemic errors would be likely to occur. The converse applied for /t-d/; the large gap was associated with significantly more phonetic errors.

Voicing influenced percentage errors ($p = .07$) in both aphasic groups, with more errors occurring on voiceless phonemes. Error type and voicing did not interact, indicating similar error patterns for both voiced and voiceless phonemes, that is, more phonemic (A and B) than phonetic gap errors.

Influence of Severity of Phonological–Articulatory Disturbance

Whether the severity of the phonological–articulatory disturbance paralleled the general severity of aphasia was examined. The general clinical severity ratings were based on information from all language modalities rather than phonological–articulatory performance alone. Mild and moderate Broca's aphasics exhibited lower mean percentages of errors than the severe Broca's, but interindividual variability was large in the mild and moderate groups. Therefore, the trend in the Broca's group was for severity of phonological–articulatory errors to parallel overall severity of aphasia, with individual exceptions. Since all patients in the conduction group were mild, except one, severities could not be compared. Again, great variability was evident among the five mild patients. Larger groups of subjects are needed before any reliable conclusions can be made.

The present results are suggestive of three important changes from previous conceptions: (1) VOT values are sensitive to age; (2) Broca's and conduction aphasics show similarities in their phonological–articulatory problems; and (3) dichotomous explanations of motor speech programming problems and phonemic selection problems for the misarticulation errors observed in Broca's and conduction aphasics are too simplistic. Our results are viewed as suggestive because of the small number of subjects in the normal and aphasic groups. Although larger than the comparison studies (Blumstein et al., 1980; Lisker & Abramson, 1964), we considered additional data were needed to verify the reliability of our findings. With the data available to us it was not possible to verify comparability of our aphasic groups with those of Blumstein et al. (1980). Therefore, different results could reflect group composition differences rather than, or in addition to, true behavioral differences. Finally, differences in measurement techniques could contribute to differences in results.

The results of the present study are not intended to describe or to explain fully "apraxia of speech." As Rosenbek, Kent, and LaPointe (this volume, Chap. 1) point out, a complex understanding of apraxia will probably come about from studying it from several approaches and synthesizing results. That is, acoustical parameters such as phoneme duration, rate, and extent of formant transition, and spectral energy of the noise burst must be viewed with respect to their saliency for aphasic and apraxic subjects' perception and production at several levels of speech complexity (syllable, word, phrase length, or longer). Only when these acoustic cues are related to micropatterns of neurophysiological processing in brain-damaged patients will the impact of any one of these cues be understood. Further, the data reported here deal with only one approach and extend beyond what traditionally have been described as "apraxic" subjects.

SUMMARY

VOT measurements were made for the initial stop consonants /p,t,k,b,d,g/ of CVC monosyllabic words in Broca's and conduction aphasic and normal control subjects. Results suggested that VOT in normal subjects was sensitive to age. Broca's and conduction aphasics demonstrated patterns for mean VOT values similar to normals — that is, voiceless stops were characterized by VOT lag while voiced stops were characterized by VOT lead or simultaneous burst, with shifts to the right along the VOT continuum as place of articulation proceeded from labial to velar. Broca's and conduction aphasics both demonstrated phonetic and phonemic errors, with greater frequency of phonemic errors. The pattern of errors was similar for both groups: phonemic B and phonetic gap errors were significantly more frequent than phonemic A errors. Type of error interacted with place of articulation and more errors occurred on voiceless phonemes. Our data were compared with those in the literature, indicating some inconsistencies and the need for additional research. The limitations of a motor speech programming impairment or a phonemic selection problem as explanations of the phonological-articulatory problems observed in Broca's and conduction aphasics were discussed.

NOTES

[1]The term phonological-articulatory is used to encompass both the articulatory system and the phonological system since impairment in either or both may underlie the perceived articulation errors associated with apraxia of speech. It is not meant to imply that both systems are always impaired.

[2]This procedure also had the effect of eliminating any voiced/voiceless or voiceless/voiced error productions which might have been missed previously.

[3]The ranges shown represented 95% of the distributions in contrast to the 90% ranges used to define "standard" values for the normal controls.

REFERENCES

Blumstein, S. E. *A phonological investigation of aphasic speech.* The Hague: Mouton, 1973.

Blumstein, S. E., Cooper, W. E., Goodglass, H., Statlender, S., & Gottlieb, J. Production deficits in aphasia: A voice-onset time analysis. *Brain and Language,* 1980, *9,* 153–170.

Blumstein, S. E., Cooper, W. E., Zurif, E. B., & Caramazza, A. The perception and production of voice-onset time in aphasia. *Neuropsychologia,* 1977, *15,* 371–383.

Booth, J. C., Leeper, H. A., & Shewan, C. M. *Stop consonant discrimination in aphasics and normals using an adaptive discrimination technique.* (In preparation)

Burns, M. S., & Canter, G. J. Phonemic behavior of aphasic patients with posterior cerebral lesions. *Brain and Language,* 1977, *4,* 492–507.

Corso, J. F. Sensory processes in man during maturity and senescence. In J. M. Ordy & K. R. Brizzee (Eds.), *Neurobiology of aging — an interdisciplinary life span approach.* New York: Plenum Press, 1975.

Fink, B. R. Spring mechanisms in the human larynx. *Acta Otolaryngologica,* 1974, *77,* 295–304.

Goodglass, H., & Kaplan, E. *The assessment of aphasia and related disorders.* Philadelphia: Lea and Febiger, 1972.

Hixon, T. J. Personal communication, March 1982.

Hixon, T., Mead, J., & Goldman, M. Dynamics of the chest wall during speech production: Function of the thorax, rib cage, diaphragm, and abdomen. *Journal of Speech and Hearing Research,* 1976, *19,* 297–356.

Hollien, H., & Shipp, T. Speaking fundamental frequency and chronologic age in males. *Journal of Speech and Hearing Research,* 1972, *15,* 155-159.

Itoh, M., Sasanuma, S., Tatsumi, I. F., & Kobayashi, Y. Voice onset time characteristics of apraxia of speech. *Annual Bulletin Research Institute of Logopedics and Phoniatrics,* 1979, *13,* 123–132.

Itoh, M., Sasanuma, S., & Ushijima, T. Velar movements during speech in a patient with apraxia of speech. *Brain and Language,* 1979, *7,* 227-239.

Jaffe, D. W. *Acoustic analysis of voice onset time characteristics of apraxic, aphasic and non-brain injured adults.* Unpublished masters thesis, University of Massachusetts, 1977.

Johns, D. F., & Darley, F. L. Phonemic variability in apraxia of speech. *Journal of Speech and Hearing Research,* 1970, 13, 556–583.

Kahane, J. C. Anatomic and physiologic changes in the aging peripheral speech mechanism. In D. S. Beasley & G. A. Davis (Eds.), *Aging: Communication processes and disorders,* New York: Grune & Stratton, 1981.

Kent, R. D., & Burkard, R. Changes in the acoustic correlates of speech production. In D. S. Beasley & G. A. Davis (Eds.), *Aging: Communication processes and disorders,* New York: Grune & Stratton, 1981.

Kertesz, A., & Poole, E. The aphasia quotient: The taxonomic approach to measurement of aphasic disability. *Canadian Journal of Neurological Sciences,* 1974, *1,* 7–16.

LaPointe, L. L., & Johns, D. F. Some phonemic characteristics in apraxia of speech. *Journal of Communication Disorders,* 1975, *8,* 259–269.

Lisker, L., & Abramson, A. S. A cross-language study of voicing in initial stops: Acoustical measurements. *Word,* 1964, *20,* 384–428.

Lisker, L., & Abramson, A. S. Some effects of context on voice onset time in English stops. *Language and Speech,* 1967, *10,* 1-28.

Martin, A. D., & Rigrodsky, S. An investigation of phonological impairment in aphasia, I. *Cortex,* 1974, *10,* 317-328.

Meyerson, M. The effects of aging on communication. *Journal of Gerontology,* 1976, *31,* 29-38.

Netsell, R. *A perceptual-acoustic-physiological study of syllable stress.* Unpublished Ph.D. dissertation, University of Iowa, 1969.

Ryan, W. J. Acoustic aspects of the aging voice. *Journal of Gerontology,* 1972, *27,* 265-268

Schow, R., Christenson, J., Hutchinson, J., & Nerbonne, M. *Communication disorders of the aged.* Baltimore, MD.: University Park Press, 1978.

Schuell, H. *Differential diagnosis of aphasia with the Minnesota Test.* Minneapolis: University of Minnesota Press, 1965.

Shankweiler, D., & Harris, K. S. An experimental approach to the problem of articulation in aphasia. *Cortex,* 1966, *2,* 277-292.

Shewan, C. M. Phonological processing in Broca's aphasics. *Brain and Language,* 1980, *10,* 71-88.

Stevenson, P. W. Responses to speech audiometry and phonemic discrimination patterns in the elderly. *Audiology,* 1975, *14,* 185-231.

Sweeting, P. M., & Baken, R. J. *Voice onset time and vowel duration in the normal aged population.* Paper presented at the annual convention of the American Speech and Hearing Association, November 1978.

Tonkovich, J. D., & Marquardt, T. P. The effects of stress and melodic intonation on apraxia of speech. In R. H. Brookshire (Ed.), *Clinical aphasiology: Proceedings of the conference 1977.* Minneapolis: BRK, 1977.

Trost, J. E. *A descriptive study of verbal apraxia in patients with Broca's aphasia.* Unpublished Ph.D. dissertation, Northwestern University, 1970.

Trost, J. E., & Canter, G. J. Apraxia of speech in patients with Broca's aphasia: A study of phoneme production accuracy and error patterns. *Brain and Language,* 1974, *1,* 63-79.

Turner, J. M., Mead, J., & Wohl, M. E. Elasticity of human lungs in relation to age. *Journal of Applied Physiology,* 1968, *25,* 664-671.

Weismer, G. Sensitivity of voice-onset-time (VOT) measures to certain segmental features in speech production. *Journal of Phonetics,* 1979, *7,* 197-204.

Weismer, G. Control of the voicing distinction for intervocalic stops and fricatives: Some data and theoretical considerations. *Journal of Phonetics,* 1980, *8,* 427-438.

ACKNOWLEDGMENT

The authors would like to acknowledge S. Moody for testing patients, J. Moon for assistance with the spectrographic analysis, and A. Donner for statistical consulting. This research was supported by a grant from the Ontario Heart Foundation to the authors.

8

Simplification and Gesture Reduction in Phonological Disorders of Apraxia and Aphasia

Eric Keller

Clinicians and researchers alike are often astonished at the lack of elaboration of contemporary theories of the phonetic and phonological breakdown in aphasia and apraxia of speech.[1,2] Although such disorders occur at the very level of linguistic processing that seems the most accessible to in-depth analysis, relatively little research has been performed in this domain. A number of detailed descriptive studies have been published (e.g., Blumstein, 1973; Hécaen & Consoli, 1973; Keller, 1975; Lecours & Lhermitte, 1969; Martin & Rigrodsky, 1974; Schnitzer, 1972; Shankweiler & Harris, 1966; Shankweiler, Harris, & Taylor, 1968; Trost & Canter, 1974); but few studies have attempted to come to grips with the essential nature of this disorder.

Particularly vexing is the lack of a coherent explanatory hypothesis. In part, this may be due to the apparent lack of pattern of the phonological breakdown in aphasia and apraxia of speech. The inconsistency and unpredictability of apraxic disorders was aptly characterized by Johns and Darley (1970), especially in comparison to the consistency and predictability seen in dysarthric disorders. For instance, phonological disorders of apraxic speakers (and it may be added, of aphasic ones, see Blumstein, 1973) are characterized by a variety of types of errors, such as substitutions ("literal paraphasias"), repetitions, additions, and omissions of phonemes or groups of phonemes. The speech of dysarthric speakers, on the other hand, is predominantly characterized by a phonetic disorder affecting the entire speech chain ("distortion"). As another example, where dysarthric patients show consistent speech distortions from one stimulus presentation to another or from one attempt at a given target utterance to the next attempt, apraxic and aphasic patients show marked variability in phonological errors over multiple attempts or stimulus presentations. Under such variable conditions, it has been difficult to formulate a coherent hypothesis concerning the underlying pathology.

A notable exception is Blumstein's (1973) proposal of a global hypothesis for apraxic and aphasic phonological substitutions in terms of markedness theory. She showed (on the basis of an apparently nonstandardized sample of consonant substitutions)[3] that a higher percentage of marked consonants tended to be substituted by unmarked consonants than vice versa (p. 52). This would have paralleled the observed tendency toward earlier acquisition of unmarked consonants in first-language acquisition, as well as the strong tendency toward the more common usage of unmarked consonants in most of the world's languages.

However, the unmarking tendency did not generalize uniformly to other samples. In a standarized sample of vowel substitutions, no significant tendency toward unmarking was evident (Keller, 1978, p. 272). Furthermore, two problems would have remained even if a tendency toward unmarked phonemes had been documented in the second study. First, a finding that aphasics seem to "prefer" unmarked to marked phonemes would have shifted the weight of the question from the nature of the pathology onto the nature of markedness. The question would then have to be answered as to what cognitive or motoric aspect of unmarked sounds causes them to be easier to produce than marked sounds under conditions of speech neuropathology. The second problem is that only between 52 and 70 percent of substitutions in Blumstein's sample were in the predicted direction. Assuming that these percentages are not artifacts of the possible nonstandardization of the sample, how are the remaining 48 to 30% of substitutions to be explained? There seems to be a clear need to develop hypotheses with greater generality, and thus with greater predictive power.

A number of theoretical considerations suggest certain alternative global hypotheses concerning the phonological pathology of apraxic patients. We shall consider here two such hypotheses, that of *Phoneme Sequence Simplification* and that of *Gesture Reduction*. It will be important to define our terms before considering the previous research and the theoretical basis of these hypotheses.

Phoneme Sequence Simplification

Phoneme sequence simplification is the omission of one or more of the constituent phonemes of a phoneme sequence (such as consonant clusters or diphthongs),[4] or the insertion of uncalled-for phonemes (such as intrusive schwas). This tendency has the effect of reducing the number of consonant-consonant (CC) and vowel-vowel (VV) sequences in the patient's speech and of augmenting the occurrence of single phonemes and of CV sequences. As we will see, such a deviation from the norm could have both cognitive and motoric advantages to the patient. One theoretical alternative to simplification is complication. This would be the addition of phonemes to existing phonemes or phoneme sequences to form phoneme sequences of greater complexity than those used in nonpathological speech.

Gesture Reduction

Gesture reduction is the shortening of the extent of an articulatory gesture in a transition from one phoneme to another. As an example, when the diphthong /aj/ is pronounced as /ae/, it may be assumed that the long articulatory lingual gesture from /a/ to /j/ was reduced to a shorter gesture tracing the trajectory from /a/ to /e/. It is possible that the speech of some neuropathologically impaired patients is characterized by a systematic tendency to reduce the extent of speech gestures between articulatory targets.

A number of alternative behaviors are also possible. Most importantly, patients' articulatory gestures could be systematically exaggerated ("gesture extension"); for instance, if the VC sequence /ku/ is replaced by the sequence /ka/, the trajectory can be assumed to be lengthened or extended. Also, patients could show gestures that are deviant from the norm in the sense that their gestures tend to be both reduced and extended, that is, that their shorter gestures would tend to be shortened while their longer gestures would tend to be lengthened. We will refer to this possibility as "gesture peripheralization." Or finally, patients' articulatory gestures could deviate toward a single gesture length which is neither reduced nor extended, but of average extent ("gesture centralization").

If it were to turn out that patients both simplify their articulations and reduce the extent of their gestures, the two hypotheses could be coalesced into a single concept, the Ease of Transition hypothesis. This hypothesis predicts that phonological disorders in certain neuropathologies are characterized by the use of phoneme-to-phoneme transitions which are "easier" to perform than those of target transitions. This means that patients would on the one hand use fewer "difficult" transitions (simplification) and on the other hand would reduce the length of the transition gestures they did perform (gesture reduction).

What Extant Data Suggests

This set of hypotheses has to my knowledge not been tested against a large corpus of aphasic or apraxic speech. However, a number of theoretical considerations and observations in the literature suggest that they are worth examining in detail.

A number of sources have reported simplification, for example, Trost and Canter (1974) report that phoneme omission is the most frequent type of error in consonant clusters, accounting for 31.2% of all such errors. Johns and Darley (1970) report that 18% of their total of 1289 errors from 10 apraxic patients were intrusive schwas (most of which can be presumed to have occurred in the middle of consonant clusters). Both of these tendencies have the effect of reducing the complexity of phoneme sequences and of increasing the frequency of CV sequences. Nevertheless, phoneme sequence simplification has been considered to be a poor candidate for an overall hypothesis to explain phonological disorders in aphasia and apraxia. Shankweiler and Harris (1966) note, for instance, that apraxics at times produce "particularly difficult strings of consonant clusters which do not occur in English words and were nearly impossible to imitate" (p. 289). It remains to be established whether it is simplification or complication that is more typical of aphasic and apraxic phonological disorders.

The status of the reduction of articulatory gestures is equally uncertain. Some indication that muscular gestures may be modified in systematic fashion comes from an early empirical study by Alajouanine, Ombredane, and Durand (1939). The authors report a weakness of the articulators, as evidenced by the respiratory insufficiency of one of their patients. This, according to their analysis, corresponds to the paralytic aspect of the articulatory breakdown in this type of disorder; other aspects noted by the authors are the dystonic aspect, an opposite tendency toward "excessive, exaggerated articulatory movements, in terms of their force and their duration"[5] (p. 116), and an apraxic aspect, evident in the substitution of one movement for another, such as an articulation performed during the inspiration phase of respiration rather than during the expiration phase.

Also, some evidence from articulatory phonetic investigations with x-ray microbeam seems to indicate that apraxic subjects show some overshoot in their movements. Lower lip movements in a repetition of the nonsense syllable /pa/ can be seen to be somewhat greater than those of a normal subject (Itoh, Sasanuma, Hirose, Yoshioka, & Ushijima, 1980, Figure 6, p. 72). However, it remains to be established whether gesture reduction or gesture extension is more typical of vocal tract activity in running speech. Also, it is important to examine the behavior of articulatory organs other than the lower lip to establish if all articulatory organs behave in a comparable manner of if they show differing pathological behaviors.

The examination of difficulties associated with phoneme-to-phoneme transitions is also well-motivated, since a number of authors have suggested that such transitions are the source of difficulties comparable to those of the emission of a specific phoneme. Alajouanine et al. (1939), for instance, characterize the "désintégration phonétique" at both the level of "the emission of elementary phonemes" and at the level of "the passage from one phoneme to another"[5] (p. 115). Luria associates phoneme-to-phoneme transition difficulties with a similar type of patient, suggesting that these difficulties involve a "pathological inertia" (Luria, 1966, p. 139). Although he acknowledges that the physiological mechanism underlying this disorder is not yet clear, he thinks that this disorder is part of a general impairment of the "kinetic melody" of movement, typical of a type of Broca's aphasia he calls "efferent motor aphasia." According to this author, difficulties similar to those seen in phoneme-to-phoneme transitions are also seen in the grapheme-to-grapheme transitions of this type of patient (Luria, 1966, p. 208).

Some recent theoretical considerations provide further motivation for examining the present hypotheses. Kelso and Tuller (1981), among others, suggest that articulatory control is most usefully viewed in terms of the temporal and spatial relations existing between (1) agonist and antagonist muscle groups, (2) different articulatory organs of the vocal tract, and (3) articulatory organs and their spatial environment. This network of interrelations serves to reduce the total number of degrees of freedom of the system, facilitating rapid and highly coordinated complex movements of some sixty articulatory muscles. As an example of a spatial relationship one may cite the vertical interaction between the jaw and the lip in lip closure gestures (see Kuehn & Moll, 1976), while the delay characteristics existing between upper vocal tract articulators and vocal folds in plosive articulations (VOT, or voice onset time) represent an example of a temporal relationship.

A number of studies seem to indicate that in apraxia of speech (or Broca's aphasia), such spatial and temporal relationships are deficient. For instance, the observations of Itoh et al. (1980) and of Blumstein, Cooper, Goodglass, Statlender, and Gottlieb (1980) suggest that timing relationship between articulatory organs are impaired. Specifically, Blumstein et al. (1980) report that a sample of Broca's aphasics failed to clearly differentiate VOTs for voiced and unvoiced stops, indicating that the timing relations between the linguopalatal articulatory valve and the laryngeal valve were impaired.

By extension, it appears likely that phoneme-to-phoneme transitions are rendered more difficult by the breakdown of preestablished timing and spatial relationships. Under such conditions, the apraxic patient must control a system with less predictable interactions between articulators and their environment, which by definition must result in much reduced processing speed (see Kelso & Tuller, 1981, p. 230). This may account for the reduced speech rate of Broca's aphasics.

Further, such patients may tend to reduce difficulties associated with the unpredictability of the system by (1) favoring transitions with looser temporal constraints over those with tighter temporal constraints (i.e., transitions between consonants and vowels, rather than transitions between consonants, or between vowels) and by (2) favoring transitions with a lesser degree of articulatory change over those with a greater degree of articulatory change. These adaptations to a state of impaired temporal and spatial relationships would permit the patient to produce a relatively greater rate of speech under conditions of impaired relationships. In other words, simplification and gesture reduction are reasonable, even likely predictions for apraxia of speech within our contemporary conception of speech motor control.

Aphasic (or nonapraxic) neuropathology, by contrast, does not seem to affect temporal relations between the actions of articulatory organs. Blumstein et al. (1980), for instance, noted a good distinction of voiced and unvoiced VOTs for their sample of Wernicke's aphasics, although the distribution of VOTs was still somewhat abnormal. Similarly, the speech rate of Wernicke's aphasics is about normal, reflecting possibly the fact that these patients control an articulatory system with about as many degrees of freedom as that of a normal speaker. In this view, the phonological errors of Wernicke's patients would have their origin in a different type of impairment than do phonological errors of Broca's aphasic people. Accordingly, it is possible that the simplification and gesture reduction hypotheses only apply to Broca's aphasic and not to

Wernicke's aphasic speakers. The position of conduction aphasics is unsure; in the Blumstein et al. (1980) study, the behavior of some of their patients resembled that of Broca's patients and the behavior of the remaining patients resembled that of Wernicke's patients. Recent phonological investigations of substitution tendencies between consonants tend to place conduction aphasia more in the domain of aphasia than of apraxia, since the predictability of substitution patterns in conduction aphasia is even less than that of Broca's aphasia (Nespoulous, in press).

In the present study, simplification and gesture reduction will be tested by means of global indicators of differences between normal and pathological speech utterances of Broca's, conduction, and Wernicke's aphasic speakers. First, comparisons will be made between percentages of phonemic sequences and simple phonemes in normal and pathological speech to assess the probability of simplification. Second, an articulatory gesture analysis of phoneme-to-phoneme transitions in normal and pathological phoneme sequences will be performed to examine the probability of reduction. The analyses will be based on about 18,500 articulations and 30,500 phoneme-to-phoneme transitions from a total of 25 patients.

A comment is in order concerning the difficulty of determining articulatory movement from transcribed speech. It is evident that there is considerable uncertainty concerning the exact placement of articulators, on the one hand because of the pronounced variability in articulatory placement in neuropathological speech, and on the other hand, due to the relatively great imprecision of transcriptions of such speech. The present study has attempted to compensate for these difficulties by (1) examining a very large corpus of articulations, (2) by requiring exacting standards of transcription, and (3) by utilizing conservative measures of phoneme-to-phoneme transition distances.

METHOD

Patients And Tasks

This study is based on samples of aphasic speech from patients with two language backgrounds, Canadian or American English on the one hand, and Canadian or Parisian French on the other hand. For simplicity's sake, the two samples will be referred to as the English and the French sample, respectively.

The English sample was elicited from seven Broca's aphasic and two conduction aphasic patients. This group was assessed and classified on the basis of the results of a neurological examination, a neuropsychological examination, and an aphasia battery. Eight patients were tested by means of the Western Aphasia Battery (Kertesz & Poole, 1974; essentially a shortened and modified version of Goodglass and Kaplan, 1972) and one Broca's aphasic patient (AB) was tested with the Schuell Aphasia Examination (Schuell, 1957). Profiles for the seven Broca's aphasic subjects showed relatively depressed standard scores for fluency, as compared to their performance on comprehension and naming tasks. Broca's subjects showed varying degrees of arthric (phonetic) distortion of their speech. By contrast, the standardized fluency scores of the two conduction aphasic subjects were superior to those obtained in the comprehension and naming tasks and their speech was free of arthric distortion. Furthermore, the two conduction aphasic subjects showed their poorest performance in the repetition tasks. All seven English-speaking patients scored above the 50th percentile in comprehension. Patients were tested at least one month post insult.

Etiologically, all of the Broca's aphasics had experienced unconfirmed cardiovascular accidents (CVAs), one of the conduction aphasics (JR) had suffered a confirmed CVA (CT scan: increased uptake in the left postero parietal region), and the other conduction aphasic (TK) had experienced a hematoma (operative evidence: aneurysm in the left sylvian fissure). One of the Broca's aphasics and one of the condition aphasics were female. Mean age for the Broca's aphasics was 59.4 (SD 8.6) and for the condition aphasics, 50.5 (SD 2.1). All patients were right-handed by self-report. Two of the Broca's aphasics (AB and GP) had French as their native language. On informal testing, both showed comprehension for French, but neither patient wished to speak their native language; both had lived in an English-speaking environment since their teens. Patients' socioeconomic backgrounds were varied; prior to insult, three patients had held blue-collar jobs, four had been in white-collar jobs, and two had been professionals. For further information on these patients, see Keller (1975).

Tasks for the English-speaking patients included spontaneous speech in informal interviews and the repetition of single words. Repetition stimuli presented in addition to those of the aphasia battery were adjusted for frequency of usage and word length to adjust for patients' varying levels of competence. Recordings were made in quiet surroundings, using a Shure lavalier microphone and a UHER Report 4200 tape recorder running at 19 cm/sec.

The French sample was elicited from five Broca's aphasics, eight conduction aphasics, and three Wernicke's aphasics, assessed by means of a neurological examination, a neuropsychological examination, and the Examen d'aphasie of the Centre de rééducation du langage et de recherche neuropsychologique, Hôtel-Dieu de Montréal.[6] Patients were grouped according to criteria presented in Lecours (1975; summarized in Note 3).

Etiologically, the patients showed a predominance of left-hemispheric cerebrovascular accidents (13 out of 16); one patient (a conduction aphasic) had a post-traumatic left subdural hematoma, and one (a Broca's aphasic) had a left-hemispheric focalized infectious disease. Mean age for Broca's aphasics was 56.0 (SD 7.1), for conduction aphasics it was 56.1 (SD 20.3), and the mean age of Wernicke's aphasics was 60.0 (SD 9.2). All patients were tested at least one month postonset (mean: 10.7; SD 17.1). One of the conduction aphasics (DJ) was recorded in Paris, the remaining patients were tested in Montreal.

Data from this group is based on patients' performance on the aphasia battery. Tasks include spontaneous speech as collected in informal conversation and in story telling (Little Red Riding Hood), automatized sequences (days, months, numbers from 1 to 10), naming (30 pictures), and the repetition of meaningful and nonsense words. Recordings were made in quiet surroundings using a UHER microphone and UHER tape recorder Model 4400 running at 19 cm/s.

TRANSCRIPTION AND ANALYSES

Transcription of the English Sample

Transcription of the English sample was performed by three linguistics students, trained in phonetic transcription, from the University of Toronto and Carleton University, Ottawa. Judges were given an initial training period to explain transcription criteria. Complete sequences of attempts at single words, plus respective targets, whether realized or not, were transcribed by means of a computer-adapted version of the Pike (1947) transcription system; task and utterance context were also noted. A broad, phonemic transcription was used. The phonemes [j] and [w] were transcribed and counted as consonants if they preceded a vocoid articulation and as vowels if they did not. The target had to be present in the successive aproximation or had to be clearly inferrable from the context for the successive approximation to be included in the sample. A total of 5627 consonantal and 4493 vocalic articulations were used in the patients' successive approximations and a total of 2197 consonantal and 1667 vocalic articulations constituted their targets (total: 13,984 articulations).

The transcriptions were twice checked against the original recordings by the author, with a time difference of half a year. A subsample of 497 consonants and 323 vowels was used to assess interjudgmental agreement on the transcription. The successive approximations for the subsample were selected randomly and in equal proportions from the nine patients and were transcribed a second time by one of the student transcribers; she was unaware of the hypotheses of this study. Agreement between the second transcription and the final transcription was 87.1% for consonants and 76.5% for vowels. Disagreements appeared to be related to the arthric component of the pathology, since agreement rates were better for those patients who showed the least phonetic distortion.[7] Furthermore, an analysis indicated that most disagreements involved a difference of a single feature and that they showed no systematic bias.

Transcription of the French Sample

Transcription of the French sample was performed by four students from various universities in Montreal who had undergone extensive training in the transcription of aphasic speech. Complete successive approximations were transcribed using a computer-adapted version of the International Phonetic Alphabet in a broad, systematic phonetic transcription, 17 consonants, 16 vowels, and three semiconsonants or semivowels were distinguished, the Canadian French dialectal allophones [I] and [U] were transcribed as [i] and [u]. The phonemes [j] and [w] were transcribed and counted as consonants if they preceded a vocoid articulation and as a vowel if they did not. Canadian French diphthongs were transcribed as [aj, au, ou, ẽj, ãu, ɑ̃j]. The target had to be clearly identifiable to the transcriber for the successive approximation to be included in the sample. Task, target utterance, as well as linguistic and nonlinguistic information preceding or following the attempts were also coded. A total of 4445 contoid and 4093 vocoid articulations were used in the patients' successive approximations and a total of 1505 contoid and 1429 vocoid articulations constituted their targets (total: 11,472 articulations). All transcriptions were checked at least twice by a native speaker of Canadian French, the first author of a previous study making use of this data base and the final judge of all disagreements in transcription (Yves Joanette; see Joanette, Keller, and Lecours, 1980). Most disagreements on transcription were resolved in listening sessions involving both the original transcriber and the final judge.

The analysis phase involved a number of computer programs designed to assist in the testing of the various hypotheses. BASIC-80 programs for tabulation, interactive good/bad scoring, gesture distance calculation, and statistical evaluation were run on a Sorcerer Z-80 microcomputer.

Gesture Distance Computation

According to the second hypothesis of this study, articulatory phoneme-to-phoneme gestures are shorter in aphasia and apraxia than they are in normal speech. To test this hypothesis, a multiple-valve model of the speech tract was applied to the data. It was felt that conventional phonetic feature systems were not applicable to the present hypothesis. All of the commonly used systems were conceived for purposes different from that of gesture distance calculation, such as psychoacoustical or systematic phonetic distinction of language sounds (e.g., Chomsky & Halle, 1968; Jakobson, Fant, & Halle, 1951; Ladefoged, 1975). By contrast, the present study required a model of vocal tract behavior capable of predicting probable gesture distances. Therefore, a model was developed along the lines of that of Dew and Jensen (1977), and taking into account concepts and data reported by such authors as Henke (1966), Fujimura (1972), Daniloff (1973), Netsell (1973), Kent and Minifie (1977), Harshman, Ladefoged, and Goldstein (1977), MacNeilage (1979) and Perkell (1980). Additional aspects of the model have been developed in our laboratory over a number of years (Keller & Labelle, manuscript).[8] Six major principles were incorporated.

1. Valves and Dimensions. The model describes the motor behavior of four major valves in the speech tract, the labial, the linguopalatal, the velar, and the laryngeal valves (see Dew & Jensen, 1977; see Table 8-1 for English and Table 8-2 for French). For purposes of idealized distinctive description, speech gestures can be assumed to involve a single movement dimension in the case of the velar and the laryngeal valves, and multiple, functionally independent dimensions in the case of the labial and linguopalatal valves. With respect to the multidimensional valves, two dimensions for speech gestures are distinguished in the labial valve, labial closure, and labial protrustion ("rounding"), while three dimensions are distinguished in the linguopalatal valve; linguopalatal closure, contact, and reference. "Linguopalatal closure" is the degree of approximation between the closest portions of the tongue and the palate. "Linguopalatal contact" is the type of contact existing between the tongue and the palate (e.g., total contact between the tongue rim and the palate for /t/ or /n/, contact between the central portion of the tongue and the palate for /l/, or insignificant contact for vowels, etc.). Finally, "linguopalatal reference" is the area of greatest approximation between the two articulators, or what is commonly referred to as "place." Vocal tract motor activity within each dimension is assumed to be multivalued (i.e., not binary), with the exception of the activity of the velar valve. This implies that relatively detailed gesture distances can be computed for the postulated dimensions.

TABLE 8-1
A coarticulatory vocal tract model for English

		LAB. VALVE						LINGUO-PALATAL VALVE																	VEL		LAR VAL			
		CLOSURE				PRO		CLOSURE							CONTACT					PAL REFER										
API	COMPUTR	CLOSED	FRICATV	APPROAC	OPEN	PROJECT	NPROJEC	CLOSED	PARTIAL	CLOSE	HIGH	MID	MID-OPN	OPEN	TOTAL	CENTRAL	FRICATV	RETROFL	INSIGNF	DENTAL	ALVEOLR	ALV-PAL	PALATAL	VELAR	CLOSED	OPEN	CLOSED	VIBRATG	FRICATV	OPEN
i	i				+		+		+										+		+	+			+	+		+		
I	I				+		+			+									+		+	+			+	+		+		
e	e				+		+				+								+		+	+			+	+		+		
ε	E				+		+					+							+		+	+			+	+		+		
æ	@				+		+						+						+		+	+			+	+		+		
a	a				+		+							+					+		+	+	+	+	+	+		+		
ɔ	)				+	+	+						+						+		+	+	+	+	+	+		+		
o	o				+	+						+							+				+	+	+	+		+		
U	U				+	+					+								+				+	+	+	+		+		
u	u				+	+				+									+				+	+	+	+		+		
ə	*				+		+						+						+			+	+		+	+		+		
j	y				+		+		+										+		+	+			+	+		+		
w	w			+		+				+									+				+	+	+	+		+		
p	p	+				+	+		+	+	+	+	+	+		+	+	+	+	+	+	+	+	+	+					+
b	b	+				+	+		+	+	+	+	+	+		+	+	+	+	+	+	+	+	+	+			+		
m	m	+				+	+	+	+	+	+	+	+	+		+	+	+	+	+	+	+	+	+		+		+		
f	f		+			+	+		+	+	+	+	+	+		+		+	+	+	+	+	+	+	+					+
v	v		+			+	+		+	+	+	+	+	+		+		+	+	+	+	+	+	+	+			+		
θ	T			+	+	+	+		+								+			+					+					+
t	t			+	+	+	+	+							+					+	+	+			+					+
ð	D			+	+	+	+		+								+			+					+			+		
d	d			+	+	+	+	+							+					+	+	+			+			+		
n	n			+	+	+	+	+							+					+	+	+				+		+		
s	s			+	+	+	+		+								+			+					+					+
z	z			+	+	+	+		+								+			+					+			+		
ʃ	S			+	+	+	+		+								+				+				+					+
ʒ	Z			+	+	+	+		+								+				+				+			+		
k	k			+	+	+	+	+							+								+	+	+					+
χ	x			+	+	+	+		+								+						+	+	+					+
g	g			+	+	+	+	+							+								+	+	+			+		
ŋ	G			+	+	+	+	+							+								+	+		+		+		
l	l			+	+	+	+		+							+				+	+	+			+			+		
r	r			+	+	+	+		+									+					+	+	+			+		
h	h			+	+	+	+			+	+	+	+	+				+	+	+	+	+	+	+	+	+			+	
ʔ	?			+	+	+	+			+	+	+	+	+				+	+	+	+	+	+	+	+	+	+			

Note. Top line: the four valves (LAB. VALVE = labial valve, LINGUOPALATAL VALVE, VEL = velar valve, LAR VAL = laryngeal valve). Second line: dimensions for the labial and the linguopalatal valves (CLOSURES, PRO = protrusion, CONTACT, PAL REFER = palatal reference). Succeeding lines: dimension specifications, listed in downward direction.

TABLE 8-2
A coarticulatory tract model for French, Abbreviations as in Table 8-1

		LAB. VALVE						LINGUO-PALATAL VALVE																	VEL		LAR VAL			
		CLOSURE				PRO		CLOSURE							CONTACT					PAL REFER										
API	COMPUTR	CLOSED	FRICATV	APPROAC	OPEN	PROJECT	NPROJEC	CLOSED	PARTIAL	CLOSE	HIGH	MID	MID-OPN	OPEN	TOTAL	CENTRAL	FRICATV	ROLLED	INSIGNF	DENTAL	ALVEOLR	ALV-PAL	PALATAL	VELAR	CLOSED	OPEN	CLOSED	VIBRATG	FRICATV	OPEN
i	i				+		+		+										+		+	+			+			+		
y	y				+	+			+										+		+	+			+			+		
I	I				+		+			+									+		+	+			+			+		
Y	Y				+	+				+									+		+	+			+			+		
e	e				+		+				+								+		+	+			+			+		
ø	0				+	+					+								+		+	+			+			+		
ɛ	E				+		+					+							+		+	+			+			+		
ɛ̃	5				+		+					+							+		+	+				+		+		
œ	9				+	+						+							+			+	+		+			+		
œ̃	1				+	+						+							+			+	+			+		+		
a	a				+		+							+					+		+	+			+			+		
ɑ	A				+		+							+					+				+	+	+			+		
ã	@				+		+							+					+		+	+	+	+		+		+		
ɔ	)				+	+	+						+						+				+	+	+			+		
ɔ̃	(				+	+	+						+						+				+	+		+		+		
o	o				+	+						+							+				+	+	+			+		
U	U				+	+					+								+				+	+	+			+		
u	u				+	+				+									+				+	+	+			+		
ə	*				+		+						+						+			+	+		+			+		
j	j				+		+		+										+		+	+			+			+		
ɥ	8			+		+			+										+		+	+			+			+		
w	w			+		+				+									+				+	+	+			+		
p	p	+				+	+		+	+	+	+	+	+		+	+		+	+	+	+	+	+	+					+
b	b	+				+	+		+	+	+	+	+	+		+	+		+	+	+	+	+	+	+			+		
m	m	+				+	+	+	+	+	+	+	+	+		+	+		+	+	+	+	+	+		+		+		
f	f		+			+	+		+	+	+	+	+	+		+			+	+	+	+	+	+	+					+
v	v		+			+	+		+	+	+	+	+	+		+			+	+	+	+	+	+	+			+		
t	t			+	+	+	+	+							+					+	+	+			+					+
d	d			+	+	+	+	+							+					+	+	+			+			+		
n	n			+	+	+	+	+							+					+	+					+		+		
s	s			+	+	+	+		+								+				+				+					+
z	z			+	+	+	+		+								+				+				+			+		
ʃ	S			+	+	+	+		+								+					+			+					+
ʒ	Z			+	+	+	+		+								+					+			+			+		
k	k			+	+	+	+	+							+								+	+	+					+
g	g			+	+	+	+	+							+								+	+	+			+		
ɲ	N			+	+	+	+	+							+							+	+			+		+		
l	l			+	+	+	+		+							+				+	+				+			+		
ʀ	R			+	+	+	+		+								+	+						+	+					+
r	r			+	+	+	+		+									+			+				+			+		+
h	h			+	+	+	+			+	+	+	+	+					+	+	+	+	+	+	+	+			+	
?	?			+	+	+	+			+	+	+	+	+					+	+	+	+	+	+	+	+	+			

2. *Coarticulation*. For an adequate calculation of theoretical gesture distances, provision must be made for the coarticulatory behavior of the various valves. This means that the model must incorporate both a Specification of articulatory position and the Domain of the specifications which the valve may assume in various coarticulatory contexts. For instance, a labial closure is required (and thus "specified") for the /p/-phase of the syllable /pa/. However the tongue gesture for the /p/-phase is not as well-specified. To some degree, the tongue will anticipate the position it will have to occupy during the succeeding /a/-phase. Similarly, it would anticipate the high front /i/ position during the /p/-phase of the syllable /pi/. The tongue has such coarticulatory liberty during the production of /p/ because the closure dimension of the linguopalatal valve can assume a relatively wide range of specifications without transgressing the perceived phoneme boundaries of /p/. In other words, the Domain of possible specifications is relatively large for linguopalatal closure while it is small for labial closure. At the entry for /p/ in Tables 8-1 and 8-2, this is represented by a series of pluses for the closure dimension of the linguopalatal valve, and by a single plus for labial closure. Table 8-3 illustrates the model's predictions for the possible speech gestures used in the English word "pie."

TABLE 8-3
Vocal tract activity domains for the word /paj/ "pie," using the coarticulatory model of Table 8-1

		LAB. VALVE						LINGUO-PALATAL VALVE																	VEL		LAR VAL			
		CLOSURE				PRO		CLOSURE							CONTACT					PAL REFER										
API	COMPUTR	CLOSED	FRICATV	APPROAC	OPEN	PROJECT	NPROJEC	CLOSED	PARTIAL	CLOSE	HIGH	MID	MID-OPN	OPEN	TOTAL	CENTRAL	FRICATV	RETROFL	INSIGNF	DENTAL	ALVEOLR	ALV-PAL	PALATAL	VELAR	CLOSED	OPEN	CLOSED	VIBRATG	FRICATV	OPEN
p	p	+				+	+		+	+	+	+	+	+		+	+	+	+	+	+	+	+	+	+					+
a	a				+		+							+					+		+	+	+	+	+	+		+		
j	y				+		+		+										+		+	+			+	+		+		

3. *Trajectories*. The model in its present elaboration makes no prediction on the likely path or trajectory of speech gestures within the specified domains; it merely characterizes domains of possible speech gesture trajectories. For example, the linguopalatal valve could

theoretically move from "close'" to "open" during the /pa/-phase of /paj/,"pie," especially if the word follows another word ending with a high vowel (e.g., "my pie"), or it could stay in open position throughout most of the /p/-phase, as in "ma pie" (expressed in more traditional terminology, the tongue may either perform a lowering movement during the lip closure of /p/ or remain in low position through the production of /p/). In a further elaboration of the model for normal speech, context-sensitive, likely-path calculation could be used to refine gesture predictions. However, such a calculation was considered to be inappropriate for the aphasic and apraxic utterances of the present sample. This is because first, the phonological context was not phonetically transcribed in the present sample and it was therefore impossible to calculate likely paths for initial and final transitions. Second, trajectories do not necessarily follow the most efficient, temporally coordinated path under conditions of neuropathology (see cineradiographic data from Itoh et al., 1980).

4. Distances. Given this model of domain specifications, the calculation of gesture distances is performed as follows: For each dimension of the four valves, the transition from one phoneme to the next involves a gesture trajectory either between two mutually exclusive domains or between two overlapping domains (overlap can be partial or complete). If the domains are mutually exclusive, trajectory distance is calculated between the two nearest points of the two domains. If they overlap, a distance of 0 is assumed. It will be noted that this distance estimate is conservative, since greater distances are theoretically possible in both conditions; for instance, it may be that the articulatory valve in fact performs a movement between the two farthest points of two mutually exclusive domains, or that it moves from one to the other exclusive portion of two partially overlapping domains. However, it was felt that the results of this study would be more compelling if they were analyzed by means of the most conservative interpretation of this vocal tract model.

An example of a distance calculation according to the present model is given in Table 8-3. In a fully articulated vowel sequence /aj/ (as in "pie"), the tongue has to travel from the low position of /a/ to the high postion of /j/. This involves a trajectory between the two mutually exclusive domains of "open linguopalatal closure" for /a/ and "partial linguopalatal closure" for /j/. Since this involves five steps from "open" through "mid-open," "mid," "high," "close," to "partial," the gesture distance is calculated to be 5 for the linguopalatal closure dimension. However, with respect to the dimension "palatal reference" (degree of fronting, or "place"), the domain of the vowel /a/ overlaps that of the semivowel /j/. A gesture distance of 0 is thus calculated for this dimension. Also, since there is total overlap at the levels of the two labial dimensions, as well as for the velar and for the laryngeal valve, a gesture distance of 0 is calculated for these latter dimensions.

5. *Universality and language specificity.* The present model is both universal and language specific in conception. In comparing the phoneme specifications for English and French, for instance, it will be seen that the basic conception of the model remains the same from one language to the other; the same valves and movement dimensions are assumed. However, specification and domains for similar phonemes differ from one language to the other. For instance, North American English uses a retroflex /r/, while French uses a rolled or fricative /r/. This difference has been incorporated into the model by assuming retroflex palatal and velar specifications for English /r/ and rolled or fricative velar specifications for French /r/ (alveolar for /R/).

6. *Spatial conception.* The present model distinguishes only spatial parameters and does not distinguish properties not directly assicated with gesture trajectory. As a result, such sounds as /i:/, /i/, and /y/ all have the same spatial vocal tract specification. For the distinction of these sounds, it is assumed that there exist further psycholinguistic specifications involving their duration of articulation and their intrasyllabic position. Yet for the purpose of gesture distance calculation, such differences can be neglected.

RESULTS

The Simplification Hypothesis

In order to test the simplification hypothesis, frequencies of phoneme sequences and of single phonemes in attempts were compared to those found in targets. Recall that "attempts" are actual utterances, while "targets" are reconstructed, phonologically correct utterances. The simplification hypothesis can be assumed to be supported if attempts show a disproportionally high number of single phonemes and a disproportionally low number of phoneme sequences, relative to respective distributions in targets.

This is a global measure of simplification, contrasting with the more commonly applied substitution measures, in which individual phonemes or phoneme sequences in attempts are compared to their counterparts in respective targets. This global measure was chosen both for computational simplicity and because substitution measures of simplification are very difficult to apply in the many cases where attempt utterances are incomplete or severely deviant from respective target utterances.

Proportions between phoneme sequences and simple phonemes were calculated separately for the two samples, for consonants and vowels, and for patients and patient groups. Distributional differences were assessed by means of two-by-two chi-square analyses, comparing phoneme sequences and simple phonemes in targets and attempts.

Table 8-4 gives raw frequencies and percentages of phoneme sequences

TABLE 8-4

Frequencies of phoneme sequences and single phonemes in corpus, presented according to language, type of aphasia, attempt or target, and type of articulation (consonantal and vocalic)

	Consonantal		*Vocalic*	
	Phoneme Sequences	*Single Phonemes*	*Phoneme Sequences*	*Single Phonemes*
English				
Broca				
Targets	557 (26.4%)	1556 (73.6%)	230 (14.3%)	1378 (85.7%)
Attempts	999 (18.6%)	4375 (81.4%)	400 (9.3%)	3902 (90.7%)
Conduction				
Targets	15 (17.9%)	69 (82.1%)	5 (15.6%)	27 (84.4%)
Attempts	43 (17.0%)	210 (83.0%)	24 (12.6%)	167 (87.4%)
French				
Broca				
Targets	50 (27.2%)	134 (72.8%)	2 (1.2%)	171 (98.8%)
Attempts	77 (16.1%)	401 (83.9%)	6 (1.4%)	409 (98.6%)
Conduction				
Targets	350 (30.7%)	789 (69.3%)	8 (0.7%)	1085 (99.3%)
Attempts	869 (24.8%)	2638 (75.2%)	33 (1.0%)	3252 (99.0%)
Wernicke				
Targets	40 (22.0%)	142 (78.0%)	2 (1.2%)	161 (98.8%)
Attempts	96 (20.9%)	364 (79.1%)	7 (1.8%)	386 (98.2%)

Note. Chi-square values for these frequencies are included at the bottom of Table 8-5.

TABLE 8-5
Results of a chi-square analysis to assess evidence for simplification or complication

	Consonantal			*Vocalic*		
Patient Type	*Result*	$X^2(1)$	*Signif.*	*Result*	$X^2(1)$	*Signif.*
E-DH BRO	SIMPL.	1.89	n.s.	SIMPL.	0.81	n.s.
E-GP BRO	SIMPL.	54.58	.001	SIMPL.	5.55	.05
E-ID BRO	SIMPL.	0.02	n.s.	SIMPL.	18.00	.001
E-BW BRO	SIMPL.	7.76	.01	SIMPL.	4.35	.05
E-AW BRO	SIMPL.	3.41	n.s.	SIMPL.	3.59	n.s.
E-AB BRO	SIMPL.	8.44	.01	SIMPL.	5.44	.05
E-EL BRO	SIMPL.	10.81	.01	SIMPL.	4.09	.05
E-TK CON	COMPL.	0.07	n.s.	SIMPL.	1.55	n.s.
E-JR CON	SIMPL.	0.04	n.s.	SIMPL.	0.17	n.s.
F-BD BRO	i.d.			i.d.		
F-BR BRO	SIMPL.	4.46	.05	i.d.		
F-PL BRO	SIMPL.	1.86	n.s.	i.d.		
F-AL BRO	i.d.			i.d.		
F-CP BRO	SIMPL.	0.33	n.s.	i.d.		
F-CR CON	SIMPL.	0.32	n.s.	i.d.		
F-LN CON	SIMPL.	5.91	.05	i.d.		
F-BR CON	SIMPL.	0.20	n.s.	COMPL.	0.002	n.s.
F-DJ CON	SIMPL.	0.33	n.s.	i.d.		
F-LS CON	SIMPL.	3.15	n.s.	i.d.		
F-CR CON	SIMPL.	7.77	.05	i.d.		
F-CD CON	SIMPL.	0.35	n.s.	i.d.		
F-LB CON	SIMPL.	3.78	n.s.	SIMPL.	0.03	n.s.
F-LR WER	SIMPL.	2.19	n.s.	i.d.		
F-GN WER	COMPL.	0.24	n.s.	i.d.		
F-ML WER	COMPL.	0.37	n.s.	i.d.		
TOT ENGL. BRO	SIMPL.	55.63	.001	SIMPL.	30.79	.001
TOT ENGL. CON	SIMPL.	0.03	n.s.	SIMPL.	1.38	n.s.
TOT FRCH. BRO	SIMPL.	10.49	.01	i.d.		
TOT FRCH. CON	SIMPL.	15.72	.001	COMPL.	0.66	n.s.
TOT FRCH. WER	SIMPL.	0.10	n.s.	i.d.		

Note. Results for analyses conducted on the transcriptions of individual patients appear at the top and results of analyses conducted on the combined transcriptions of patients with various types of aphasia appear at the bottom. Simplification denotes a lesser proportion of phoneme sequences in attempts than in targets, complication denotes the reverse. Abbreviations: (Patient:) E English patients, F French patients. (Type:) BRO Broca's aphasia, CON conduction aphasia, WER Wernicke's aphasia. (Result:) SIMPL. simplification, COMPL. complication, i.d. insufficient data in one or more cell, n.s. not significant.

and single phonemes for the various types of patients and the two kinds of phonemes. It can be observed that phoneme sequences are regularly more frequent in targets than in attempts. Significance levels are reported at the bottom of Table 8-5. Differences were statistically significant for consonantal and vocalic articulations of English Broca's aphasics and for consonantal articulations of French Broca's and conduction aphasics. All of these differences supported the hypothesis in that there were significantly more phoneme sequences in targets than in attempts.

The top of Table 8-5 shows results and significance levels for individual patients, Twelve out of a possible 50 comparisons reached significance (there was insufficient data available for the application of a X^2 analysis in 14 of the 50 comparisons). All significant differences supported the simplification hypothesis, as did all but two of the nonsignificant comparisons.

We conclude that the simplification hypothesis was well-supported in the case of English-speaking Broca's aphasics and with respect to the consonants of French-speaking Broca's and conduction aphasics. Also, English conduction aphasics show some simplification, although their values did not reach significance. By contrast, the distributions of single phonemes and phoneme differences were not significantly different for targets and attempts in the case of Wernicke's aphasics who did not show clear tendencies toward simplification or complication. All significant differences were associated with simplification; no significant complication tendency was recorded.

French vocoid articulations showed no significant tendencies. Insufficient data for vowel sequences often precluded a chi-square analysis. This is in part because diphthongs are relatively rare in Canadian French (nonexistent in Parisian French); in the present French sample, for instance, vowel sequences form just 1% of all vocoid articulations.

Altogether, the results support the simplification hypothesis for Broca's aphasia and the French sample of conduction aphasia. The hypothesis does not seem applicable, however, to Wernicke's aphasia. The position of the relatively small sample of utterances gathered from two English conduction aphasics is equivocal. It is possible that a larger sample of errors from a greater number of patients of this type could clarify the position of conduction aphasia.

The Gesture Reduction Hypothesis

The gesture reduction hypothesis was tested by three comparisons involving the calculation of gesture distances in phoneme-to-phoneme transitions according to the vocal tract model presented above. First, all transitions found in targets were compared to those found in attempts. Second, separate comparisons were made for consonant and vowel sequences in targets and attempts. And third, a comparison was made between phoneme sequences judged to be either phonotactically acceptable or unacceptable; this analysis exploits the fact that aphasics often produce non-existing consonant clusters or diphthongs, as in /kbi:/ for "clip", /vrbɔ:w/ for "snowball" or /ju:Imandə/ for "remember". The sequences /kb-/,/vrb-/ and /u:I-/ are not commonly used in English and are thus classified as "phonotactically unacceptable."

Under the reduction hypothesis, it was expected that gesture distances between phonemes would be lesser in patients' attempts and in phonotactically unacceptable sequences (in "pathological transitions") than they would be in targets or in phonotactically acceptable sequences (in "normal transitions"). This corresponds to "movement undershoot". As indicated in the introduction, four alternative possibilities were distinguished in this study.

First, there is extension, the opposite tendency of reduction. This would involve a tendency toward greater gesture trajectories in pathological transitions than in normal transitions, that is, a tendency toward "movement overshoot." Second, there is peripheralization, a combination of reduction and extension. This tendency would be evident if some pathological transitions showed evidence of "undershoot," while others by the same patient showed "overshoot." Then there is centralization, the opposite tendency to peripheralization. In this condition, all pathological transitions would tend toward gestures of average length. And finally, it is possible that patients' gestures are statistically abnormal but showed no clear tendency.This pattern was entitled "no tendency.."

Analysis 1: Targets Versus Attempts of Whole Sample

It was first examined if gesture distances for all phoneme-to-phoneme transitions found in the corpus differed for reconstructed normal target utterances and pathological attempt utterances. As an example, consider frequencies for the transitions of English broca's aphasics shown in Table 8-6. These patients used 10,738 transitions in their attempt utterances, and 4523 transitions in target utterances. Each of these 15,261 transitions was analyzed according to the 7 movement dimensions of the vocal tract model.

Of the target transitions, 3421 (or 75.6%) involved no distinctive gesture change in labial closure ("gesture distance 0"); 257 (or 5.7%) of target transitions involved a distance of one step in labial closure (e.g., from "open" to "approaching," as in /ow/); 343 (7.6%) transitions involved a distance of two steps(e.g., from"open" to "fricative," as in /If/); and 502

TABLE 8-6
Gesture distance analysis

	Gesture Distance							*Total Trans*
	0	*1*	*2*	*3*	*4*	*5*	*6*	*(%)*
Labial Valve								
Closure								
Targets	3421	257	343	502				452
	(75.6)	(5.7)	(7.6)	(11.1)				(100)
Attempts	8053	591	736	1358				10738
	(75.0)	(5.5)	(6.9)	(12.6)				(100)
Protrusion								
Targets	4320	203						4523
	(95.5)	(4.5)						(100)
Attempts	10343	395						10738
	(96.3)	(3.7)						(100)
Ling.-Pal. Valve								
Closure								
Targets	1308	754	602	320	842	596	101	4523
	(28.9)	(16.7)	(13.3)	(7.1)	(18.6)	(13.2)	(2.2)	(100)
Attempts	3261	1683	1340	784	1631	1522	517	10738
	(30.4)	(15.7)	(12.5)	(7.3)	(15.2)	(14.2)	(4.8)	(100)
Contact								
Targets	1561	540	579	553	1290			4523
	(34.5)	(11.9)	(12.8)	(12.2)	(28.5)			(100)
Attempts	4065	1049	1268	1084	3272			10738
	(37.9)	(9.8)	(11.8)	(10.1)	(30.5)			(100)
Reference								
Targets	3319	993	125	86				4523
	(73.4)	(22.0)	(2.8)	(1.9)				(100)
Attempts	8345	2005	227	161				10738
	(77.7)	(18.7)	(2.1)	(1.5)				(100)
Velar Valve								
Targets	4297	226						4523
	(95.0)	(5.0)						(100)
Attempts	10303	435						10738
	(95.9)	(4.1)						(100)
Laryngeal Valve								
Targets	3016	43	1464					4523
	(66.7)	(1.0)	(32.4)					(100)
Attempts	6886	309	3530					10738
	(64.1)	(2.9)	(32.9)					(100)

Note. Shown are gesture distance frequencies for all phoneme-to-phoneme transitions of targets and attempts of English Broca's aphasics. Percentages are shown in parentheses. See Table 8-7 for deduced tendencies, chi-square values, and statistical significance of these comparisons. Abbreviation: TRANS transitions.

(11.1%) transitions involved a distance of three steps (e.g., from "closure" to "open," as in /paj/). By comparison, transition distances for attempts involved, respectively, 75.0% for Distance 0, 5.5% for Distance 1, 6.9% for Distance 2, and 12.7% for Distance 3.

TABLE 8–7
Chi-square evaluation of articulatory distances in phoneme-to-phoneme transitions (1): All transitions in targets versus all transitions in attempts

	Labial Valve		*Linguopalatal Valve*			*Vel.*	*Lar.*
	CLO	*PRO*	*CLO*	*CON*	*REF*		
ENG							
B	9.00* (3) E	5.54* (1) R	83.88*** (6) N	44.16*** (4) P	34.28*** (3) R	6.87** (1) R	60.16*** (3) E
C	2.15 (3) C	4.32* (1) R	9.11 (6) N	1.21 (4) N	1.51 (3) C	0.89 (1) R	4.50* (1) R
FR							
B	2.19 (3) E	0.15 (1) E	4.52 (6) N	8.78 (4) N	3.18 (2) R	1.30 (1) R	4.15* (1) E
C	3.43 (3) E	0.03 (1) R	8.05 (6) R	7.51 (4) R	1.25 (2) P	0.09 (1) P	2.71 (1) E
W	1.20 (3) R	0.93 (1) E	4.87 (6) N	1.50 (4) N	1.21 (2) C	0.87 (1) E	4.19* (1) E

TOT	A	S	A	S	A	S	A	S	A	S	A	S	A	S
R	1	—	3	2	1	—	1	—	2	1	3	1	1	1
E	3	1	2	—	—	—	—	—	—	—	1	—	4	3
P	—	—	—	—	—	—	1	1	1	—	1	—	—	—
C	1	—	—	—	—	—	—	—	2	—	—	—	—	—
N	—	—	—	—	4	1	3	—	—	—	—	—	—	—

Note. See Table 8–6 for a sample comparison of the results for English Broca's aphasics. For each row, the top line shows chi-square values and significance and the bottom line shows the tendency and the degrees of freedom. Tendencies are as follows (see text for details): E extension, R reduction, P peripheralization, C centralization, N no tendency. Other abbreviations: CLO closure, PRO protrusion, CON contact, REF linguopalatal reference, VEL. velar valve, LAR. laryngeal valve, ENG English sample, FR French sample, B Broca's aphasics, C conduction aphasics, W Wernicke's aphasics, TOT tendency totals, A all tendencies, S significant tendencies. Significance: *** = $p < .001$; ** = $p < .01$; * = $p < .05$.

It can be seen that the reduction hypothesis is not supported by this example. Slightly more target transitions than attempt transitions involved the shorter distances of 0, 1, and 2 steps, while there are somewhat fewer target transitions than attempt transitions at the greatest distance of 3. In other words, the "weight" of the pathological transitions tended toward the greatest distance in this example; this was thus judged to be a case of gesture extension. The tendency was significant by chi-square test at $p < .05$ ($X^2(3) = 9.00$) (see Table 8-7).

Chi-square analyses for the comparison of all transitions in targets and attempts of the entire sample were not supportive of the simplification hypothesis (Table 8-7). Out of a total of 35 comparisons, only 11 showed significant differences between normal and pathological gesture distance distributions. Five of these were tendencies toward reduction, four were tendencies toward extension, one involved a peripheralization, and one was a nondirectional abnormal distribution. Nonsignificant tendencies showed a similar distribution as did significant tendencies.

It is interesting to note that there was not much evidence in favor of peripheralization or centralization, despite the fact that these are possible tendencies in 5 out of the 7 vocal tract dimensions. Only 4 out of a possible 25 comparisons showed nonsignificant tendencies toward peripheralization or centralization.

Analysis 2: Targets and Attempts in Phoneme Sequences

While the first analysis involved transitions between all adjoining phonemes of the corpus, the second analysis involved only transitions within phoneme sequences, separately for consonant and vowel sequences (see Table 8-8). Given the small overall differences between distance distributions for targets and attempts evident in the previous analysis, it was considered possible that greater differences could be found within sequences, since intrasequence transitions could potentially pose greater articulatory difficulty than the average phoneme-to-phoneme transition.

In this analysis, differences between distance distributions were compared by means of Cochran's extension to the common chi square (Cochran, 1954, p. 137). This test takes advantage of the directionality of a distribution within a set of ranked categories and is particularly useful in those cases where a large number of cells show small expected values. Both of these conditions apply in the present data; each vocal tract dimension is directional, that is, its categories are ranked in terms of distance. Also, a great number of cells showed expected values below 5 in this analysis. A disadvantage of this test is that it is relatively insensitive to peripheralization and centralization tendencies; this risk was deemed

TABLE 8-8
Chi-square evaluation of articulatory distances in phoneme-to-phoneme transitions (2): Phoneme sequences in targets versus phoneme sequences in attempts

		Labial Valve		*Linguopalatal Valve*			*Vel.*	*Lar.*
		CLO	*PRO*	*CLO*	*CON*	*REF*		
E–B								
	C	0.00	0.00	6.17*	1.29	0.00	3.03	0.02
		E	N	E	E	C	R	C
	V	31.-75***	0.46	15.-47***	0.00	2.19	0.00	0.00
		R	E	N	N	R	N	N
E–C								
	C	0.47	0.00	0.47	0.88	0.92	0.65	8.56**
		R	N	E	E	C	R	E
	V	0.42	3.89*	1.12	0.00	3.89*	0.00	0.00
		R	E	N	N	E	N	N
F–B								
	C	0.56	0.00	0.44	0.01	3.87*	0.02	2.56
		E	N	R	N	R	R	R
	V	i.d.	i.d.	i.d.	i.d.	i.d.	i.d.	i.d.
F–C								
	C	1.18	0.00	5.07*	1.37	0.44	0.00	0.03
		R	N	E	E	E	N	R
	V	1.05	2.60	0.01	0.00	2.86	0.21	0.00
		E	R	N	N	R	E	N
F–W								
	C	0.16	0.00	0.91	0.19	0.00	0.87	0.18
		R	N	E	N	N	E	E
	V	i.d.	i.d.	i.d.	i.d.	i.d.	i.d.	i.d.

TOT	A	S	A	S	A	S	A	S	A	S	A	S	A	S
R	5	1	1	—	1	—	—	—	3	1	3	—	2	—
E	3	—	2	1	4	2	3	—	2	1	2	—	2	1
P	—	—	—	—	—	—	—	—	—	—	—	—	—	—
C	—	—	—	—	—	—	—	—	2	—	—	—	1	—
N	—	—	5	—	3	1	5	—	1	—	3	—	3	—

Note. Cochran's (1954) extension to the common chi square was used (1 degree of freedom for each value). In each row, the top line shows chi-square values and significance and the bottom line shows the tendency. Abbreviations: CLO closure, PRO protrusion, CON contact, REF linguopalatal reference, VEL. velar valve, LAR. laryngeal valve, E-B English Broca's aphasics, E-C English conduction aphasics, F-B French Broca's aphasics, F-C French conduction aphasics, F-W French Wernicke's aphasics, C consonant sequences, V vowel sequences, E extension, R reduction, P peripheralization, C centralization, N no tendency, i.d. insufficient data, A all tendencies, S significant tendencies. Significance: ***p ⟨.001; **p ⟨.01; *p ⟨.05.

acceptable, given the lack of evidence for these tendencies in the previous analysis.

Results of this analysis are roughly parallel to those of the previous analysis. Only 8 of a possible 56 comparisons showed significant differences between distributions in attempts and in targets.

Analysis 3: Acceptable Versus Unacceptable Phoneme Sequences

As a final test of the gesture reduction hypothesis, phonotactically acceptable sequences were compared with phonotactically unacceptable sequences. It was considered possible that the previous analyses obscured pathological tendencies through the presence of a great many correct articulations in the target utterances. This probably reflects a general bias towards normal articulations in transcribed corpora of aphasic and apraxic speech, since correct articulations are a necessary guide to the identification of pathological articulations.

For this analysis, all phoneme sequences in the corpus were evaluated by means of an interactive computer program. A phoneme sequence was judged to be acceptable if another word of the same language could be found which incorporates the given phoneme sequence in the same intraword position (initial, medial, or final). If none could be found, it was judged unacceptable. Intraword positions for aphasic utterances were established according to the position the sequence would take within the target word. With respect to French sequences, use was made of the phonetic dictionary of Quebec French (Pupier, 1977) to assess acceptability.

It was assumed that gesture reduction could be a contributing factor in the production of a phonotactically unacceptable sequence. This is particularly evident in English vowel sequences with substitute diphthongs involving shorter gesture trajectories than target diphthongs. Common examples are: /da:e/ for /dawn/ "down," or /hoə-/ for /hawEvər/ "however". Relatively short gesture trajectories are also evident in other types of phonotactically unacceptable phoneme sequences. Noted were a few examples of apparent try-out movements (e.g. /ao-/ in /aordIna-jzefʃən/ for "organization," or /fəa-/ for "factory"), as well as some cases of prolongation or the repetition of phonemes (e.g. /mœttIkdli:/ for "dramatically" or /ne:e/ for "name"/. In all of these cases, phoneme-to-phoneme transitions can be seen to involve relatively short gesture trajectories.

Phoneme-to-phoneme trajectory distances were calculated for each articulatory valve, separately for consonant and vowel sequences, language samples, and patient groups (see Table 8-9). Results tended to be in support of the gesture reduction hypothesis in the case of Broca's and con-

TABLE 8-9

Chi-square evaluation of articulatory distances in phoneme-to-phoneme transitions (3): Phonotactically acceptable phoneme sequences versus phonotactically unacceptable phoneme sequences

	Labial Valve		*Linguopalatal Valve*			*Vel.*	*Lar.*
	CLO	*PRO*	*CLO*	*CON*	*REF*		
E-B							
C	0.68	0.00	4.47*	0.15	0.73	20.54***	5.56*
	N	N	E	N	N	R	N
V	27.89***	1.32	20.96***	0.00	2.75	0.00	0.00
	R	R	N	N	R	N	N
E-C							
C	i.d.	i.d.	i.d.	i.d.	i.d.	i.d.	i.d.
V	i.d.	i.d.	i.d.	i.d.	i.d.	i.d.	i.d.
F-B							
C	1.77	0.00	0.07	10.22**	4.48*	0.00	0.34
	R	N	R	N	R	E	R
V	0.64	0.63	5.65*	0.00	3.11	2.43	0.00
	R	R	R	N	R	E	N
F-C							
C	0.32	0.00	0.16	12.23***	3.77	5.71*	0.05
	N	N	R	R	R	E	R
V	5.09*	1.66	12.08***	0.00	3.47	9.67**	0.00
	R	E	R	N	R	E	N
F-W							
C	0.69	0.00	0.06	2.00	0.11	0.04	1.90
	N	N	R	R	C	R	R
V	0.00	1.00	1.71	0.00	3.44	1.40	0.00
	N	R	N	N	R	E	N

TOT	A	S	A	S	A	S	A	S	A	S	A	S	A	S
R	4	2	3	—	5	2	2	1	6	1	2	1	3	—
E	—	—	1	—	1	1	—	—	—	—	5	2	—	—
P	—	—	—	—	—	—	—	—	—	—	—	—	—	—
C	—	—	—	—	—	—	—	—	1	—	—	—	—	—
N	4	—	4	—	2	1	6	1	1	—	1	—	5	1

Note. Cochran's (1954) extension to the common chi square was used (1 degree of freedom for each value). In each row, the top line shows chi-square values and significance and the bottom line shows the tendency. Abbreviations: CLO closure, PRO protrusion, CON contact, REF linguopalatal reference, VEL. velar valve, LAR. laryngeal valve, E-B English Broca's aphasics, E-C English conduction aphasics, F-B French Broca's aphasics, F-C French conduction aphasics, F-W French Wernicke's aphasics, C consonant sequences, V vowel sequences, E extension, R reduction, P peripheralization, C centralization, N no tendency, i.d. insufficient data, A all tendencies, S significant tendencies. Significance: ***$p < .001$; **$p < .01$; *$p < .05$.

duction aphasics, but they showed no significant tendency in the case of Wernicke's aphasics. Seven of the 13 significant differences between acceptable and unacceptable sequences represent cases of gesture reduction. Three of the four exceptions to this rule involve nondirectionally significant differences. Also, 25 of the reported 56 tendencies (significant and nonsignificant) represent gesture reduction.

Wernicke's aphasics showed no significant tendency in this analysis. This accords with their tendency toward nonsignificant differences evident in the previous two analyses. The only significant difference reported for these patients in the three analyses involves a tendency toward extension in laryngeal valve gestures (see Table 8-7).

No clear differences were evident in the behavior of different vocal tract valves in this analysis. While there had been some tendency toward extension in the larynegeal valve in the previous two analyses, this tendency was not manifested in the present analysis.

DISCUSSION

Two hypotheses concerning phonological breakdown in apraxia and aphasia were investigated in this study. It was found that data from Broca's and conduction aphasia in two languages provided good support for the hypothesis of phoneme sequence simplification, while they gave moderate support for the hypothesis of gesture reduction in phoneme-to-phoneme transitions. No clear support for either tendency was evident for Wernicke's aphasia.

Specifically, it was found that Broca's and conduction aphasics tended to reduce the proportion of phoneme sequences (e.g., consonant clusters and diphthongs) in their speech. As a result, there was a higher proportion of single vowels and single consonants in their attempt utterances than could be found in their respective target utterances. This finding supports the simplification hypothesis; these patients tended to favor transitions between consonants and vowels (i.e., CV or VC sequences) over those between two consonants or between two vowels (ie., CC or VV sequences). Expressed in terms of motor speech theory, these patients appeared to favor phoneme-to-phoneme transitions with looser timing requirements over transitions with tighter timing requirements found inside consonant clusters or diphthongal sequences.

Also, it was found that phonotactically unacceptable phoneme sequences of Broca's and conduction aphasics tended to involve phoneme-to-phoneme transitions of lesser gesture extent than the phontactically acceptable phoneme sequences of the same patient subsample. This finding is in support of the gesture reduction hypothesis; it appears that phonotactically unacceptable sequences may be at least in part the result of patients favoring transitions involving less articulatory change than is found in normal speech.

However, it was not the case that phoneme-to-phoneme transition distances were reduced in aphasic utterances as a whole. Overall, Broca's and conduction aphasics showed tendencies toward both reduction and extension, but only the results of English Broca's aphasics reached significance. These tendencies can be interpreted in the sense that in disorders characterized by apraxia, phoneme-to-phoneme transitions involve a general breakdown of spatial relationships between adjoining articulations. This may be conceptually related to the breakdown in temporal relationships between gestures documented for these patients by other research (see introduction).

The fact that Wernicke's aphasics did not show a tendency toward simplification, nor show any clear evidence toward gesture reduction, lends further support to the present interpretation of the results in terms of an apraxic disorder: The phonologically abnormal sequences of these patients probably have a different origin than those of patients marked by an apraxia of speech.

To integrate these findings into a general theory of articulatory disorders in neuropathology, we will review the three major aspects of articulatory disorders of gross neurological origin, and will attempt to see how the present findings can be integrated into our understanding of these three aspects. We shall assume that two or three of these aspects can be found to coexist and interact to various degrees in a single patient, or that a single aspect can be seen to dominate the patient's articulatory behavior. The descriptions which follow are formulated in terms of the latter case, a patient who is primarily affected by a single aspect of neurogenic articulatory impairment.

The dysarthric (or arthric) aspect is characterized by a general modification of the speech quality. Phonemes usually remain phonemically distinctive and are used phonotactically within utterances as they are in normal speech. Prominent perceived speech pathologies are distorted phonemes, monotonous tone: altered voice, hypernasality, and altered rate of speech (slowed speech or great rushes of speech) (for full list of pathologies, see Darley, Aronson, & Brown, 1969). Misarticulations are not generally corrected by the patient. Both neuroanatomical lesion evidence and experimental kinematic and electrophysiological data from x-ray, fiberoptics, and EMG suggest that different types of pathology may interfere with different subcomponents of this aspect of articulatory breakdown. Parkinsonism (basal ganglia lesion) has, for instance, been observed to result in articulatory movements that decrease in amplitude and velocity, spastic dysarthria (upper motor neuron lesion) has been shown to reduce speed of production and to decrease maximum velocity of articulator movement, and ataxic dysarthria (cerebellar lesion) has been shown to result in irregular rhythm of production and in greatly varying extent and precision of displacement (see Hirose & Kiritani, 1979; Hirose & Sawashima, 1979; Hirose, Kiritani, Ushijima, Yoshioka, & Sawashima, 1978, for Parkinsonism; Hirose, Kiritani, & Sawashima, 1980, for upper motor lesion; Hirose & Sawashima, 1979; Hirose & Kiritani, 1979, for cerebellar lesion).

The apraxic aspect is externally marked by such phenomena as the substitution, the omission, and the addition of phonemic, subphonemic, or supraphonemic units (features, phonemes, phoneme sequences, syllables, etc.). Attempts at self-correction tend to be both frequent and successful (Joanette et al., 1980). Difficulties of phoneme selection (paradigmatic difficulties) as well as difficulties of phoneme-to-phoneme transition (syntagmatic difficulties) are in evidence. These patients make predominantly paradigmatic substitutions (consonants: Blumstein, 1973; vowels: Keller, 1978) and they are particularly prone to errors when asked to repeat stimulus material that is paradigmatically difficult (e.g., that contains relatively infrequent phonemes, such as /ʃ/ or /ʋ/; Derouesne, Beauvois, & Ranty, 1977; Guyard, Sabouraud, & Gagnepain, 1981). Also, patients of this type show experimental evidence of temporal discoordination between various components of the vocal tract when producing sounds requiring the coordination of a number of vocal tract valves (x-ray microbeam: Itoh et al., 1980; VOT: Blumstein et al., 1980; see also Johns & LaPointe, 1976).

Syntagmatically, the apraxic aspect of the disorder slows down phoneme-to-phoneme transitions. As was demonstrated in this study, patients favor articulatorily less demanding transitions between consonants and vowels, and sometimes produce nonexisting phoneme sequences, in part because of a tendency to constrain the degree of change in the speech tract valves. Finally, productive apraxic disorders seem to be independent of perceptual phonological disorders, at least with respect to vocoid articulations (Keller, Rothenberger, & Goepfert, 1982).

The aphasic aspect is marked by the fluent production of utterances that are likely to resemble the target in their syllabic structure but which contain numerous subphonemic, phonemic, or supraphonemic substitutions. Attempts at self-correction tend to be infrequent and unsuccessful (Joanette et al., 1980). These patients show a somewhat greater proportion of contextual, or syntagmatic, errors (Blumstein, 1973) and in repetition show particular difficulty with stimuli that are syntagmatically confusing at the intersyllabic level (e.g., "caramel" vs. "camera;" Derouesne et al., 1977; Guyard et al., 1981). Experimental evidence from

VOT shows relatively good proficiency at interarticulator coordination (Blumstein et al., 1980).

This analysis of articulatory disorders permits an approximate classification of the three types of patients presented in this study. It would seem that Broca's aphasics show, with respect to their articulatory impairment, an admixture of primarily apraxic and secondarily spastic dysarthric phenomena. Wernicke's aphasics show primarily aphasic phenomena, and conduction aphasics show both apraxic and aphasic phenomena. The interpretation of conduction aphasia appears to be in accord with experimental data on VOT distinction (Blumstein et al., 1980) and with analyses of their phonological breakdown (Nespoulous, in press).

Extrapolating from the presented research one step further, it is possible to relate these deficits to a general model of speech production (see Keller, 1979). On the basis of a number of criteria (such as the presence of anticipation errors, the structure of pauses, oral performance in shadowing experiments, etc.), it is reasonable to assume that speech production involves two temporally overlapping stages of processing, planning and execution. Variable-length portions of speech are planned in a time frame reflecting difficulty of processing at that level (e.g., memory access difficulty); these utterances are executed at a rhythm reflecting articulatory constraints as well as social and communicative conditions prevailing at the time of speech production. As was suggested in Keller (1979), the main reason for the existence of the two distinct processing stages is the presence of different time requirements for the two types of processing.

The aphasic aspect of articulatory neuropathology probably relates to the planning aspect of the speech production process. It is likely that this is a difficulty of lexical access, since phonologically grossly abnormal (i.e., jargonaphasic) utterances tend to occur when patients are looking for appropriate words (Buckingham & Kertesz, 1974, p. 61). Also, certain differences between phonological errors in Broca's aphasia and in Wernicke's aphasia are more easily accounted for if it is assumed that at least a good proportion of these errors are difficulties in lexical access. For instance, Blumstein (1973, p. 46) reports only 6.6% addition and 24.4% omission errors for Broca's aphasics, but 13.8% addition and 30.3% omission errors for Wernicke's aphasics. The production of erroneous lexemes that are often longer or shorter than target lexemes suggests an incomplete or erroneous activation of a lexical representation, rather than an incorrect processing of a correctly (and thus completely) specified lexical representation. Similarly, difficulties associated with syntagmatic processing at the intersyllabic level (e.g., "camera" vs.

"caramel") are more readily understood in terms of planning processes which serve to establish sequential precedence than in terms of execution processes which presumably operate on sequentially specified phonological utterances.

The apraxic aspect of articulatory neuropathology can be assumed to affect spatial and temporal relationships between muscle groups responsible for a single vocal tract valve and/or between a number of vocal tract valves. Such disturbances were seen to affect phoneme selection and phoneme-to-phoneme processing. It is conceivable that this type of disorder occurs at the interface between planning and execution, and results from a difficulty in maintaining temporal and spatial relations during the neural activation of preplanned utterances. Under this hypothesis, some elements are activated (i.e., sent into the execution process) sequentially when they should be concurrent, or are activated concurrently when they should be sequential (temporal relationship impaired). Or then, activation of agonist and antagonist neuronal pathways may be unbalanced, resulting in gesture reduction or extension (spatial relationship impaired). Or finally, preactivated (i.e., planned) elements are not sufficiently distinct from nonpreactivated elements, resulting in the erroneous activation of an unplanned element (selectional distinction impaired). All three types of impairment can lead to a perceived phoneme substitution. Since the usual temporal, spatial, and/or paradigmatic relationships are disrupted, the system has to control additional degrees of freedom. This causes a slowdown of execution processing and, in a certain proportion of cases, a favoring of "easier" phoneme-to-phoneme transitions.

The dysarthric aspect of articulatory neuropathology affects a specific aspect of execution processing, such as upper motor neuron, cerebellar, or lower motor neuron processing. As a result, the complete speech chain is "filtered" by the given pathology, producing speech that is best described as spastic, ataxic, or flaccid, respectively. This may have the effect of disturbing low-level contextual relationships affecting phoneme-to-phoneme transitions. For instance, spastic dysarthria may involve an impairment of spatial relationships, while ataxic dysarthria could be an impairment of the relationship between previous articulatory gestures and gestures about to be executed.

Although most of this conceptualization is at present untested, it forms a useful frame of reference for future research. For instance, planned experiments using ultrasound measurement techniques for tongue and larynegeal activity (Keller & Ostry, in press) will examine the disruption of temporal and spatial relationships in apraxic and dysarthric speech. Also, further analyses of the lexical impairment in Wernicke's aphasia are planned using the present data base. With these techniques, it should be possible to distinguish between a number of theoretical alternatives presented here and to verify their empirical usefulness.

NOTES

[1]In this text, the terms "phonetic" and "phonological disorders" are used descriptively. Phonetic disorders are speech impairments that affect the manner of producing individual phonemes (through distortion, excessive forcefulness, nonsystematic prolongation, harshness of voice, etc.) without transgressing perceived phoneme boundaries. Such disorders are known in the French literature as "arthric disorders" ("troubles arthriques" or "la composante arthrique"). Although seen in the dysarthrias in their pure form (see Darley, Aronson, & Brown, 1969, 1975), they also coexist with other speech and language disorders, particularly with phonological disorders, in aphasia and apraxia of speech. Phonological disorders are speech disorders involving the substitution, the omission, and the addition of phonemes or other submorphemic units (phonetic features, consonant clusters, diphthongs, or syllables). Disorders of this type are seen in all types of aphasia and in apraxia of speech.

[2]In this text, aphasiological terminology follows the usage of the two major U.S. aphasiological traditions. Behaviorally, the term "apraxia" and "aphasia" are distinguished as they are in the Midwestern U.S. aphasiological tradition (e.g., Darley, 1977). Aphasia is defined as an "impairment, due to brain damage, of the capacity to... formulate language symbols," while Apraxia of speech is "an articulatory disorder resulting from impairment... of the capacity to program the positioning of speech muscles and the sequencing of muscle movements for the volitional production of phonemes" (Wertz, 1978, p. 2). The behavioral distinction between aphasia and apraxia of speech corresponds well to the theoretical distinction between the planning phase and the execution phase proposed for normal speech production (Foss & Hakes, 1978; Keller, 1979, 1982). Within such a psycholinguistic framework, aphasic pathological language behavior can be seen as an interference in the planning phase and apraxia of speech can be considered to occur at the interface between planning and execution. The behavioral distinction of the two terms does not imply their syndromic distinction; as Wertz (1978) emphasizes, most patients show varying degrees of coexisting behaviorally classified disorders (p. 9). Syndromic distinction follows the East coast tradition (and that generally adhered to by European authors and by my Montreal colleagues). Broca's aphasia, conduction aphasia, and Wernicke's aphasia are thus defined as in Goodglass and Kaplan (1972), Lecours (1975), and Joanette, Keller, and Lecours (1980). Broca's aphasics are patients with nonfluent oral expression, but showing a reasonably preserved comprehension. These patients present phonemic as well as phonetic deviations. Conduction aphasics are patients with somewhat more fluent oral expression, a marked deficit of repetition, but showing a reasonably preserved comprehension. These patients show numerous phonemic paraphasias in their oral expression, but lack phonetic deviations. Wernicke's aphasics are patients with fluent oral expression, but with a considerable comprehension deficit. These patients may present deviations of all types, except for phonetic distortions. A high proportion of moderately impaired patients whose language corresponds to these profiles show destinctive lesion localization; Broca's aphasics present more anterior lesions while conduction and especially Wernicke's aphasics show more posterior lesions. Although these profiles and their neurological implications adequately characterize the major proportion of the moderately impaired patients, a minority of moderately impaired and the majority of the severely impaired aphasic patients are not adequately categorized by this syndromic classification. All patients of the present study satisfy this classification.

[3]Standardization of spontaneous speech and repetition samples must account for the unequal frequency of various phonemes in running speech. A formula which will accomplish this is given in Keller (1978, p. 268).

[4]In this text, the term "phonemic sequence" denotes either a consonant or a vowel sequence. A consonant sequence can be a consonant cluster or it can be a set of identical consonants, such as /tt/. Similarly, a vowel sequence can be a diphthong or it can be a set of identical vowels, such as /ee/.

[5]Translation from French by the present author.

[6]Examen de l'aphasie du Centre de rééducation du langage et de recherches neuropsychologiques, Hôtel-Dieu de Montréal, available from: La Librairie de l'Université de Montréal, C.P.

[7]Interjudgmental agreement figures on the phonetically distorted speech of Broca's aphasics may be improved by filtering and speech extension techniques. The recordings of one patient with considerable arthric impairment (EL) were filtered by means of a frequency equalizer and interjudgmental agreement for the vowels of this patient was three quarters of a standard deviation above the mean for vowels.

[8]This presentation of the vocal tract model follows the requirements of a methodological description of the present research and is not meant to be an exhaustive motivation and treatment of the model. The domain specifications presented in Tables 8-1 to 8-3 represent a preliminary working hypothesis, rather than a final version of the model. Work is presently underway to motivate further working principles of the model and to bring it into line with published data and with information gathered by means of our ultrasound measuring technique for lingual articulation (Keller & Ostry, in press).

REFERENCES

Alajouanine, T., Ombredane, A., & Durand, M. *Le syndrome de desintegration phonétique dans l'aphasia.* Masson et Cie., 1939.

Blumstein, S.E. *A phonological investigation of aphasic speech.* The Hague: Mouton, 1973.

Blumstein, S. E., Cooper, W. E., Goodglass, H., Statlender, S., & Gottlieb, J. Production deficits in aphasia: A voice onset time analysis, *Brain and Language*, 1980, *9*, 153–170.

Buckingham, H. W., Jr., & Kertesz, A. A linguistic analysis of fluent aphasia. *Brain and Language*, 1974, *1*, 43–62.

Chomsky, N., & Halle, M. *The sound pattern of English.* New York: Harper & Row, 1968.

Cochran, W. G. Some methods for strengthening the common chi-square tests. *Biometrics*, 1954, *10*, 417–445.

Daniloff, R. G. Normal articulation processes. In F.D. Minifie, T.J. Hixon, & F. Williams (Eds.), *Normal aspects of speech, hearing, and language,* Englewood Cliffs, NJ: Prentice Hall, 1973.

Darley, F. L. A retrospective view: Aphasia. *Journal of Speech and Hearing Disorders*, 1977, *42*, 161–169.

Darley, F. L., Aronson, A. E., & Brown, J. R. Differential diagnostic patterns of dysarthia. *Journal of Speech and Hearing Research,* 1969, *12*, 246–269.

Darley, F. L., Aronson, A. E., & Brown, J. R. *Motor speech disorders.* Philadelphia, PA: Saunders, 1975.

Desrouesne, J., Beauvois, M. F., & Ranty, C. Deux composantes dans l'articulation du langage oral: Preuve expérimentale de leur indépendance, *Neuropsychologica*, 1977, *15*, 143–153.

Dew, D., & Jensen, P. J. *Phonetic processing*. Columbus, OH: Merrill, 1977.

Foss, D. J., & Hakes, D. T. *Psycholinguistics*. Englewood Cliffs, NJ: Prentice-Hall, 1978.

Fujimura, O. Acoustics of speech. In J.H. Gilbert, (Ed.), *Speech and cortical functioning*. New York: Academic Press, 1972.

Goodglass, H., & Kaplan, E. F. *The assessment of aphasia and related disorders*. Philadelphia: Lea and Febiger, 1972.

Guyard, H., Sabouraud, O., & Gagnepain, J. A procedure to differentiate phonological disturbances in Broca's aphasia and Wernicke's aphasia. *Brain and Language*, 1981, *13*, 19–30.

Harshman, R., Ladefoged, P., & Goldstein, L. Factor analysis of tongue shapes. *Journal of the Acoustical Society of America*, 1977, *62*, 693–707.

Hécaen, H., & Consoli, S. Analyse des troubles du langage au cours des lésions de l'aire de Broca. *Neuropsychologia*, 1973, *11*, 377–388.

Henke, W. L. *Dynamic articulatory model of speech production using computer simulation*. Ph. D. dissertation, Massachusetts Institute of Technology, 1966.

Hirose, H., & Kiritani, S. Velocity of articulatory movements in normal and dysarthric subjects. *Research Institute of Logopedics and Phoniatrics*, 1979, 13, 105–112.

Hirose, H., Kiritani, S., & Sawashima, M. Patterns of dysarthric movements in patients with amyotrophic lateral sclerosis and pseudobulbar palsy. *Research Institute of Logopedics and Phoniatrics*, 1980, *14*, 263–272.

Hirose, H., Kiritani, S., Ushijima, T., Yoshioka, H., & Sawashima, M. Patterns of dysartric movements in patients with Parkinsonism. *Research Institute of Logopedics and Phoniatrics*, 1978, *12*, 73–86.

Hirose, H., & Sawashima, M. Disturbance of the rhythmic structure of speech in the dysarthrias. *Research Institute of Logopedics and Phoniatrics*, 1979, *13*, 113–122.

Itoh, M., Sasanuma, S., Hirose, H., Yoshioka, H., & Ushijima, T. Abnormal articulatory dynamics in a patient with apraxia of speech: X-ray microbeam observation. *Brain and Language*, 1980, *11*, 66–75.

Jakobson, R., Fant, C. G. M., & Halle, M. *Preliminaries to speech analysis*. Cambridge, MA: MIT Press, 1951.

Joanette, Y., Keller, E., & Lecours, A. R. Sequences of phonemic approximations in aphasia. *Brain and Language*, 1980, *11*, 30–44.

Johns, D. F., & Darley, F. L. Phonemic variability in apraxia of speech. *Journal of Speech and Hearing Research*, 1970, *13*, 556–583.

Johns, D. F., & LaPointe, L. L. Neurogenic disorders of output processing; Apraxia of speech. In H. Whitaker & H.A. Whitaker (Eds.), *Studies in Neurolinguistics*. New York: Academic Press, 1976.

Keller, E. Vowel errors in aphasia, Ph.D. dissertation, University of Toronto, 1975 (available from the author).

Keller, E. Parameters for vowel substitutions in Broca's aphasia. *Brain and Language*, 1978, *5*, 265–285.

Keller, E. Planning and execution in speech production. *Recherches Linguistiques à Montréal*, 1979, *13*, 34–51 (available from the author).

Keller, E. *Manuel de psycholinguistique*, Montreal: UQAM, Département de linguistique, 1982.

Keller, E., & Labelle, M. *Modèle coarticulatoire pour l'action du conduit vocal.* Montreal: Université du Québec a Montréal (manuscript available from the author).

Keller, E., & Ostry, D. J. Computerized pulsed-echo ultrasound measurements of tongue dorsum movements. *Journal of the Acoustical Society of America*, in press.

Keller, E., Rothenberger, A., & Goepfert, M. Perceptual discrimination of vowels in aphasia. *Archiv Fun Psychiatrie und Nervenkrankheiten*, 1982, *231*, 339-357.

Kelso, J. A. S., & Tuller, B. Toward a theory of apratic syndromes. *Brain and language,* 1981, *12*, 224-245.

Kent, R. D., & Minifie, F. D. Coarticulation in recent speech production models. *Journal of Phonetics*, 1977, *5*, 115-133.

Kertesz, A., & Poole, E. The aphasia quotient: The taxonomic approach to measurement of aphasic disability. *Canadian Journal of Neurological Science*, 1974, *1*, 7-16.

Kuehn, D. P., & Moll, K. L. A cineradiographic study of VC and VC articulatory velocities. *Journal of Phonetics*, 1976, *4*, 303-320.

Ladefoged, P. *A course in phonetics*. New York: Harcourt Brace Jovanovich, 1975.

Lecours, A. R. Aphasie, *Encyclopédie médico-chirurgicale*, 17019 *A10*, 1-20, 1975.

Lecours, A. R., & Lhermitte, F. Phonemic paraphasias: Linguistic structures and tentative hypotheses. *Cortex*, 1969, *5*, 193-228.

Luria, A. R. *Higher cortical functions in man*. New York: Basic Books, 1966.

Martin, A. D., & Rigrodsky, S. An investigation of phonological impairment in aphasia, part 2: Distinctive feature analysis of phonemic commutation errors in aphasia. *Cortex*, 1974, *10*, 329-346.

MacNeilage, P. F. Speech production. In E. Fisher-Jorgensen, J. Rischel, & N. Thorsen (Eds.), *Proceedings of the Ninth International Congress of Phonetic Sciences*, University of Copenhagen, 1979.

Nespoulous, J. L. La dichotomie "phonétique-phonémique" a-t-elle une valeur nosologique? In P. Messenli (Ed.), *L'expression orale*. Paris: C.N.R.S., in press.

Netsell, R. Speech physiology. In F.D. Minifie, T.J. Hixon, & F. Willaims (Eds.), *Normal aspects of speech, hearing, and language*. Englewood Cliffs, NJ: Prentice Hall, 1973.

Perkell, J. S. Phonetic features and the physiology of speech production. In B. Butterworth, (Ed.), *Language production*. New York: Academic Press, 1980.

Pike, K. L. *Phonemics*. Ann Arbor, MI: The University of Michigan Press, 1947.

Pupier, P. *Dictionnaire phonologique informatisé du franqais-québecois*. Montréal: Université du Québec à Montréal, 1977.

Schnitzer, M. L. Generative phonology — Evidence from aphasia. *Pennsylvania State Studies*, 1972, *1*, 95-104.

Schuell, H. A short examination for aphasia. *Neurology*, 1957, *7*, 625-634.

Shankweiler, D., & Harris, K. S. An experimental approach to the problem of articulation in aphasia. *Cortex*, 1966, *2*, 277-292.

Shankweiler, D., Harris, K. S., & Taylor, M. L. Electromyographic studies of articulation in aphasia. *Archives of Physical Medicine & Rehabilitation*, 1968, *49*, 1-8.

Trost, J., & Canter, G. J. Apraxia of speech in patients with Broca's aphasia: A study of phoneme production accuracy and error patterns. *Brain and Language*, 1974, *1*, 63-79.

Wertz, R. T. Neuropathologies of speech and language: An introduction to patient management. In D.F. Johns (Ed.), *Clinical management of neurogenic communication disorders.* Boston, MA: Little, Brown, 1978.

ACKNOWLEDGMENTS

I am indebted to many friends, colleagues, assistants, students, and subjects for their help in this project. Dr. Y. Joanette and Dr. A. R. Lecours permitted me to reutilize our common data base, Dr. A. Kertesz and Dr. S. E. Blumstein allowed me to copy the tape recordings of some of their patients, and Ms. F. Ezerzer, L. Walsh, F. Ryner, and J. Moore provided me with access to aphasic and apraxic patients in the Toronto region. The tedious transcription job was performed, for English patients, by J. Naughton, A. Greenwood, and L. Moran, and for French patients, by A. Viau, C. Lévesque, L. Bourret, M.-C. Charest, and F. Courtois. Various theoretical and methodological aspects of the project were refined in fertile discussions with Dr. J.-N. Nespoulous, Université de Montréal, Dr. D. J. Ostry, McGill University, Ms. M. Mandel, McGill University, and Ms. A. Simon, Université de Montréal, and through the many useful suggestions of Dr. G. Breton, Concordia University. Financial assistance was available through grants from the Université du Québec à Montréal, the FCAC programme of the Québec government, the National Science and Engineering Council of Canada, and the Medical Research Council of Canada. I have also benefited from a research leave from the Université du Québec a Montréal while conducting this study.

9

Response to Treatment in Patients with Apraxia of Speech

Robert T. Wertz In Association With
the Study Group of The Veterans Administration
Cooperative Study on Aphasia
M.J. Collins, D. Weiss, J.F. Kurtzke, T. Friden, R.H. Brookshire, J. Pierce, P. Holtzapple,
D.J. Hubbard, B.E. Porch, J.A. West, L. Davis, V.Matovitch, G.K. Morley, and E. Resurreccion.

INTRODUCTION

Studies of the efficacy of therapy for improving speech in adult patients suffering from apraxia of speech are scattered throughout the literature. Typically, these are reports on a single case or a few cases submitted to a variety of treatments. The large *"N"* studies include those of Rosenbek, Lemme, Ahern, Harris, and Wertz, (1973) who reported on response to treatment in three patients and Deal and Florance (1978) who provided data on four patients. Single-subject reports are typified by the use of a variety of methods.These include speech specific techniques (Holtzapple & Marshall, 1977; Rosenbek, 1978); intrasystemic reorganization (Keith & Aronson, 1975; Tonkovich & Marquardt, 1977); intersystemic reorganization (Rosenbek, Collins, & Wertz, 1976; Simmons, 1978; Skelly, Schinsky, Smith, & Fust, 1974); stimulus and language driven methods (Hand, Tonkovich, & Aitchison, 1979; Houston-Weidel, 1976; Rosenbek, 1978; Simmons, 1980; Wilson, 1977); preverbal, rehearsal strategies (Bugbee & Nichols, 1980; Warren, 1977); and a variety of miscellaneous techniques such as environmental manipulation (Florance, Rabidoux, & McCauslin, 1980), biofeedback (McNeil, Prescott, & Lemme, 1976), and alternative modes of communication (Rabidoux, Florance, & McCauslin, 1980; Skelly et al., 1974).

Unlike the group study designs used to determine the efficacy of treatment for aphasia, what we know about whether treatment works for the apraxic patient comes from single-subject and small sample designs. Therefore, we know more about the treatments, the conditions under which the treatments were administered, and the patient's response to treatment. The efforts to date may lack quantity, but they are clothed in quality. Unfortunately, support for the efficacy of treatment with apraxic patients from large "*N*" studies is hidden in means of patient performance who were labeled aphasic. Thus, we know little about the patients in Kertesz and McCabe's (1977); Basso, Capitani, and Vignolo's (1979); and Wertz, Collins, Weiss, Kurtzke et al.'s (1981) samples who may have suffered apraxia of speech in addition to their aphasia.

Wertz and Rosenbek (1978) have listed the advantages and disadvantages in single-subject and group designs. What is restricted in one method is permitted by the other. Both are necessay to provide bits and pieces of truth about a disorder and whether it responds to treatment. For example, what we know about treatment for the apraxic patient from the single-subject literature is that the patients reported were, indeed, apraxic; that they received a well-described treatment of a specified amount and duration; and that they improved or did not improve on the specific criterion measures administered. What the single-subject reports do not tell us is the natural history information about the disorder, how it may change if treated in a group design, and how patients demonstrating it may be abused when submitted to the controlled conditions imposed by a group design. Thus, the single-subject research tells us about patients who suffer a disorder, and group research tells us about the disorder.

The purpose of this chapter is to report the response to treatment by patients demonstrating apraxia of speech and aphasia who participated in the Veterans Administration Cooperative Study, A Comparison of Individual and Group Treatment for Aphasia. Our previous report (Wertz et al., 1981) submerged these patients in group mean data by combining them with patients who demonstrated only aphasia. By examining patients in our sample who demonstrated apraxia of speech coexisting with aphasia, we willl attempt to provide, for apraxia of speech, what Darley (1972) requested for aphasia, "More data... applying to clearly specified samples... subjected to clearly specified regimens of therapy... for specified periods" (p. 8).

METHODS AND PROCEDURES

Five Veterans Administration Medical Centers — Albuquerque, Kansas City, Minneapolis, New Orleans, and New York — participated in the study. Patients who met selection criteria were assigned randomly to one of two treatment groups. Group A received traditional, individual treatment administered by a speech-language pathologist who used direct, stimulus-response manipulation of speech and language deficits. Group B received group treatment conducted by a speech-language pathologist who stimulated language through social interaction with no direct manipulation of speech and language deficits.

Selection Criteria

In an attempt to control several variables believed to influence response to treatment, all study patients were required to meet the following selection criteria: status, veteran; sex, male; age, 40–80 years; literacy, premorbid ability to read and write English; etiology, first thromboembolic cerebrovascular accident (CVA); localization, damage confined to the left hemisphere; medical status, no coexisting major medical complications; sensory status, auditory acuity no worse than a 40-dB speech reception threshold in the poorer ear; visual acuity no worse than 20/100 corrected in the poorer eye; and tactile function demonstrated by adequate sensory and motor ability in one hand to write and gesture; time postonset, 4 weeks at entry; and language severity, 15th to 75th overall percentile performance on the Porch Index of Communicative Ability (PICA) (Porch, 1967) at entry.

Study Patients

Potential study patients were obtained by screening the neurology, medical, and surgical wards in the five cooperating medical centers. During a 3½-year period, 1071 patients were screened. Sixty-seven of these met all selection criteria and were entered into the study. Of the 67 patients entered, 19 were judged to demonstrate apraxia of speech coexisting with aphasia (AOS) at entry. An additional 10 patients were suspected of demonstrating apraxia of speech coexisting with aphasia, but judges were sufficiently uncertain, so these patients were classified "apraxia of speech undetermined" (AOS Undetermined) at entry.

If a patient met all selection criteria, he was asked to participate in the study. If he agreed, he was assigned randomly to Group A, individual treatment, or Group B, group treatment. A 44-week treatment trial, 4-48 weeks postonset (WPO) was planned. However, attrition was high — approximately 50% of all patients entered dropped out prior to completing

TABLE 9-1
Sample size of patients judged to display apraxia of speech coexisting with aphasia or apraxia of speech undetermined at entry and in each treatment cohort

	Number of Patients				
				Dropouts	
Cohort	*Group A*	*Group B*	*Total*	*A*	*B*
Entry (4 Weeks Postonset)	17	12	29	—	—
15 Week (11 Weeks of Treatment)	14	12	26	3	0
26 Week (22 Weeks of Treatment)	12	11	23	2	1
37 Week (33 Weeks of Treatment)	9	9	18	3	2
48 Week (44 Weeks of Treatment)	9	8	17	0	1

Note. A cohort is defined by the number of weeks of treatment completed. For example, patients in the 15-week Cohort completed 11 weeks of treatment, from the 4th to 15th week postonset. Patients in longer cohorts are included in shorter cohorts.

the 44-week treatment period. Of the 29 patients who demonstrated AOS or who were judged AOS Undetermined, 12 (41%) dropped out prior to completing the 44-week treatment period.

To preserve data, we fractionated the itital sample of AOS and AOS Undetermined patients into the cohorts shown in Table 9-1. Each is defined by the number of weeks of treatment received. Twenty-nine patients were judged to display AOS or AOS Undetermined at entry. Seventeen were randomized to Group A treatment, and 12 were randomized to Group B treatment. Of these, 26 patients, 14 in Group A and 12 in Group B, completed 11 weeks of treatment; 23 patients, 12 in Group A and 11 in Group B, completed 22 weeks of treatment; 18 patients, 9 in each group, completed 33 weeks of treatment; and 17 patients, 9 in Group A and 8 in Group B, completed 44 weeks of treatment. Patients in longer cohorts, (e.g., the 48-Week Cohort) are also represented in shorter cohorts, for example, the 15-, 26-, and 37-Week Cohorts.

Attrition was not significantly related to the treatment received. The most common reason for dropping out was geographical. Some study patients lived sufficiently far from the treatment centers to require they remain in the hospital or travel long distances for treatment. Of the 12 dropouts, 9 did so because they elected to return home or tired of the long journey for treatment, one became too ill to participate in treatment, one suffered a second CVA, and one died.

Age, education, and language severity at intake are shown in Table 9-2. No significant differences ($p \langle .05$) between treatment groups were observed for age, education, or language severity at intake. All patients displayed right hemiplegia. A retrospective classification of patients at intake (Wertz, Kitselman, & Deal, 1981) on the Boston Diagnostic Aphasia Examination (BDAE) system (Goodglass & Kaplan, 1972) revealed 10 patients displayed Broca's aphasia, three displayed Global aphasia, one displayed Conduction aphasia, one displayed Anomic aphasia, one displayed Transcortical Motor aphasia, six displayed mixed aphasia, and seven were unclassifiable.

TABLE 9-2
Descriptive data at intake (4 weeks postonset) for age, education, and language severity for each treatment group

	Treatment Group		
Variable	*A (N = 17)*	*B (N = 12)*	*Combined*
Age in Years			
Mean	58.76	59.00	58.88
Range	46–73	45–79	45–79
Education in Years			
Mean	11.00	10.92	10.96
Range	6–16	5–19	5–19
PICA Overall Percentile			
Mean	40.8	43.0	41.7
Range	15–72	15–71	15–72

Evaluation Battery

A battery of measures was administered at intake and every 11 weeks thereafter up to 48 weeks postonset or until a patient dropped out of the study. These included: a standardized, complete clinical neurologic examination to determine neurologic status and severity; sensory screening to determine auditory, visual, and tactile acuity; Porch Index of Communicative Ability (PICA) (Porch , 1967) to determine the presence and severity of aphasia; Token Test (De Renzi & Vignolo, 1962) to determine auditory comprehension ability; Word Fluency Measure (Borkowski, Benton, & Spreen, 1967) to determine word-finding ability; a motor speech evaluation adapted from Wertz and Rosenbek (1971) to determine the presence and severity of apraxia of speech and dysarthria; Coloured Progressive Matrices (Raven, 1962) to determine "nonverbal intelligence"; a conversation rating, developed for this study; and an informant's rating of "functional language" use adapted from Sarno (1969) to determine "functional" language ability.

The motor speech evaluation required the examiner to judge whether each patient displayed apraxia of speech, did not display apraxia of speech, or whether the presence of apraxia of speech could not be determined. For patients judged to be apraxic, the examiner rated the severity of apraxia of speech on a 7-point rating scale, where "1" indicated mild apraxia of speech and "7" indicated severe apraxia of speech. The conversation rating also utilized a 7-point scale, where "1" indicated "normal" conversational ability and "7" indicated no conversational ability. The rating was based on a 3- to 5-minute conversation with the patient about his general condition and events occurring within the previous week.

A cooperating neurologist in each participating medical center conducted the neurologic examination. The informant's rating of "functional language" use was completed by each patient's representative, a family member or friend. All other measures were administered and scored by a speech pathologist. Patient performance on these latter measures was videotaped and scored "blind" by two speech pathologists who had no knowledge of treatment group assignment in order to control bias and obtain reliability.

Reliability between the two "blind" scorers was above +.95 on all measures except the motor speech evaluation. Judge reliability for determining the presence of apraxia of speech ranged from +.69 to +.87 across evaluation dates, and reliability for determining the severity of apraxia of speech ranged from +.65 to +.93 across evaluation dates.

Treatment

A treatment therapist was employed in each participating medical center to administer all therapy given in both treatment groups. This was an attempt to control for a potential therapist variable, at least, within a given participating center. All study patients received 8 hours of treatment each week they were in the study.

Group A received 4 hours of direct therapist contact in traditional, individual, stimulus-response type treatment of speech and language deficits in all communicative modalities. For example, specific auditory comprehension, reading, speaking, and writing tasks were selected by the therapist and presented to the patient, and the patient's responses were corrected when incorrect or inappropriate. Because all patients displayed aphasia coexisting with apraxia of speech, treatment was administered to combat both disorders. Specific treatments for apraxia of speech included: retraining points of articulation and sequences of articulatory movements; developing ability to use visual cues to program articulatory movements; training in the use of compensatory movements, such as the instrusive schwa, equal and even stress, and so forth; drill involving repetition and reading words, phrases, and sentences of graded difficulty for the patient in which the length of utterance and distance between successive phonemes was gradually increased. The individual, face-to-face treatment was supplemented with 4 hours each week of drill using workbooks and machine-assisted methods (e.g., tape recorder, language master). Therapeutic emphasis, on aphasia or on apraxia of speech, was determined by the clinician.

Group B patients received 4 hours of direct therapist contact in a group of three to seven patients designed to facilitate language use in a group setting with no direct manipulation of speech or language deficits. For example, patients were encouraged to enter into group discussion on current events or topics selected by the therapist or the group. No specific tasks designed to improve auditory comprehension, reading, speaking, or writing were presented. No direct attempt was made to improve or correct incorrect responses. However, taciturn patients were asked questions and encouraged to participate in the discussion. This was supplemented by 4 hours each week of group recreational activities including films, guest speakers, craft activities, and games.

Both types of treatment were elaborated in a Treatment Protocol to maximize differences between Group A and Group B therapy and to ensure essentially the same types of treatment were being administered in the five treatment centers.

RESULTS

Results are organized into three areas. First, we will report change in apraxia of speech. Second, we will report change on the primary language measure, the PICA. And third, we will compare how change in apraxia of speech related to change in aphasia.

Change in Apraxia of Speech

Change in the diagnosis of AOS was rampant during the treatment trial. This is shown in Tables 9-3 and 9-4. Of the 26 patients who received at least 11 weeks of treatment and two or more evaluations, only six who were diagnosed as demonstrating AOS at intake, two in Group A and

TABLE 9-3
Classification of patients in each treatment group, A and B, at each evaluation date, shown in weeks postonset

	Evaluation Date									
	4		*15*		*26*		*37*		*48*	
Classification	*A*	*B*	*A*	*B*	*A*	*B*	*A*	*B*	*A*	*B*
AOS	11	8	10	8	7	6	6	4	6	4
AOS Undetermined	6	4	3	2	1	2	0	4	0	3
No AOS	—	—	1	2	4	3	3	1	3	1
Cumulative Dropouts	—	—	3	0	5	1	8	3	8	4
Number of Patients	17	12	17	12	17	12	17	12	17	12

four in Group B, maintained their diagnosis at the time they dropped out or completed the treatment trial. Of the ten patients who were classified as AOS Undetermined at intake, seven — four in Group A and three in Group B — were diagnosed as demonstrating AOS at their 15-week evaluation. The three that remained AOS Undetermined at 15 weeks postonset, two in Group A and one in Group B, were diagnosed as demonstrating AOS at their 26-week evaluation.

Six patients, four in Group A and two in Group B, were diagnosed as demonstrating AOS at intake and, on subsequent evaluations, were judged to be not apraxic. Change in diagnosis for three of these patients, one in Group A and two in Group B, occurred at 15 weeks postonset. Change in diagnosis for the other three patients, all in Group A, occurred for one at 26 postonset, and for two at 37 weeks postonset. Two additional patients, originally judged to display AOS, were diagnosed, on one subsequent evaluation to be nonapraxic; however, the diagnosis for one returned to AOS, and for the other, to AOS Undetermined on the next evaluation. Initial severity of AOS in the six patients who became nonapraxic and remained so was mild, "1" for three patients and "2" for three patients on the 7-point rating scale.

Twenty — 12 in Group A and 8 in Group B — of the 26 patients who had at least two evaluations migrated among the three possible diagnoses — AOS, AOS Undetermined, No AOS. Diagnosis changed only once across evaluation periods for the 12 patients in Group A. In Group B, diagnosis changed once for four patients, twice for two patients, and

TABLE 9–4
Change in the classification of patients in each treatment group, A and B, from one evaluation date, shown in weeks postonset, to the next evaluation date

Classification	*Intake*		*Evaluation Dates*							
	4		*15*		*26*		*37*		*48*	
	A *(N = 17)*	*B* *(N = 12)*	*A* *(N = 14)*	*B* *(N = 12)*	*A* *(N = 12)*	*B* *(N = 11)*	*A* *(N = 9)*	*B* *(N = 9)*	*A* *(N = 9)*	*B* *(N = 8)*
Diagnosis Unchanged From Previous Evaluation										
AOS	11[b]	8	6[a]	5	5[a]	5[a]	5	4	6	3
AOS Undetermined	6	4	2	1	1[a]	0	0	2	0	2
No AOS	—	—	—	—	1	2[a]	2	1[a]	3	1
Diagnosis Changed From Previous Evaluation										
AOS to AOS Undetermined	—	—	1	1	0	2	0	1	0	1
AOS to No AOS	—	—	1	2	3[a]	0	1	0	0	0
AOS Undetermined to AOS	—	—	4[a]	3[a]	2	1	0	0	0	1
AOS Undetermined to No AOS	—	—	0	0	0	1	0	0	0	0
No AOS to AOS	—	—	—	—	0	0	1	0	0	0
No AOS to AOS Undetermined	—	—	—	—	0	0	0	1	0	0

[a] = One patient dropped out prior to the next evaluation.
[b] = Three patients dropped out prior to the next evaluation.

three times for two patients. Patients whose diagnosis changed were not typified by their severity of coexisting aphasia or their severity of apraxia of speech.

Change in the severity of apraxia of speech is shown in Table 9-5. Nineteen patients either remained apraxic or became nonapraxic. Six dropped out of the study prior to demonstrating any change in AOS, and four remained AOS Undetermined at the time they dropped out. Mean initial severity of AOS on the 7-point rating scale at the time it was diagnosed was 3.50 in Group A and 3.40 in Group B for patients who remained apraxic. Severity ranged from 3 to 4 in Group A and 2 to 5 in Group B. At the time of the patients' last evaluation, mean severity was 2.50 in Group A and 3.00 in Group B. Six of the eight patients in Group A improved one level on the 7-point scale, one patient improved two levels, and one patient displayed no change in severity of AOS. One of the five patients in Group B improved two levels on the 7-point rating scale, and the other four patients displayed no change in severity of AOS. T tests indicated improvement was significant in Group A ($p<.01$) and nonsignificant in Group B ($p<.05$).

TABLE 9–5
Change in the diagnosis and severity of Apraxia of Speech in each treatment group, A and B, prior to dropping out or completing the treatment trial

			*Mean Severity**					
			At Diagnosis		*Last Evaluation*		*Mean Change*	
Classification	*A*	*B*	*A*	*B*	*A*	*B*	*A*	*B*
Remained AOS	8	5	3.50	3.40	2.50	3.00	1.00	.40
AOS Resolved	4	2	1.50	1.50	0	0	1.50	.50
Dropped Out Prior to Change	5	1	3.80	3.00	—	—	—	—
AOS Remained Undetermined at Dropout	1	3	—	—	—	—	—	—

*Severity on 7-point rating scale (1 = mild, 7 = severe).

Change in Aphasia

For the purpose of this report, we will use PICA performance as the measure of change in aphasia. Table 9-6 shows PICA performance in each treatment group at intake, 4 weeks postonset, and at each subse-

TABLE 9-6
Change in coexisting aphasia, measured by PICA percentiles, in patients diagnosed as AOS and AOS Undetermined at entry, four weeks postonset

	PICA Percentiles							
	Overall		*Gestural*		*Verbal*		*Graphic*	
Time Postonset	$\overline{X}$	*Range*	$\overline{X}$	*Range*	$\overline{X}$	*Range*	$\overline{X}$	*Range*
4 Weeks Postonset								
Group A (*N*=17)	40.8	15–72	45.3	15–70	37.6	5–70	39.7	9–82
Group B (*N*=12)	43.0	15–71	43.5	8–68	43.0	19–58	46.3	17–79
15 Weeks Postonset								
Group A (*N*=14)	60.6	31–85	60.4	39–85	55.7	22–88	66.6	39–89
Group B (*N*=12)	55.4	16–84	54.0	16–88	53.3	17–84	59.7	7–83
26 Weeks Postonset								
Group A (*N*=12)	71.6	55–94	71.1	51–93	64.8	38–85	74.1	46–96
Group B (*N*=11)	59.3	12–83	57.6	12–93	53.1	1–71	63.7	2–88
37 Weeks Postonset								
Group A (*N*=9)	75.5	59–93	73.6	61–94	68.5	47–88	79.9	51–94
Group B (*N*=9)	64.1	19–87	67.5	19–93	58.6	10–89	64.3	3–87
48 Weeks Postonset								
Group A (*N*=9)	76.6	60–98	76.1	55–91	69.7	50–92	79.2	46–99
Group B (*N*=8)	67.1	32–87	73.2	32–96	57.5	13–78	70.2	45–87

quent evaluation. There were no significant differences ($p < .05$) between treatment groups on any PICA measure at intake. Each group displayed significant change ($p < .05$) in their PICA Overall percentile from one evaluation to the next — 4–15, 15–26, 26–37 — except the last comparison — 37–48, where neither group displayed significant change. There were no significant differences in the PICA Overall percentile between groups at any evaluation date except at 26 WPO, where Group A was significantly better ($p < .10$) than Group B. Thus improvement in aphasia tended to occur early in the treatment trial, by 37 weeks postonset, and the type of treatment had little influence on improvement.

Table 9-7 shows PICA group mean change scores for the 14 patients in Group A and the 12 patients in Group B who received two or more evaluations. All measures changed significantly ($p < .01$) from intake to the last evaluation in both groups. Significant differences between groups were few, and those that did occur were slight. Group A made significantly more change ($p < .10$) than Group B in the PICA Verbal and Graphic percentiles. A comparison of group mean change scores indicates that Group A made more improvement in PICA Overall, Verbal, and Graphic scores, and Group B made more improvement in the PICA Gestural score. The pattern of improvement in the three PICA modalities differed between groups. Group A made more change in Graphic performance followed by Verbal and Gestural performance. Group B made more change in Gestural performance followed by Graphic and Verbal performance.

TABLE 9–7
Mean change in coexisting aphasia measured by PICA percentiles at intake (4 WPO) and at last evaluation in each treatment group

	Group A (N = 14)			*Group B (N = 12)*			
PICA Measure	*Pre*	*Post*	*Dif.*	*Pre*	*Post*	*Dif.*	*A–B Dif.*
Overall	42.9	70.8	27.9*	43.0	64.6	21.6*	6.3
Gestural	48.5	69.2	20.7*	43.5	66.5	23.0*	−2.3
Verbal	37.8	63.1	25.3*	43.0	58.4	15.4*	9.9**
Graphic	41.7	76.1	34.4*	46.3	68.1	21.8*	12.6**

*Significant at $p < .01$.
**Significant at $p < .10$.

Relationship between Change in Apraxia of Speech and Change in Aphasia

To determine the relationship between severity of apraxia of speech and severity of aphasia and change in apraxia of speech and change in aphasia, correlations were computed. These are shown in Table 9-8. Severity of apraxia of speech, as measured on the 7-point rating scale at intake, 4 weeks postonset, was correlated with PICA Overall, Gestural, Verbal, and Graphic percentile performance at intake to determine the relationship between the severity of the two disorders. The relationship between change in the two disorders was determined by correlating change scores on the apraxia rating scale and change in PICA percentile performance that occurred between the intake evaluation and each patient's final evaluation. Of course, the PICA Overall and Verbal percentiles are influenced by the presence of apraxia of speech. The Gestural and Graphic percentiles provide a measure of coexisting aphasia that is less influenced by the presence of apraxia of speech.

TABLE 9-8
Correlations for treatment groups, A and B, between severity of apraxia of speech at intake and PICA percentile performance at intake and between improvement in apraxia of speech and improvement in PICA percentile performance

	Apraxia of Speech			
	Severity at Intake		*Amount of Improvement*	
PICA Performance	*A (N = 17)*	*B (N = 12)*	*A (N = 13)*	*B (N = 8)*
Overall	−.57*	−.28	−.15	+.06
Gestural	−.15	−.14	−.51	+.64
Verbal	−.83**	−.55*	+.43	+.58
Graphic	−.16	−.28	−.21	−.45

*Significant at $p < .05$.
**Significant at $p < .01$.

There was a significant negative relationship ($p < .05$) at intake between the severity of AOS and the severity of aphasia as measured by the PICA Overall percentile in Group A, but not in Group B. The negative correlation results from severe AOS being represented by high ratings on the rating scale — 4 to 7 — and severe aphasia being represented by low PICA percentiles. No significant relationships ($p < .05$) for either group were observed when severity of AOS was compared with PICA Gestural and Graphic percentiles. Both groups displayed significant correlations,

$p < .01$ for Group A and $p < .05$ for Group B, when severity of AOS at intake was compared with PICA Verbal performance at intake. These data imply that the severity of AOS is not significantly related to the severity of aphasia except when the measure of aphasia includes oral-expressive language performance.

No significant relationships were observed for change in the two disorders. Because change scores were used in these comparisons, one would expect positive correlations if change in one was related to change in the other. All comparisons for Group A except change in AOS and change in the PICA Verbal percentile were negative. All comparisons for Group B except change in AOS and change in the PICA Graphic percentile were positive. Positive correlations between change in AOS and change in PICA Verbal performance could be expected, because the latter measure probably is influenced by change in AOS. What was not expected was the difference in correlations for the two groups on the comparison between change in AOS and change in PICA Gestural performance. While neither reached significance, the result was negative for Group A, −.51, and positive for Group B, +.64. This difference may have resulted from the different treatments, direct manipulation of AOS in Group A and no direct manipulation of AOS in Group B; the difference in the scales used to determine change in the two measures; or the small sample size. However, the absence of significant relationships indicates that change in one disorder can or cannot occur independent of change in the other.

DISCUSSION

Our results tell us not only about our patients, but also about ourselves. We were able to determine how our patients who displayed apraxia of speech responded to treatment and how that response may have been influenced by coexisting aphasia. In addition, we observed how good we were at giving our patients a diagnosis. Both observations deserve discussion.

Appraising Apraxia of Speech

We wonder why we were unable to diagnose AOS in 10 of our 29 patients at intake. Patients in the VA Cooperative Study were selected because they were aphasic. Of the 67 who met all selection criteria, 29 were identified as displaying apraxia of speech or suspected of displaying apraxia of speech. This constitutes 43% of the sample. It seems high, but we know of no reports on the incidence of AOS for comparison. The classification of these patients according to the traditional types of aphasia appears reasonable. All but two, the Anomic and the Conduction patients, were nonfluent. And, apraxic-like errors can be found in the types — Broca's, Global, Conduction, Transcortical Motor, Mixed — represented in our sample. Seven of the 29 patients, 24%, were not classifiable at 4 weeks postonset. A comparison of those patients who were diagnosed as displaying AOS with those who were labeled AOS Undetermined indicates 3 of the 19 patients in the AOS group, 16%, could not be classified, and 4 of the 10 patients in the AOS Undetermined group, 40%, could not be classified.

Severity of coexisting aphasia did not appear to influence our ability to label. While the mean PICA Overall percentile for patients who received a diagnosis was higher, 45th percentile, than the mean for those who did not, 35th percentile, we were able to diagnose AOS in severely aphasic patients, down to the 15th percentile. However, the severity of apraxia of speech, once identified, may explain our difficulty in making an early diagnosis. Those patients who were labeled AOS at intake had a mean severity of 2.6 on the 7-point scale. Those identified as AOS Undetermined at intake displayed a mean severity of 3.8 when the diagnosis was eventually made. Only 3 of the 19 patients who had an early diagnosis displayed a severity of 4 or 5 on the 7-point scale. Six of the 10 patients who had to wait for a diagnosis showed an eventual severity of 4 to 6.

Our method for appraising AOS and determining its severity can be considered traditional. The appraisal measure (Wertz & Rosenbek, 1971) included tasks traditionally used to detect the presence of AOS — repetition of syllables, monosyllabic words, multisyllabic words, words of increasing length, and sentences. The stimuli were loaded with sounds demonstrated to be difficult for apraxic patients. The measure did not include picture description or reading, however, we were able to observe each patient's spontaneous speech on the conversation measure. Perhaps our observations were biased by the abundance of behavior that flowed from the repetition tasks. And perhaps our difficulty in applying the label resulted from the data collected. Some (Rosenbek, 1978; Wertz, 1978) have stressed the need for useable data in detecting the presence of AOS. The ambiguous patient needs to be pushed through a series of steps on each task — repeated performance, performance after auditory and visual cues — to elicit useable data. A single response to a stimulus, sometimes, does not permit those patients who provide minimal verbal productions to tell the clinician the problem lies in motor speech and not auditory comprehension or some aspect of oral-expressive aphasic deficit. Our attempts to obtain useable data, while tenacious, were not always successful.

Finally, ambiguity in diagnosis may have resulted from patient variability and severity. Thirteen of the 26 patients who received at least two evaluations were classified as AOS Undetermined on at least one of their evaluations. Those that migrated from one classification to another tended to reside at the ends of our severity scale. Some were extremely mild and displayed only a few, inconsistent apraxic errors. Others were quite severe and provided little verbal output on which we could hang a label.

Group designs require putting patients in bins, even if the bin is called undetermined. Single-subject designs permit selecting only that patient who displays the behavior of interest. The latter tells us about patients who display a disorder. The former tells us about the disorder. What we learned about AOS in a random sample of aphasic patients is that its presence, its variability, and its persistence is probably influenced by the tools and the talents we use to appraise it.

Response to Treatment

Nineteen patients remained in the treatment trial long enough to determine whether treatment had any influence on improving apraxia of speech. Six patients became nonapraxic, eight patients improved in their severity of AOS, and five patients did not improve in their severity of AOS. All improved in the severity of their coexisting aphasia. Patients who became nonapraxic were mild, 1–2 on the 7-point severity scale, at the time of diagnosis. Patients who improved ranged from 2 to 4 in their initial severity. Patients who did not improve ranged from 2 to 5 in their initial severity. Improvement in patients who remained apraxic, therefore, was not related to initial severity. In those patients who did improve or became nonapraxic, improvement ranged from one to two levels on the 7-point severity scale, and the amount of improvement was not related to initial severity.

The type of treatment appeared to influence whether patients improved. More patients improved and improvement was greater in Group A, individual stimulus-response treatment, than in Group B, group treatment. These results imply the way to treat AOS is to treat it aggressively by direct manipulation and not by general, group discussion. This is consistent with what has been recommended (Rosenbek, 1978).

Apraxia of Speech and Aphasia

All of our patients displayed coexisting aphasia. And all experienced significant improvement in their aphasia. Except for verbal performance, the initial severity of AOS was not significantly related to initial severity of aphasia. Further, improvement in AOS was not significantly related to improvement in aphasia. Improvement in PICA Verbal percentiles was positively correlated with improvement in aphasia in both treatment groups. This could be expected, because PICA Verbal performance is probably influenced by the presence and severity of AOS as well as the severity of aphasia. What we did not expect was the discrepancy between the two treatment groups when improvement in PICA Gestural performance was correlated with improvement in AOS. Group A revealed a negative correlation, and Group B revealed a positive correlation. Neither was significant, but the difference is puzzling. The PICA Gestural percentile results from performance on a variety of tasks — gesture, auditory comprehension, reading and matching. Group B made more improvement in their Gestural percentile than in any other modality. Group A made less improvement in their Gestural percentile than in any other modality. Group A made significant change in AOS. Group B did not. One could infer that the type of treatment has little influence on improvement in the behaviors represented in the PICA Gestural percentile, but the type of treatment has a significant influence on improvement of apraxia of speech. However, until tested with larger samples and improved measures in a more controlled investigation, one would not want to back that inference with health or home.

Our results do suggest that the initial severity of AOS is not significantly related to the initial severity of aphasia. Further, change in one disorder does not appear to be significantly related to change in the other.

CONCLUSIONS

If it matters what you call it, and some believe it does, there is a need to improve our ability to appraise apraxia of speech and its severity. Over one-third of our sample had to wait for a diagnosis. And, even after the diagnosis was made, it was not etched. We vacillated with 20% of our sample.

Most patients who display apraxia of speech improve. Seventy-four percent of our sample improved the severity of their apraxia of speech during the treatment trial. The type of treatment appeared to influence whether improvement occurred or not. Four of the five patients who did not improve received group treatment with no direct manipulation of their motor speech deficit.

The presence of coexisting aphasia, its severity, and its improvement appeared to have no significant relationship with the presence, severity, and improvement in apraxia of speech. In our sample, change or the lack of it in one disorder occurred or did not occur independent of the severity of and change in the other disorder.

Our results do not support the efficacy of treatment for patients suffering apraxia of speech, nor do they deny it. The absence of a randomly assigned no treatment group does not permit us to speak to the question of whether treatment works. Most of our apraxic patients improved. But, all were treated.

REFERENCES

Basso, A., Capitani, E., & Vignolo, L. Influence of rehabilitation on language skills in aphasic patients. A controlled study. *Archives of Neurology*, 1979, *36*, 190–196.

Borkowski, J. G., Benton, A. L., & Spreen, O. Word Fluency and brain damage. *Neuropsychologia,* 1967, *5,* 135–140.

Bugbee, J. K., & Nichols, A. C. Rehearsal as a self-correction strategy for patients with apraxia of speech. In R. H. Brookshire (Ed.), *Clinical aphasiology: Proceedings of the conference.* Minneapolis: BRK, 1980. pp. 279–284.

Darley, F. L. The efficacy of language rehabilitation in aphasia. *Journal of Speech and Hearing Disorders*, 1972, *37*, 3–21.

Deal, J. L., & Florance, C. L. Modification of the eight-step continuum for treatment of apraxia of speech in adults. *Journal of Speech and Hearing Disorders*, 1978, *43*, 89–95.

De Renzi, E., & Vignolo, L. A. The Token Test: A sensitive test to detect receptive disturbances in aphasia. *Brain*, 1962, *85*, 665–678.

Florance, C. L., Rabidoux, P. S., & McCauslin, L. S. An environmental manipulation approach to treating apraxia of speech. In R. H. Brookshire (Ed.), *Clinical aphasiology: Proceedings of the conference.* Minneapolis: BRK, 1980. pp. 285–293.

Goodglass, H. & Kaplan, E. *The assessment of aphasia and related disorders. Phila*delphia: Lea and Febiger, 1972.

Hand, C. R., Tonkovich, J. D., & Aitchison, J. Abonormal syntactic compensations utilized by a patient with chronic Broca's aphasia. In R. H. Brookshire (Ed.), *Clinical aphasiology: Proceedings of the conference.* Minneapolis: BRK, 1979. pp. 261–269.

Holtzapple, P. A., & Marshall, N. The application of multiphonemic articulation therapy with apraxic patients. In R. H. Brookshire (Ed.), *Clinical aphasiology: Proceedings of the conference.* Minneapolis: BRK, 1977. pp. 46–58.

Houston-Wiedel, I. M. The basic foundation approach for decreasing aphasia and verbal apraxia in adults. In R. H. Brookshire (Ed.), *Clinical aphasiology: Proceedings of the conference.* Minneapolis: BRK, 1976. pp. 209–223.

Keith, R. L., & Aronson, A. E. Singing as therapy for apraxia of speech: Report of a case. *Brain and Language*, 1975, *2*, 483–488.

Kertesz, A., & McCabe, P. Recovery patterns and prognosis in aphasia. *Brain,* 1977, *100,* 1–18.

McNeil, M. R., Prescott, T. E., & Lemme, M. L. An application of electromyographic biofeedback to aphasia/apraxia treatment. In R. H. Brookshire (Ed.), *Clinical aphasiology: Proceedings of the conference.* Minneapolis: BRK, 1976. pp. 151–171.

Porch, B. E. *Porch Index of Communicative Ability.* Palo Alto, CA: Consulting Psychologists Press, 1967.

Rabidoux, P. C., Florance, C. L., & McCauslin, L. S. The use of a Handi Voice in the treatment of a severely apractic nonverbal patient. In R. H. Brookshire (Ed.), *Clinical aphasiology: Proceedings of the conference.* Minneapolis: BRK, 1980. pp. 294–301.

Raven, J. C. *Coloured Progressive Matrices.* London: Lewis, 1962.

Rosenbek, J. C. Treating apraxia of speech. In D. F. Johns (Ed.), *Clinical management of neurogenic communicative disorders.* Boston: Little, Brown, 1978. pp. 191–241.

Rosenbek, J. C., Collins, M. J., and Wertz, R. T. Intersystemic reorganization for apraxia of speech. In R. H. Brookshire (Ed.), *Clinical aphasiology: Proceedings of the conference.* Minneapolis: BRK, 1976. pp. 255–260.

Rosenbek, J. C., Lemme, M. L., Ahern, M. B., Harris, E. H., & Wertz, R. T. A treatment for apraxia of speech in adults. *Journal of Speech and Hearing Disorders*, 1973, *38*, 462–472.

Sarno, M. T. *Functional communication profile.* New York: Institute of Rehabilitation Medicine, New York University Medical Center, 1969.

Simmons, N. N. Choice of stimulus modes in treating apraxia of speech: A case study. In R. H. Brookshire (Ed.), *Clinical aphasiology: Proceedings of the conference.* Minneapolis: BRK, 1980. pp. 302–307.

Simmons, N. N. Finger counting as an intersystemic reorganizer in apraxia of speech. In R. H. Brookshire (Ed.), *Clinical aphasiology: Preceedings of the conference.* Minneapolis: BRK, 1978. pp. 174–179.

Skelly, M., Schinsky, L., Smith, R. W., & Fust, R. S. American Indian sign (AMERIND) as a facilitator of verbalization for the oral verbal apraxic. *Journal of Speech and Hearing Disorders*, 1974, *39*, 445–465.

Tonkovich, J. D. & Marquardt, T. P. The effects of stress and melodic intonation on apraxia of speech. In R. H. Brookshire (Ed.), *Clinical aphasiology: Proceedings of the conference.* Minneapolis: BRK, 1977. pp. 97–102.

Warren, R. L. Rehearsal for naming in apraxia of speech. In R. H. Brookshire (Ed.), *Clinical aphasiology: Proceedings of the conference.* Minneapolis: BRK, 1977. pp. 80–90.

Wertz, R. T. Neuropathologies of speech and language: An introduction to patient management. In D. F. Johns (Ed.), *Clinical management of neurogenic communicative disorders.* Boston: Little, Brown, 1978. pp. 1–101.

Wertz, R. T., Collins, M. J., Weiss, D., Kurtzke, J. F., Friden, T., Brookshire, R. H., Pierce, J. et al. Veterans Administration cooperative study on aphasia: A comparison of individual and group treatment. *Journal of Speech and Hearing Research*, 1981, *24*, 580–594.

Wertz, R. T., Kitselman, K. P., & Deal, L. A. *Classifying the aphasias: Contributions to patient management.* Paper presented to the Academy of Aphasia, London, Ontario, 1981.

Wertz, R. T., & Rosenbek, J. C. Group designs for the study of aphasia. In R. H. Brookshire (Ed.), *Clinical aphasiology: Proceedings of the conference.* Minneapolis: BRK, 1978. pp. 1–10.

Wertz, R. T., & Rosenbek, J. C. Appraising apraxia of speech. *Journal of the Colorado Speech and Hearing Association*, 1971, *5*, 18–36.

Wilson, P. B. Temporal relationships in therapy for apraxia. In R. H. Brookshire (Ed.), *Clinical Aphasiology: Proceedings of the conference*. Minneapolis: BRK, 1977. pp. 119–123.

ACKNOWLEDGMENT

This research was supported by funds provided by the Veterans Administration Cooperative Studies Program.

10

Sequential Treatment of Split Lists: A Case Report

Leonard L. LaPointe

INTRODUCTION

Research on intervention in apraxia of speech faces some of the same hurdles as that in aphasia. In intervention research few empirical studies can tolerate close scrutiny of design evaluation without revealing flaws that frequently confound interpretation of results. Confounding variables are problematic and legendary. Traditional approaches have attempted to match large experimental and control groups and evaluate any resulting differential response to a treatment package by inferential statistics. Identifying and matching subject variables for large groups is difficult even if one can afford the costs of gathering data and following subjects.

The ethical considerations of withholding treatment have proven problematic as well and have inhibited or prevented some research. The last decade, though, has seen not only more carefully designed group empirical research, but also the development of an emerging technology of research design with emphasis on the individual. Single case time-series, or within subject experimental design for neurogenic communication disorders was advocated as early as 1974 (LaPointe) in aphasia, and evolving interest has spawned a number of variations on the theme (Davis, 1978; Salvatore, 1978; LaPointe, 1978). Despite this surge of advocacy, very few examples of applications of these principles are apparent in research on intervention in either aphasia or apraxia of speech.

Design Features

The features of single-*N* and multiple-*N* time-series designs are adequately outlined in a number of works, including that of Kratochwill (1978) and McReynolds and Kearns (1982). Cautions about weakness and potential threats to internal and external validity of single-subject designs also are well presented in these sources. Some writers advocate complex mathematical approaches that sometimes require hundreds of observations to overcome validity threats, but Hayes (1981) and Tryon (1982) have recently suggested that simplified and economical designs are available for evaluating intervention effects.

The forerunner of most of this type of research and the foundation upon which it is built is the basic AB design. (A = baseline measurement; B = intervention measurement). With this approach to quantifying clinical change, controlled observations are taken repeatedly over a time period in order to establish the nature and degree of change in a behavior of interest. At some planned point in the data series, an intervention is selected and introduced and change in whatever is being measured is noted. This fundamental AB design is the least powerful of the time-series design choices, and it has been modified and improved.

Withdrawal and reversal phases of intervention with observation of the subsequent effect on the measured dependent variable became the first variations on the AB theme. Later modifications were dubbed multiple baseline, multiple schedule, concurrent schedule, changing criterion, alternating treatment, sequential multiple-*N*–multiple-*I*, stratified multiple-*N*–single-*I*, and inverted designs. The evolution and situational relevance of these approaches is outlined in Hersen and Barlow (1976), Kratochwill (1978), and McReynolds and Kearns (1982). The emerging literature is fraught with new labels and the simultaneous birth of research design concepts from different disciplines has resulted in some redundancy and confusion in design names. Despite labeling differences many common features can be seen across designs.

Multiple Baseline Designs

A variant of basic time-series withdrawal or reversal approaches is the multiple baseline design. In all versions of this design, data are collected simultaneously across two or more baseline series. For neurogenic communication impairment, it has been proposed to measure changes across behaviors, individuals, and settings and as a means of determining the nature and degree of generalization from trained to nontrained items (LaPointe, 1978). One use of the multiple baseline design is to demonstrate an intervention effect by showing that a change in response accompanies introduction of a specified treatment package at different points in time. A variant on this approach for judging the effect of two or more treatments or for determining the result of treatment versus no treatment is called the alternating treatments design by McReynolds and Kearns (1982).

A major advantage of this design is that it promotes simultaneous measurement of two or more behaviors. It could be argued that a withdrawal phase should be added to strengthen the design's validity as a measure of intervention effect. Designs such as these could contribute information on both the degrees and level of change attributable to treatment packages.

It would be instructive to observe, for example, the sequential effect of application of a treatment package on a subject whose performance was measured on a verbal production task during alternating phases of treatment. This study reports the result of such an approach. The purpose of this study is to demonstrate the application of a multiple baseline design and to present evidence on the effects of a sequentially applied treatment package on the phonological production of a single individual who suffered aphasia and apraxia of speech.

METHODS AND PROCEDURES

Subject

At the time of admission, F.B. was a 52-year-old right-handed male veteran. He was employed as a truck driver and salesman for a local wholesale beer distributor. He was referred to our services 6 days after he suffered a left middle cerebral artery thromboembolic cerebrovascular accident (CVA) which left him with a mild right hemiparesis and nonfluent aphasia, complicated by severe phonologic selection and sequencing impairment (apraxia of speech).

F.B. had a history of diffuse atheromatous vascular disease, hypertension since 1949, myocardial infarction in 1970, and a long history of right lower extremity claudication with femoral artery bypass in 1974. He suffered an apparent transient ischemic attack (TIA) in 1976 and subsequently underwent right carotid endarterectomy. Prior to the most recent CVA, F.B. had complained of a left vertex headache almost daily for a month. On the night prior to admission he complained that his speech was "not-right." On the morning of admission he awoke at approximately 6:00 a.m., made breakfast, was noted by his family to speak infrequently, and approximately 1½ hours later while standing, appeared dazed and developed a droop of the right face, weakness in the right extremities, and complete cessation of speech output.

A brain scan demonstrated an area of increased uptake in the "left frontal central temporal area," felt to be consistent with a CVA. A 16-channel electroencephalogram (EEG) demonstrated normal background with slow wave focus over the left anterior and midtemporal regions. He was hospitalized for 24 days and received occupational, physical, and speech-language therapy during his inpatient stay. Since he was a local resident he was scheduled for four, 1-hour speech-language therapy sessions per week upon his discharge.

During his hospitalization F.B. was administered a variety of tests to evaluate his communication function. These include our standard intake recording protocol, a variety of tasks that sample speech from vowel imitation to conversational speech; the Boston Diagnostic Aphasia Examination; the Porch Index of Communicative Ability; the Reading Comprehension Battery for Aphasia; an Oral and Limb Apraxia Battery; and the Fischer-Logemann Test of Articulation Competence. Table 10-1 summarizes the results of these measures.

Approximately three months after F.B.'s CVA and after considerable clearing of his aphasia he was enrolled in the program described in this paper. The focus of treatment was on his residual phonologic selection and sequencing impairment. In the phase of his treatment reported here, we were primarily concerned with establishment and maintenance of accurate and consistent phonologic production and this was attempted by use of a variety of techniques of imitation, modeling, integral stimulation, explanation, and phonetic placement.

Stimuli

In order to accomplish these treatment objectives and to explore the nature of rates of change of treated and nontreated stimuli, 50 photographs of everyday objects (i.e., milk, watch, money, sink, toilet, etc.) were selected and organized for scoring and progress plotting on Base-10 Response Forms. Table 10-2 lists the stimuli selected.

All photographs were approximately 5 by 7 inches in size and were reproduced in black and white. The pictures were presented in a confrontation naming format and F.B.'s response to each item was scored for accuracy on a pass (+) or fail (−) basis. A response was considered accurate if all phones were present, judged to be within normal limits, and

TABLE 10-1
Results of speech - language measures administered to F.B.

Test			
Boston Diagnostic Aphasia Examination		Subtest	Raw Scores
	A.	Word Discrim.	69
		Body Parts	18
		Commands	10
		Complex Ideat.	8
		Oral Agility	7
		Verbal Agility	4
		Auto. Seq.	0
		Recit.	0
		Rep. Words	0
	B.	Repeat Phrases	0
		Word Reading	0
		Responsive Naming	0
		Conf. Naming	0
		Body Part Naming	0
		Sent. Reading	0
	C.	Symbol-Word Discrim.	9
		Word Recog.	6
		Comp-Oral Spelling	0
		Word-Pict. Matching	10
		Reading Sentences/ Paragraphs	5
		Mechanics of Writing	2
		Serial Writing	39
		Primer Dictation	8
		Spelling to Dictation	0
		Written Conf. Naming	3

Porch Index of Communicative Ability	Overall	Gestural	Verbal	Graphic
Score	12.2	14.6	11.4	9.7
Percentile	72	96	52	72

Oral and Limb Apraxia Battery	Percentage Correct	
	Oral Nonspeech	Limb Gesture
	41	91

Fischer–Logemann Test of Articulation Competence	
	Predominance of inter- and prevocalic errors on fricatives, affricates, glides, consonant blends; initiation problems; audible and silent groping for articulatory postures.

TABLE 10–2
Stimuli depicted in fifty photographs

1.	ketchup	11.	iron	21.	piano	31.	fence	41.	light
2.	coke	12.	couch	22.	bed	32.	shovel	42.	broom
3.	milk	13.	radio	23.	TV	33.	hammer	43.	aspirin
4.	tie	14.	toaster	24.	chair	34.	nails	44.	mop
5.	watch	15.	stove	25.	shower	35.	rake	45.	bowl
6.	razor	16.	scale	26.	window	36.	saw	46.	mousetrap
7.	wallet	17.	camera	27.	door	37.	pliers	47.	calendar
8.	jacket	18.	sink	28.	toilet	38.	flashlight	48.	soap
9.	money	19.	bathtub	29.	oven	39.	rug	49.	towel
10.	keys	20.	clock	30.	lamp	40.	letter	50.	kleenex

in proper order. Any phonologic substitution, distortion, addition, omission, or phonologic process resulting in production judged outside normal limits was scored as a minus (−). Additionally, if abnormal delay in initiation or audible groping or posturing of the articulators was noted, the response was scored as a minus (−). On multisyllabic words, if the response was phonologically intact but stress was misplaced it was still regarded as correct and assigned a plus (+). During each session responses to each of the 50 photographs were measured and recorded. The 50 items were then divided into two sets of 25, one of which first served as the trained (odd numbered items) and one the untrained set (even numbers).

Baseline measurements were made on all items for three successive sessions prior to initiation of training. During the baseline phase, average performance on each 25 item list was similar. Table 10-3 presents baseline scores.

TABLE 10–3
Baseline scores in percentage of correct responses for trained and untrained lists

	Baseline 1	*Baseline 2*	*Baseline 3*	*Mean of Three Baseline Measures*
Odd Numbers	4	16	8	9
Even Numbers	8	8	12	9

After baseline measurement the treatment phase was begun and during each session responses to each of the 50 photographs (both the trained and untrained lists) were measured and recorded.

During the 17 sessions of Phase 1 the odd numbered items were treated. In Phase 2 training was reversed. That is, training was focused on the even numbered items, those that were untrained for the first 17 sessions, and the odd numbered items were left untrained.

Treatment Package

At the beginning of each session throughout the treatment phases, performance on all 50 items was measured. Then a treatment package was instituted on the trained set only. The treatment package consisted of the following steps:

1. If correct: Repeat each item five times for stabilization.
2. If incorrect:
   A. Clinician indicates error locus with explanation of error type.
   B. Clinician models correct production and elicits correct production by imitation, integral stimulation, demonstration, or phonetic placement.
   C. If correct production is not achieved, go on to next item. If achieved, F.B. repeats word with correct production five times, slowly.
   D. F.B. repeats five times at approximately double speed.
   E. Expansion: F.B. embeds corrected word in phrase provided by clinician.
   F. Go on to next item. Apply treatment package to all items in trained set.

Reliability

Scoring reliability was evaluated in two ways: Periodic tape recordings of performance on all 50 photographs were made during the course of treatment. From these recordings subsequent measurements in inter- and intrascorer reliability could be made. To establish interscorer reliability the services were enlisted of another certified speech-language pathologist who had extensive experience in the evaluation and treatment of neurogenic communication impairment.

Scoring criteria were explained, several practice items were scored, and a representative session (Phase 1, Session 17) of F.B.'s initial responses to all list items was played. The author and second scorer then scored each response for subsequent analysis of agreement. For interscorer reliability, agreement of score assignment was achieved on 39 of 50 items (78%). Intrascorer agreement was determined by comparing the author's assigned scores from the tape recording of Session 17 to the scores orignally assigned during the session. Intrascorer agreement was achieved on 42 of 50 items (84%). These levels of inter- and intrascorer agreement were somewhat lower than anticipated. However, they were deemed adequate to proceed with analysis of the data in this study. Perhaps additional analysis of the methods, validity, and selection of scoring criteria related to judgments of clinical performance are warranted. Refinements of reliability analysis have been suggested previously by Hopkins and Hermann (1977) and by Kearns (1981).

RESULTS

Figure 10-1 is an illustration of the linear function slopes that were constructed to fit the responses of F.B. for all conditions during the duration of the study trial. This figure does not include the baseline phase of the treatment trial. The illustration represents 17 sessions of

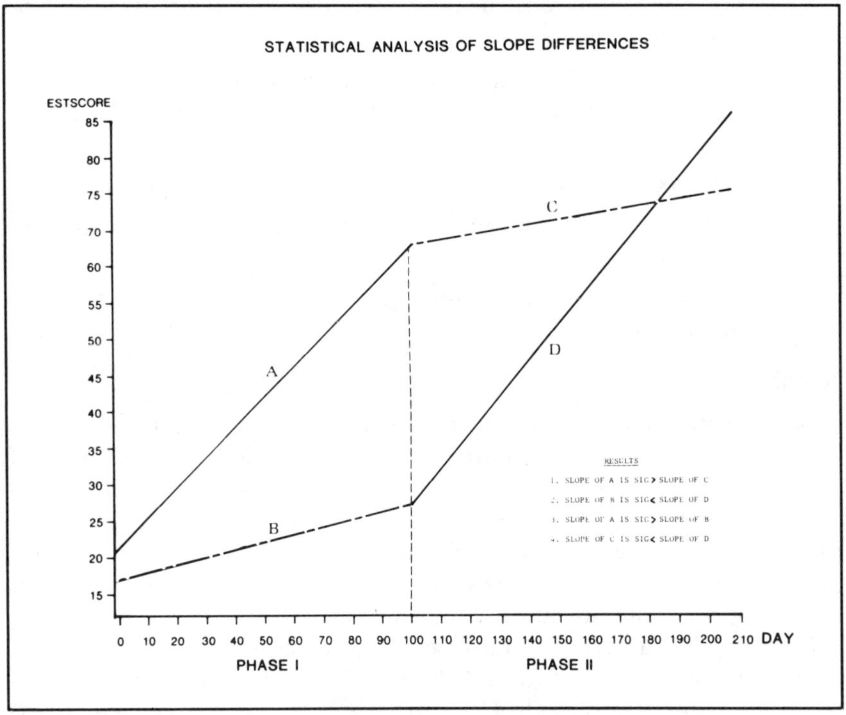

FIGURE 10-1
Linear function slopes fit to the subject's responses for all conditions. Results: 1. slope of A is sig>slope of C; 2. slope of B is sig<slope of D; 3. slope of A is sig>slope of B; 4. slope of C is sig<slope of D.

observations for both trained and untrained lists for Phase 1 and 17 sessions of observations during Phase 2 during which training emphasis was reversed on the stimulus sets. The abscissa represents the duration of the treatment trial in days. Phase 1 lasted 100 days. Seventeen sessions of four sessions per week were extended throughout the 100-day duration of Phase 1. Some alteration in the regularity of sessions per week was dictated by F.B. and the author's illness, travel, and convenience. The ordinate of Figure 10-1 represents performance level in percentage of correct responses. In Phase 1, A represents performance on the trained set and B represents performance on the untrained set. After 17 sessions (100 days) treatment on the split lists of stimuli was reversed and so in Phase 2, C represents the untrained list (previously trained during Phase 1) and D represents performance on the trained list (previously untrained during Phase 1). Visual inspection of these slopes reveals differences in acceleration rates of trained and untrained sets. The slopes of the trained sets appear steeper, and this of course reflects faster rates of change and the achievement of higher levels of performance accuracy on the set of stimuli being trained over the course of the study trial.

In order to determine whether or not these slope differences were statistically significant, analysis using measures appropriate to single-subject experimentation were conducted by the Biostatistics Unit of the Department of Statistics at the J. Hillis Miller Health Center of the University of Florida. Full and reduced model F tests and simple linear regression analysis strategies appropriate to single-subject experiment were conducted and the results are listed in Figure 10-1. Slope A, the trained set of stimuli during Phase 1, is significantly greater than Slope B ($p = < .0001$). After reversal in Phase 2, Slope C (now untrained) is significantly less steep than Slope D (now trained). Further, when performance on a given 25-item list is followed across phases throughout the duration of the treatment trial, Slope A is significantly greater than change in performance on the same items (Slope C) during the untrained phase ($p = < .0003$). Similarly, Slope B (untrained) is significantly less steep than performance on the same items (Slope D) under the training phase ($p = < .0003$).

From these data we can conclude that for the duration of this treatment trial for F.B., with the methods and particular treatment package selected for this study, progress was faster and performance reached higher levels of accuracy for the trained than for the untrained lists. Research that uses single-subject time-series methodologies to address the tangle of questions related to the nature and degree of effectiveness of our intervention strategies is in the embryonic stages in its application to people who have neurogenic disruptions of communication. No doubt future refinements and discoveries will allow us to hone our edge of sophistication to levels that will make some of these early efforts look quaint. We should view these findings with the tentativeness that scientific caution deserves. In the meantime though, we should gain solace from the realization that emerging research strategies can offer very tangible contributions to the mounting evidence that what we do does some good.

REFERENCES

Davis, G. A. The clinical application of withdrawal, single-case research designs. In R. Brookshire (Ed.), *Clinical aphasiology: Conference proceedings.* Minneapolis: BRK, 1978. pp. 11-19.

Hayes, S. C. Single case experimental design and empirical clinical practice. *Journal of Consulting and Clinical Psychology,* 1981, *49*, 193-211.

Hersen, M., & Barlow, D. H. *Single case experimental designs: Strategies for studying behavior change.* New York: Pergamon Press, 1976.

Hopkins, B. L., & Hermann, J. A. Evaluating inter-observer reliability of interval data. *Journal of Applied Behavior Analysis*, 1977, *10*, 121-126.

Kearns, K. Inter-observer reliability procedures in applied aphasia research: A review with suggestions for change. R. Brookshire (Ed.), *Clinical aphasiology: Conference proceedings.* Minneapolis: BRK, 1981. pp. 26-34.

Kratochwill, T. R. *Single subject research: Strategies for evaluating change.* New York: Academic Press, 1978.

LaPointe, L. L. Base-10 "Programmed-Stimulation" task specification, scoring, and plotting performance in aphasia therapy. B. Porch (Ed.), *Clinical aphasiology: Conference proceedings.* Albuquerque, NM. 1974. pp. 106-127.

LaPointe, L. L. Multiple baseline designs. In R. Brookshire (Ed.), *Clinical aphasiology: Conference Proceedings.* Minneapolis: BRK, 1978. pp. 20-29.

McReynolds, L. V., & Kearns, K. P. *Single subject experimental designs in communicative disorders.* Baltimore: University Park Press, 1982.

Salvatore, A. P. Aphasia treatment: An exertise in stimulus control. In R. Brookshire (Ed.), *Clinical aphasiology: Conference Preceedings.* Minneapolis: BRK, 1978. pp. 30-36.

Tryon, W. W. A simplified time-series analysis for evaluating treatment interventions. *Journal of Applied Behavior Analysis*, 1982, *15*, 423-429.

ACKNOWLEDGMENTS

I would like to acknowledge the contributions of Barbara A. J. Matthews for help in reduction, organization, and analysis of data; and Randy Carter for aid in statistical analysis. I thank Charles R. Eisenbach II for lending me his ears and for demonstrating perseverance. I also thank F.B. who contributed time and sweat and data and laughter. Finally, I am grateful for the example and inspiration of Fred Darley, whose influence is so widespread we have no ruler big enough to measure it.

Author Index

Subject Index